Clinicians' Guide to
Inflammatory Bowel Disease

Alastair Forbes
St Mark's Hospital
Harrow,
UK

CHAPMAN & HALL MEDICAL
London · Glasgow · Weinheim · New York · Tokyo · Melbourne · Madras

Published by Chapman & Hall, 2–6 Boundary Row, London SE1 8HN, UK

Chapman & Hall, 2–6 Boundary Row, London SE1 8HN, UK

Chapman & Hall GmbH, Pappelallee 3, 69469 Weinheim, Germany

Chapman & Hall USA, 115 Fifth Avenue, New York, NY 10003, USA

Chapman & Hall Japan, ITP-Japan, Kyowa Building, 3F, 2-2-1 Hirakawacho, Chiyoda-ku, Tokyo 102, Japan

Chapman & Hall Australia, 102 Dodds Street, South Melbourne, Victoria 3205, Australia

Chapman & Hall India, R. Seshadri, 32 Second Main Road, CIT East, Madras 600 035, India

First edition 1997

Typeset in 10/12pt Palatino by Saxon Graphics Ltd, Derby
Printed in Great Britain by T. J. International (Padstow) Ltd

ISBN 0 412 78850 0

Drugs mentioned in this book are not necessarily licensed for suggested indications; prescribers should always check doses and indications in their own territories.

A catalogue record for this book is available from the British Library

Library of Congress Catalog Card Number 97-67516

 Printed on acid-free text paper, manufactured in accordance with ANSI/NISO Z39. 48-1992 (Permanence of Paper).

Contents

Foreword

The burgeoning literature on inflammatory bowel disease provides too much information too fast for the average clinician. How can he or she feel confident when answering patients' questions, advising between alternative treatments, or watching the literature for significant advances? The answer is to read this book.

Alastair Forbes combines wide clinical experience and extensive reading to synthesize a mass of information into a coherent, readable text. Marshalling over 700 references, the majority published during the period 1990–96, requires a sense of what is relevant and useful. This intellectual feat by one person achieves a global view of the topic with continuity and balance. Not only are recent papers quoted on every aspect of the subject, some in journals not usually read by gastroenterologists, but also the latest abstracts which anticipate future papers. Current concepts on aetiology and pathogenesis are covered in sufficient depth and structured in such a way that, instead of becoming lost in a labyrinth, the clinician emerges with a clear understanding of what is known and of where progress is likely.

St Mark's hospital is noted for the integration achieved between physicians, surgeons, and diagnostic departments. As a tertiary referral centre it sees the full range of clinical problems associated with inflammatory bowel disease. Dr Forbes is thus equally at home when discussing clinical variants of IBD, medical treatments, indications for and results of surgery, or the management of complications such as enterocutaneous fistula, narcotic dependence, or short bowel syndrome. Balanced practical guidance is given on difficult clinical decisions such as the indications for surgery in severe ulcerative colitis on the management of intra-abdominal sepsis in Crohn's disease. Controversial topics such as cancer surveillance are reviewed crisply and critically. Having stated the evidence available, Alastair Forbes is not afraid to sum up with his own opinion, a refreshing feature which reflects current clinical practice at St Mark's.

This volume occupies a niche between the general textbook and the large reference book. Clinicians who read it from cover to cover will be rewarded by a grasp of current knowledge about IBD that is up to date and forward looking. Those who use the book as a source of reference will find practical help with their problem and, if need be, reference to key papers.

All gastroenterologists are challenged by inflammatory bowel disease. Alastair Forbes has done his readers a service for which they should be truly grateful. I am delighted that my successor at St Mark's continues the tradition of studying these intriguing disorders which demand all one's skills as a clinician and allow one to make a real contribution to the welfare of patients.

John E. Lennard-Jones
Emeritus Professor of Gastroenterology
University of London,
St Mark's Hospital

Preface

It may be asked whether we need another book of any sort, and particularly whether a new volume on the inflammatory bowel diseases is of any use when there are several exhaustive reference texts available and increasingly comprehensive access to the latest research data from on-line and CD-ROM sources. I asked myself and my publishers these same questions when it was suggested that I should be responsible for such a compilation, and I have done so again on numerous occasions since the decision was made to go ahead. I think, immodestly, that the decision was correct, not least since the task has exposed my own ignorance of many areas in these fascinating diseases, despite the fact that they have occupied by far the largest part of my clinical, research and teaching prac-tice for the past 5 years. I hope, but doubt, that I have adequately reme-died most of these lacunae, and take full responsibility for errors of omission and commission.

I believe that there is still a role for the single-author volume and I have deliberately kept the references as inconspicuous as possible to allow for smooth reading, although I would not expect anyone to consider the book suitable for the bedside table. I have deliberately included new data (including quite a number available only in abstract form) to reduce the out-of-datedness common to so many books by the time they reach the bookshop. I recognize that this recklessness increases the risk of including statements that time will ridicule, but this too can be a valuable exercise in collective humility. I have tried to put a little extra weight on topics that it seemed to me were less well covered in the major textbooks, which is why the sections on extra-intestinal manifestations, and particularly those on intra-abdominal sepsis, fistulae and short bowel syndrome, are arguably disproportionately long. This is also a response to the frequency with which these clinical problems lead to questions and referrals to me. A high proportion of the hard data on these topics is old, and in many cases seems to get transferred from one text to another without much clarifica-tion or even elaboration as the years pass. I hope that the pragmatic stance I have taken over these issues is useful.

I anticipate the book being useful to me as a memory jogger and source for 'leads', containing as it does reference to most of the current active workers in inflammatory bowel disease, indicating their particular areas of expertise. I know that others will disagree with some of my conclusions and interpretations, and I hope that they will regard our differences as a constructive attempt on my part to be concise and yet to highlight the controversial topics, with an expressed opinion to help the more junior. I envisage the book being most useful to the gastroenterology trainee, but also to the teacher in ensuring that the important issues have been covered. The book should also provide most that the gastrointestinal surgeon needs to know about the activities of his or her medical colleagues, and will probably be helpful for the specialist nurse and the non-clinical researcher working in inflammatory bowel disease units. Most of all, I hope that my enthusiasm for the subject can be conveyed, and that once in a while the book contributes to someone's decision to explore these diseases more fully.

I am grateful for contributions made by many of my junior staff and to the help of my colleagues in other disciplines, but particularly thank Miss Claire Chadwick, Dr Aida Jawhari, Dr Steven Mann and Dr Nicholas Reading, who have helped to prepare earlier reviews on some of the topics included in the present volume; I think they will recognize their contributions.

Alastair Forbes, London

1

Epidemiology, aetiology and pathogenesis

INTRODUCTION

There are a number of inflammatory bowel diseases to be considered but for the most part this account will concentrate on ulcerative colitis and Crohn's disease. It is still debated whether these idiopathic diseases are truly distinct or merely different ends of an inflammatory spectrum. The relevant sections of this book will illustrate such differences as their genetic associations, their clinical, radiological and histological features, their complications and disease associations, and their responses to therapy. Compelling circumstantial data such as these cannot, however, quite answer the question. After all, lepromatous and tuberculoid leprosy, or chicken pox and shingles, are clinically and pathologically quite distinct, but each pair is caused by the same organism. Until we have more certain aetiological information about inflammatory bowel disease there can be no authoritative conclusion. As there are so many differences, it will be assumed that it is legitimate to describe two diseases, but with the proviso that if this is proved incorrect that the majority of the information collected here will nevertheless remain pertinent.

EPIDEMIOLOGY

In general, the sexes are affected at a similar rate and to a similar severity by both ulcerative colitis and Crohn's disease. Few studies show more than a 10% difference in incidence or prevalence between males and females. Most studies that show a difference have a small excess of females with Crohn's disease and of males with ulcerative colitis [1], although males with Crohn's disease as well as with ulcerative colitis are more often over-represented in studies from areas of lower incidence [2]. The reason for this phenomenon is not known but it may contribute to the more striking male excess in a large southern European study (n = 1255) in which there was a 2 : 1 male excess in those with ulcerative colitis presenting over the age of 65 ($n = 114$), compared to a more usual nearly equal frequency in those under 25 [3]. Intermediate ratios of 1.4 and 1.7 in the 26–35 and 36–50-year-old groups suggest that the observation is real and not a statistical quirk, but whether this is a cohort effect from an influence operating much earlier in life is unclear.

Ulcerative colitis

Reliable data on the incidence and prevalence of ulcerative colitis exist for most developed nations. There is typically an annual incidence of around 7 per 100 000 population, with a general tendency for somewhat higher figures in regions more distant from the equator (such as the Faroe Islands and Norway) than, for example, in southern Europe, Israel, South Africa and New Zealand. Within individual population groups in northern Europe and North America the frequency now appears relatively constant over time. The South Wales study, which examined 357 incident cases in a relatively stable population over the period 1968–87 [4], found that although the range of annual incidence was wide (between 3 and 9 per 100 000 for individual years) the mean annual incidence for the entire period was 6.3 per 100 000, and showed neither an upward nor downward trend. In Italy (and perhaps in other Mediterranean states) it is probable that the annual incidence is slowly rising, the Lombardia survey of 1990–94 revealing an average of 7.0 cases per 100 000 population, which is the highest figure yet recorded in Italy [5]. It is possible that a component of this increase is from improved case ascertainment, but unlikely that this is the complete explanation; longer-term observations of stable populations will no doubt clarify this in due course.

Crohn's disease

The incidence of Crohn's disease is generally lower than that of ulcerative colitis, but appears to be increasing steadily in most of the regions in which it has been studied sequentially. Collected studies from Europe and North America yield annual incidence figures mostly lying between 2 and 6 per 100 000, with rates of around 5 per 100 000 for the better population studies performed since the early 1980s. A study in northern France covering the years 1988–90, and which found a mean incidence of 4.9 per 100 000, is representative of these (although it also revealed a discordantly low incidence of ulcerative colitis) [6]. Again there is a trend for the frequency to increase with greater distance from the equator (the figure of 3.4 per 100 000 in the Lombardia study fitting this pattern [5]). Virtually every report that has been able to measure changes in incidence of Crohn's disease has shown an increase with time. This phenomenon is probably explained in part by better case ascertainment, and by assign-ment of a Crohn's disease diagnosis to some colitic patients who would previously have been considered to have ulcerative colitis. However, it is unlikely that either of these factors is sufficient to account for the magni-tude of the rise recorded by some centres, especially since the incidence of ulcerative colitis has remained constant. In Copenhagen county, for example, the incidence recorded for 1979–87 of 4.1 per 100 000 was sixfold higher than in the early 1960s [7]. The clinical features in these incident patients were relatively constant over time and did not appear to be less severe in later years; it is accordingly probable that changes in case ascer-tainment were, at most, of minor impact. The Lancashire study, based on the Victoria Hospital in Blackpool, confirmed the general upward trend, but suggested that it had ceased after 1980, with standard age-adjusted incidence figures for the quinquennia 1971–75, 1976–80, 1981–85 and 1986–90 being 3.6, 6.0, 6.4 and 6.5 per 100 000 [8]. There is a little anxiety about the veracity of a hospital- rather than community-based study, but this is unlikely to influence this observation greatly, unless more cases are being managed by general practitioners without hospital support. As the condition is better recognized and more widely discussed, this is a possi-ble but improbable explanation.

The increase in frequency of Crohn's disease seems particularly true in paediatric series. A recent paper to address this issue, in the under-16s in South Wales, is representative [9]. The incidence of Crohn's disease had risen from a mean of 1.3 cases per 100 000 from 1983 through to 1988, to 3.1 over the period 1989–93. (The incidence of ulcerative colitis remained at a mean of 0.71 per 100 000 during the entire 11-year period.) There is a resultant prevalence of Crohn's disease in the under-16s of 16.6 per 100 000, now considerably exceeding that of ulcerative colitis in the same age group (3.4 per 100 000). However, a comparable, but prospective, study performed in children aged under 16 in southern Norway [10] yielded an annual incidence of 2.2 per 100 000 for ulcerative colitis and 2.0 for Crohn's disease, in both cases rising with age, inflammatory bowel dis-ease being a rare diagnosis in the under-10s. These figures are similar to those previously reported for Scandinavia and point away from a rising incidence in this already high-incidence region, perhaps indicating that (as in Lancashire) a plateau has now been reached.

The European Inflammatory Bowel Disease Study Group recently completed its assessment of the prevalence and incidence of inflamma-tory bowel disease in 20 areas chosen for their relatively stable popula-tion and expected reliable case ascertainment, but also to reflect the geographical and political variation within western Europe. The differ-ences are less than anticipated, and although there is a tendency for both Crohn's disease and ulcerative colitis to be less frequent in southern

Europe, the overall range of incidence and prevalence is everywhere within around 25% of the mean [10a].

The influence of race and ethnicity is discussed further in relation to the aetiopathogenesis of inflammatory bowel disease (see below), but the best known association – between Jewish origin and Crohn's disease – deserves comment here also. The magnitude of the association has probably been exaggerated by study methodology, but it appears real. In one representative and reasonably matched study, a relative risk fivefold (confidence interval 2.3–17.2-fold) higher than in non-Jewish residents was documented [11].

Data are scanty for within-country comparisons of other groups but there is no doubt, whatever allowance is made for poor case ascertainment and false diagnoses of intestinal tuberculosis in developing countries, that inflammatory bowel disease is much less common in Asia, Africa and South America. The rising incidence of Crohn's disease in northern Europe is paradoxically most obvious in those of an Asian background, but there are very few data on the population groups of African origin, in whom it is probably less frequent. A small study indicated an annual incidence of Crohn's disease of between 4.5 and 5.6 per 100 000 in those of West Indian origin living in Derby, UK, which was less than the rate of 7.0 per 100 000 in the local Caucasian population (but not significantly so) [12].

Seasonal variation in the onset of inflammatory bowel disease

Patients are often convinced that new and relapsing symptoms from inflammatory bowel disease are concentrated at certain times of year; there is some clinical and epidemiological support for this. Peak times for first presentation in the autumn and early winter, and for clinical relapses in the spring and autumn, with a relative dearth of clinical events in the summer months, have been suggested by several retrospective analyses [13, 14], but not others [15]. A large prospective study of incident cases [16] argues against such any such association for Crohn's disease, but is strongly indicative of a continuing cyclical incidence for ulcerative colitis, with regular peaks in winter, and troughs in late spring. Pooling data for four consecutive years provides December with a 1.48-fold increased risk for colitis presentation, while May is favoured at a relative rate of 0.76 (overall significance for departure from uniform distribution: $p = 0.028$). The obvious question as to why the month should influence presentation with colitis is unanswered but lends further credence to the hypothesis that there is an infective trigger for presentation if not necessarily one of a truly pathogenic nature (see below). Moum and colleagues speculated [16] that winter upper respiratory tract infections, or the antibiotics often used in their treatment, are implicated, and are inclined to dismiss the more obviously gastrointestinal pathogens which are more commonly isolated during summer months in Scandinavia. It is not clear why the peak months for incidence should appear to differ from those for relapse.

AETIOLOGY AND PATHOGENESIS

Introduction

The aetiology and pathogenesis of the inflammatory bowel diseases have limited immediate bearing on clinical practice, but it is hoped that the following analysis will aid an understanding of the disease process and of the mechanisms by which some therapeutic agents may act. It should also help to provide comprehensible answers to some of the justifiable and increasingly frequent questions being asked by patients about the cause(s) of their disease.

It is conventional to consider separately the inherited factors, assumed to be controlled genetically, and the environmental and other influences which predispose to inflammatory bowel disease. It is probable, however, that (in the absence of simple Mendelian inheritance) the genetic factors act predominantly as factors which place the predisposed individual at greater risk of sustaining inflammatory bowel disease when exposed to a subsequent environmental challenge. Pragmatism dictates that until such time as the relative apportionment of these influences is known, convention is followed: inherited and environmental aspects will therefore be considered separately.

Genetics of inflammatory bowel disease

General aspects and family studies
There is a clear familial link to both major forms of inflammatory bowel disease, with supportive data from studies of twins and individual families, and from population groups [17, 18]. The risk of a second first-order family member being affected lies between 1 in 15 and 1 in 10, which is in the region of 50 times the population prevalence (see above). The concordance rate for Crohn's in twin pairs is at least at the level of that seen in other conditions (such as insulin-dependent diabetes) for which a genetic link is uncontroversial. No less than 8 of 18 individuals with a monozygotic twin affected by Crohn's disease developed the disease themselves (compared to only 1 of 26 dizygotic twins) in the study of Tysk *et al.* [17]. Extended family pedigrees make it clear that simple monogenic Mendelian type inheritance is unlikely to be relevant, even with a complex attribution of incomplete penetrance. Although the technique of segregation analysis indicates that genetic predisposition is present in as few as 10% of inflammatory bowel disease patients [19], this is probably an underestimate,

given accumulating evidence for a variety of distinct genetic sites being involved, but each with low penetrance (and perhaps also dependent on additional environmental factors for disease expression).

Concordance for type of inflammatory bowel disease is generally stronger for Crohn's disease than for ulcerative colitis. There was, for example, only one pair of identical twins in whom both had ulcerative colitis of 16 pairs where the index twin had the disease, compared to the 8 (of 18) with Crohn's in Tysk's study [17]. Recent Oxford data which concentrated on affected sibs confirm a general tendency for the nature of the disease to be concordant [20]. Thus ulcerative colitis affected both of 29 sibling pairs; Crohn's, 42 pairs; and only 12 pairs with disease were discordant.

Anticipation

Ulcerative colitis seems to occur at a younger age in familial cases in comparison with those without a family history, with a significantly different mean age at diagnosis (28.5 v. 35 years; $p < 0.02$) in at least one study [20]. There is also a strong possibility that genetic 'anticipation' occurs in Crohn's disease. This concept has been established in other fields, and refers to the phenomenon where a genetically influenced disease presents at an earlier age with each successive generation. Anticipation was sought in a recent study from Baltimore of families concordant for Crohn's disease [21]. Family members from at least two generations were included, combining the data (where relevant) with an earlier published series. The mean age of diagnosis was more than 12 years earlier in the younger generation (at 18.9 years v. 31.4 years in the Baltimore families) – a statistically significant result. This difference was also carried across three generations in the few families thus afflicted. The possible biases introduced by earlier diagnosis being prompted by an informed family milieu, or by missing late-affected offspring, are considered by the authors (in the paper and in response to subsequent correspondence) and it is probable that these are insufficient to explain the differences seen (especially since in some families the child was diagnosed before the parent). In other conditions for which genetic anticipation is recorded there is an association with paternal transmission. This may also be pertinent in Crohn's disease, not least since in the Baltimore series (in which there was a greater extent of disease in the second-generation patient in 15 of 27 parent/child pairs) in 13 of the 15 pairs the affected parent was the father. There are otherwise no other obvious phenotypic differences between familial and non-familial cases for either ulcerative colitis or Crohn's.

HLA in ulcerative colitis

HLA links have long been sought in ulcerative colitis, in part because of the original descriptions of a link with positivity for HLA B27 in patients also affected by ankylosing spondylitis (Chapter 6), and the postulates that there were autoimmune phenomena operating in colitis (see below). A variety of HLA-A and HLA-B associations were reported in the 1980s, but with marked international differences and not a little controversy. The field is not an easy one for the amateur, given continuing uncertainty, and the multiple, overlapping names used for antigens and alleles. Methodological criticisms, particularly of small studies, have been invoked to explain many of the differences between past reports, and interest has increasingly converged on the class II antigens. Alleles for the serological DR2 antigens are reproducibly over-represented on both sides of the Pacific (around 40% of colitics compared to about 20% of control populations) with under-representation of DR4 and Drw6 [22, 23]. DR2 in general, and its DR15 subtype, DRB1*1502, in particular, have been associated with a higher frequency of total colitis, the latter predicting a higher frequency of intractability, while the DR2 DRB1*1501 subtype is reportedly protective against a need for surgery [23].

A recent Oxford study, aiming to avoid many of the earlier pitfalls in HLA work, considered haplotype sharing in relation to disease expression in 29 ulcerative colitis sib pairs [20]. If colitis were devoid of genetic influence one would expect a standard 1 : 2 : 1 ratio of complete, to partial, to absent haplotype identity for affected sibs. This proved not to be the case, there being strong linkage with the DRB1, DQB haplotype ($p = 0.016$) and the DRB1 locus ($p = 0.017$). Only one pair was discordant for both haplotypes, and 15 of the 29 pairs shared two DRB1, DQB haplotypes. The 1 : 2 : 1 ratio was thus replaced by an informative 15 : 13 : 1 ratio. The authors calculated a coefficient of genetic contribution for HLA genes of at least 64%, based on a background risk of 2–4% in siblings and of 6.3% in identical twins [17]. Although the DRB1*0103 and DRB1*12 alleles figured significantly more prominently than in the controls, and DRB1*04 was apparently protective, their numerical impact was small. The DR3, DQ2 haplotype (= DRB1*0301, DQB*0201) was significantly less frequent in females with colitis and gave apparent protection against distal disease (2.3% v. 26.3% in normal controls; $p = 0.001$), but was also strongly associated with extensive colitis (in both males and females) to a frequency of 32.9% ($p < 0.01$). However, there was no association between DR3, DQ2 and the need for colectomy. Comparable data (Caucasian sib pairs but from families with multiple members affected by inflammatory bowel disease) from St Mark's fail to support this degree of haplotype sharing [24]. The explanation for this disparity is not immediately obvious, and additional large series are probably required to establish the correct interpretation.

The degree of *expression* of HLA class II antigens on peripheral blood monocytes does appear to have an inverse correlation with disease activity, and low expression is positively linked to a need for surgery [25]. This aspect is considered further in respect of pathogenesis, antigen presentation and cytokine behaviour (see below).

HLA in Crohn's disease

Positive data for HLA linkage in Crohn's disease have been fewer than in ulcerative colitis, with no enduring associations with the class I antigens, and only weak links with those of class II, exemplified by the Californian study which suggested an association with a DR1, DQw5 haplotype rather than with any individual allele [22]. However, a recent study in the German population suggests a linkage to DRB1*07. This reasonably large study (162 unrelated patients, 4251 controls) examined selected class II alleles. DRB1*07 was present in 18.4% of patients v. 10.4% of controls (relative risk, 1.9) with a corrected confidence interval (CI) between 1.66 and 2.14. The association appeared most strong in patients with disease of onset before 35 years of age (relative risk, 3.1; CI, 2.44–3.76) [26]. In Boston a significant linkage has been demonstrated with the HLA DRB3*301 allele [27] which may be in linkage disequilibrium with the allele identified in Germany. French data support class II associations, with HLA DQB1*0501 overexpressed at an odds ratio of 1.6, DRB1*01 at 1.75, and, as in the German study, an increased frequency of DRB1*07 at 1.58 [28]. Satsangi's sib-pair study showed a number of small differences which were not sufficiently robust to survive Bonferroni correction for the number of tests performed [20].

Cytokine gene polymorphism

The influence of altered cytokine expression as part of the inflammatory response and its contribution to the pathogenesis of inflammatory bowel disease will be considered later, but there is also good evidence that the cytokine milieu is regulated at the genetic level through a series of gene polymorphisms. The interleukin-1 receptor antagonist (IL-1RA) gene has attracted most attention to date, coding as it does for an endogenous antagonist of IL-1, one of the most potent inflammatory mediators. Both cytokine and antagonist are implicated in the pathogenesis of inflammatory bowel disease. The gene for IL-1RA, which is on chromosome 2, has a number of alleles. Although there was initial confidence that allele 2 was positively associated with ulcerative colitis, this was only at a comparatively low relative risk with a prevalence of 35% in ulcerative colitis versus 24% in controls [29]. Only a minority of subsequent studies have reached the same conclusion (reviewed by Satsangi and Jewell [30]), but in some of those that have, the association is very strong [31]. It remains possible that allele 2 is important in some racial and ethnic groups but not others, and perhaps in predicting those in whom colitis is, or will become, extensive. It does not appear to be a key to a general understanding of ulcerative colitis pathogenesis.

Similar reservations apply to analysis of the other cytokine gene so far studied in depth. The expression of tumour necrosis factor-α (TNF-α) in Crohn's disease has aroused interest both in pathogenesis and in the potential for its therapeutic inhibition (Chapter 3). The TNF-α gene lies between the class I and class II HLA genes on chromosome 6 and, like IL-1RA, exhibits polymorphism. By chance, it is again a number 2 allele that has aroused interest. It appears that transcription of this allele is markedly and disproportionately higher in some cell lines, but although homozygotes have a higher risk of fatal cerebral malaria(!), the influence on inflammatory bowel disease is less clear-cut [30]. Targan's group found significant linkage to a particular TNF-α haplotype in 75 patients with Crohn's disease compared both to patients with ulcerative colitis and normal controls (relative risk 4.4 to 7.4) [32]. There was also a correlation between the over-represented haplotype – TNFa2b1c2d4e1 – and HLA-DR1/DQ5, which was overexpressed in the same group's earlier study [22], but at a lower frequency. The reasonable conclusion is that the true genetic linkage is to the TNF rather than to the HLA loci, and that this might contribute to heterogeneity in TNF-α production in Crohn's disease (see below), and perhaps also to prediction of response to therapeutic manipulation (Chapter 3).

Putative inflammatory bowel disease gene foci on chromosomes 2, 3, 7, 12 and 16

There are early indications that chromosome 16 may bear a susceptibility locus for Crohn's disease. A European collaborative study of DNA obtained from families with multiple affected members has permitted a genome-wide search using markers at roughly 13 centiMorgan intervals [33]. A putative locus lying near to (probably between) D16S409 and D16S419 has been identified. The provisionally named *IBD1* gene locus therefore lies near to known genes coding for several cell adhesion molecules and for the interleukin-4 receptor, lending potential pathophysiological relevance to its site (see below). However, exciting though this new development is, the magnitude of linkage is low – only a relative risk of 1.3 – and it is acknowledged that this locus can only account for a small fraction of the overall increase in Crohn's risk in affected families. Whether the locus has a bearing on risk of inflammatory bowel disease in non-familial cases remains to be seen, but this could prove to be important (cf. the *apc* gene defect in (rare) familial polyposis coli but also in (common) sporadic colorectal carcinoma).

The systematic genome-wide search in the Oxford sib-pair study supports linkage to the same focus on chromosome 16 in Crohn's disease, and provides somewhat stronger support for linkage to marker sites on chromosomes 3, 7 and 12 for both Crohn's and ulcerative colitis, with, in each case, a statistically significant 'lod' score in excess of 3. A further marker on chromosome 2 was linked to ulcerative colitis [34].

Other possible genetically coded associations with inflammatory bowel disease

The importance of apoptosis (programmed cell death) is being examined in many areas of gastrointestinal pathology, and may be of some relevance in inflammatory bowel disease, with particular bearing on abnormalities of intestinal permeability (see below). A Canadian group [35] has begun to establish a link between a greater expression of two lymphocyte subpopulations that are known to be predisposed to apoptosis and the increased intestinal permeability in patients with Crohn's disease and their healthy relatives (see below). Normal controls and ulcerative colitis patients, who had normal permeability, had few of the apoptosis-prone lymphocytes.

There is little doubt that other inflammatory bowel disease susceptibility genes of greater or lesser importance remain to be identified and characterized.

pANCA

Some years ago a circulating antibody to a neutrophil cytoplasmic antigen (ANCA) was found in patients with inflammatory bowel disease. It was thought initially to be that identified in systemic vasculitic conditions such as Wegener's granulomatosis, but subsequent immunohistological work has shown that it is a different antigen, the site of expression in inflammatory bowel disease having a distinct perinuclear focus – hence pANCA. The identity and function of the principal antigen remain unclear. However, the so-called bactericidal permeability-increasing protein appears to be a minor target antigen for ANCA and is itself related to colonic involvement in Crohn's disease and to disease activity in ulcerative colitis [36].

There is interest in whether patients with pANCA represent a clinically or biologically distinct subgroup and whether the expression of the antibody is genetically determined. There seem to be links between pANCA positivity and certain HLA subtypes, the DR3, DQ2, TNF-α2 haplotype being particularly strongly associated in the Oxford database [37]. There have been reports of pANCA being found in healthy first-order relatives of colitics [38, 39, 40], but the Oxford group found no cases of pANCA positivity in family members that did not themselves have an inflammatory condition with which the antibody is associated [41]. It remains possible that expression and familial risk vary between populations, but probable that pANCA is not itself a crucial marker of increased genetic risk.

pANCA antibodies are very frequently found in ulcerative colitis, but rarely in patients with Crohn's disease, in whom the rates of detection are similar to those of control populations, although these rates appear themselves to vary between geographical regions. There is a strong association between the presence of antibody and concurrent primary sclerosing cholangitis (Chapter 6). It does not seem likely that the antibody has a directly harmful effect nor that neutrophils are activated by the antibody. Expression of the antibody does not seem to reflect disease activity [42], although some authors find that antibody levels slowly diminish after colectomy. Estève *et al.* join those who predict a reduction in antibody positivity postoperatively, but base this on a comparison of postoperative patients with those who have not needed surgery, thereby neglecting the possibility that pANCA positivity (rather than diminishing because of successful surgery) is actually a good prognostic marker which indicates the patient who will not need resection [43]. Whether positivity for pANCA is associated with a particular inflammatory bowel disease phenotype remains controversial, apart from the strong link with sclerosing cholangitis, but more than one group has felt that patients with Crohn's disease and pANCA behave with more ulcerative colitis-like features than those without. Vasiliauskas *et al.* have now studied 69 patients with Crohn's disease and reach the same conclusion [44]. All pANCA-positive patients had colitis, compared to only just over half of those without the antibody (or with cANCA); they were less likely to have a positive family history (17% v. 35%); less likely to have fistulating disease (28% v. 39%), and less likely to have intestinal obstruction (39% v. 65%) or to need prolonged steroid therapy (1.8 years v. 4.2 years mean duration). Clearly these factors are not entirely independent and most do not reach statistical significance, but it does seem reasonable to consider that pANCA is a marker for some of the clinical features of Crohn's disease. It is doubtful that there is a causal link.

Intestinal permeability

Intestinal permeability is increased in both Crohn's and ulcerative colitis when these are active. The global changes (as measured by excretion of orally administered polyethylene glycol, simple sugars or EDTA) reflect abnormal permeability predominantly at the site of macroscopic disease, as recently confirmed in a small but careful study [45]. There is an identifiable defect in tight junction function, with associated abnormality of sodium transport, which is not of a secretory nature, but rather the result of profound barrier dysfunction and concurrent malabsorption. This can also be demonstrated in ulcerative colitis resection specimens [46].

Abnormal permeability could simply reflect the results of tissue damage once inflammation is established, but there is increasing evidence that it occurs earlier and has aetiopathogenetic significance. The pioneering study of Hollander and colleagues demonstrated changes not only in patients with Crohn's disease, but also in their healthy relatives [47], results which were challenged by others in the field, with vigorous objections to the use of the polyethylene glycol technique for assessing permeability. However, it is probable that there is a subgroup of healthy relatives in whom permeability is increased, while other relatives (or other families) have normal permeability. A recent study by Sutherland's group was designed to test further the generality of relevance of inherited permeability differences [48]. This was effectively a stress test for permeability in which patients with Crohn's disease and their first-degree relatives were compared with controls. Permeability was measured by the widely accepted postabsorption lactulose–mannitol ratio, and all subjects were studied before and after the administration of two 1.3 g doses of aspirin. Permeability rose between the two study periods by 57% in unrelated controls, but by 110% in healthy relatives, of whom 35% were considered 'hyper-responders'. The relatives were statistically distinguishable from the controls but not from those with Crohn's disease (133% increase). The majority of patients with Crohn's disease and a sub-set of their relatives with increased permeability also prove to have an associated phenotypic alteration of circulating B cells which is absent in controls [49]. The CD45RO isoform appeared almost exclusively and specifically in those with abnormal permeability, but independently of the presence of inflammation, again indicative of a primary role for abnormal permeability. The CD45RO isoform is itself strongly related to the immune response to antigen challenge. It thus seems probable that there is a inherited increase in permeability in some families with Crohn's disease, and that this might be aetiologically relevant. These affected relatives are probably those at especial risk of Crohn's disease if exposed to necessary additional factors. In other words, the increased permeability may be legitimately considered as a genetic risk factor that predisposes to the development of inflammatory bowel disease. Sutherland's group has indicated one such possible mechanism, since exposure to quantities of aspirin similar to those used in their study [48] is a common environmental challenge (and one that would not be likely to have been ascertained epidemiologically).

Abnormalities of permeability are generally evident before other manifestations of disease when sequential observation has been performed. In an illustrative study performed in Crohn's patients in remission, a high lactulose–mannitol ratio (indicative of increased permeability) predicted relapse within a year. Relapse occurred in 70% of such patients compared to only 17% of those with an initially normal result ($p < 0.01$) [50].

Cell adhesion molecules

At the cellular level, in addition to information on tight junctions, there is an increasing literature based around the cell adhesion molecules. These molecules have a key role in the normal behaviour of cells in relation to their neighbours, whether of the same or distinct morphological type. Understandably, much of the interest to date has focused on issues of oncogenesis and metastasis [51], but the cell adhesion molecules are of no less potential relevance to abnormalities of permeability in inflammatory bowel disease, in which their disorder could easily play a primary role. Migration of circulating leucocytes into intestinal tissues is clearly an important component of the inflammatory response and leads to some of the pathological changes recognized in inflammatory bowel disease.

Leucocyte immigration is preceded by 'rolling' and subsequent adhesion – both almost certainly governed to a large extent by the endothelial cell adhesion molecules. Relevance of the epithelial cell adhesion molecules is suggested by existing data on psoriasis and the bullous skin diseases in which desmosomal integrity and normal function of the integrins are impaired [51]. Bacteria also can make use of cell adhesion molecule receptors to gain access to mammalian cells, the particular case of *Yersinia* and its postulated entry via Peyer's patches using its invasin protein to bind to integrins [52], being of interest given the similarities between some forms of yersiniosis and Crohn's disease (see below).

The vascular cell adhesion molecule (VCAM-1) has important roles in leucocyte adherence (predominantly of monocytes) to the endothelial luminal surface, but although it is constitutively expressed in the colonic vasculature, there is disagreement as to whether there are alterations in its expression in patients with inflammatory bowel disease relative to controls. Koizumi *et al.* [53] found no differences, while the Leeds group found elevated levels that correlate well with clinical activity [54]. On the contrary the endothelial leucocyte adhesion molecule, ELAM-1, which is normally absent from colonic endothelium, is consistently found in the vessels of inflamed tissues in both ulcerative colitis and Crohn's disease, and within neutrophils in crypt abscesses [53]. There is a probable positive correlation with sites of free radical damage (see below). The intercellular adhesion molecule ICAM-1, which promotes the initial T cell–macrophage interaction, is also significantly elevated in active inflammatory bowel disease, and behaves in parallel with more traditional markers of inflammation such as C-reactive protein (CRP) and orosomucoid [54, 55]. Work combining inflammatory bowel disease tissues with an endothelial cell line confirms the link with ICAM-1, and adds comparable data implicating E-selectin [56]. This study also claims a significant difference in this over-expression between Crohn's disease and ulcerative colitis, with much greater levels of the adhesion molecules in Crohn's despite apparently similar degrees of inflammation histologically. P-selectin (also known as CD62) which, like the other selectins, binds to carbohydrate ligands rather than to other proteins, is also overexpressed in the vessels of both forms of inflammatory bowel disease when active [57]. Perhaps more important, however, is the observation that it is also focally overexpressed in tissues from patients in remission. *In vitro* work has also suggested that these molecules may have a role in the evolution of the granuloma [58].

There are animal data implicating dysfunction of the cell adhesion molecules and the key intercellular junctions in models of colitis [59], and a failure of normally regulated epithelial cell adhesion behaviour has also been implicated in pathologically excessive apoptosis (anoikis) in isolated colonic crypt cells [60]. Arguably the most exciting of all in this context is the behaviour of a genetically engineered mouse chimera bearing a mutant N-cadherin, N-cadherin delta [61]. N-cadherin is an epithelial cell adhesion molecule present in normal intestine but first described in neural tissue, hence N-cadherin. When the mutant N-cadherin was expressed in the entire crypt–villus axis a transmural gastrointestinal inflammation with many features common to Crohn's disease was demonstrable. Abnormal expression of this cadherin in the crypts was also found to be associated with abnormal proliferation and adenoma formation – could this link a cell adhesion defect associated with inflammation to the increased risk of neoplasia in inflammatory bowel disease (Chapter 8)?

It is not yet possible to be sure that these various associations between disorders of cell adhesion and inflammatory bowel disease are of an initiating nature; they may occur more as the result of inflammation, of which they are simply new markers. Clinical value could follow in either event, however, since antibodies to the cell adhesion molecules exist and could probably be adapted for therapeutic use.

The microvascular aetiology for inflammatory bowel disease

Speculation that Crohn's disease is of primarily vascular origin, arising via multifocal but microscopic infarction of the relevant areas of intestine, remains controversial [62], there being a parallel suggestion that the observations made could equally be explained by a primary defect affecting the lymphatic endothelium (given the considerable difficulties in distinguishing vascular from lymphatic endothelium). The granulomas characteristic of Crohn's disease do at least appear to be associated with vascular structures. In a study of 485 granulomas from the tissues of 15 patients, 85% were intimately associated with vascular injury, suggesting that abnormality of the intestinal microvasculature plays an early (if not necessarily causative) role in the pathogenesis of Crohn's disease [63]. It does not appear that any such vasculitis is mediated in an autoimmune fashion, since even when vasculitis is demonstrable histologically there is little evidence of a humoral immune response [64]. However, there is evidence for platelets having more than an incidental role. In an interesting peroperative study of platelet aggregation and neutrophil distribution, it has been demonstrated that as blood passes from mesenteric artery to vein there is the expected loss of neutrophils into the tissues in both ulcerative colitis and Crohn's disease [65], but that in Crohn's there is also a substantial increase in platelet aggregation as blood crosses the mesenteric capillary bed. This may indicate that platelets are contributing to microinfarction and local inflammation, and also presents the possibility that this is a major influence on vascular events distant from the gut (Chapter 7).

The marginal artery and ulcerative colitis

The striking demarcation of the upper limit of ulcerative colitis (Chapter 2) might suggest a vascular explanation. In a small study, not yet replicated in other centres, *in vitro* angiography and detailed pathological examination of colitis resection specimens indicated that the point of demarcation was coincident with the proximal extent of the marginal artery – a normally small branch of the inferior mesenteric artery [66]. The observation as it stands is impressive, but it is difficult to conceptualize why this 'additional' blood supply should predispose to colitis, and difficult to understand how initially distal colitis can spread to involve more proximal sites (Chapter 2), given the embryological determination of the extent of the marginal artery, unless the vascular status merely defines the maximum possible extent of disease.

Mucus and mucins

There are deficiencies and abnormalities of the intestinal mucus layer in ulcerative colitis [67] and associated abnormality of the mucus glycoproteins, with evidence in both colitis and Crohn's disease that there may be deranged restitution of damaged mucosa, perhaps mediated by defects in normal functioning of transforming growth factor-β (TGF-β), intestinal trefoil peptide or transglutamase [68]. The colonocyte is known to be partially dependent on short-chain fatty acids, and it appears that there are reductions in both availability and utilization of butyrate in active ulcerative colitis, and, moreover, that butyrate exposure and mucin production are directly linked [69]. It is probable that the mucus loss in active colitis is the result of faecal mucinase activity [70], given differences in levels in stools from patients with ulcerative colitis and in those from Crohn's disease patients and normal controls. The links between smoking and inflammatory bowel disease also implicate mucins (see below). The impact of gastrointestinal microflora on this process remains to be determined (see below).

Infection as the cause of inflammatory bowel disease

Introduction

For many years, and arguably for the entire history of recognized Crohn's disease, infective aetiologies have been sought, and postulated pathogenic organisms promulgated by their individual enthusiastic supporters. Longest runners in this particular race are the mycobacteria, suspected even by Crohn and his colleagues. However, before considering individual organisms it may be instructive to explore a number of epidemiological pointers. Inflammatory bowel disease remains a rare diagnosis in the developing world. Although this may reflect underdiagnosis, it is highly probable that the incidence and prevalence of both ulcerative colitis and Crohn's disease are substantially lower than in developed countries. Emerging and more newly developed countries report a steadily rising incidence of inflammatory bowel disease (see above). An intriguing three-centre study performed in the UK [71] examined the childhood socio-economic circumstances of patients with inflammatory bowel disease in comparison to controls matched by age, sex and general practice registration. Access to hot running water and a separate bathroom in the first five years of life were associated with greatly *increased* risk of Crohn's disease (relative risks after correction for social class of 5.0 and 3.3, respectively) (but not of ulcerative colitis). This falls short of a causal association but might be taken to suggest that protection from 'ordinary' environmental organisms in early childhood renders some individuals more prone to Crohn's disease in later life. Countries with a high mortality from childhood diarrhoeal illnesses consistently have a low frequency of inflammatory bowel disease. An untestable supplementary assertion may be constructed that endemic gastrointestinal infection kills those who would otherwise go on to develop inflammatory bowel disease. This hypothesis is tangentially supported by observations made in several of the gene knock-out animal models considered below. If these animals are housed in germ-free environments they remain healthy, but their exposure to a normal, non-sterile environment leads inevitably to an inflammatory bowel disease-like state.

Evidence from a number of centres manifest in a variety of different fashions supports the idea that infective organisms may act as triggers for relapses of inflammatory bowel disease: this is certainly many patients' experience at an anecdotal level. Particular organisms loosely associated with this phenomenon include *Clostridium difficile*, *Campylobacter* species, toxigenic *E. coli*, *Aeromonas* species, and a *Helicobacter* species (not *H. pylori*). There is no reliable evidence that what is being described is any more than a more severe clinical manifestation of an otherwise mild gastrointestinal infection in a patient with an underlying inflammatory bowel disease. Infection may have an important role in modulation of an underlying mucosal barrier defect (see above), and thereby promote disease in a situation when the normal individual would be protected. It is striking that when injury, ischaemia or severe inflammation leads to perforation of the intestinal wall, profound adverse consequences follow, with, at the very least, the formation of a circumscribed intra-abdominal abscess, if not frank peritonitis and septicaemia. However, these life-threatening illnesses are caused by organisms that belong to the normal gut flora and which may be not only commensal but sometimes actively beneficial to the human host when in their correct location. It is not surprising that the intestinal mucosa is well equipped to contain such potential pathogens, but it is a little remarkable that normally no inflammatory response is demonstrable. Several research units have explored this lack of response and compared it to the situation in inflammatory bowel disease patients. It appears that rectal dialysates and lavage fluid from the normal intestine do not activate neutrophils despite the coexistence of the normal gut flora. Ferguson makes the pertinent point that this is probably a more significant observation than that of the chemotactic activation seen in samples from inflammatory bowel disease patients [72]. Epithelial permeability can certainly be shown to be disrupted by bacterial infection *in vitro* [73].

Newer data implicate hydrogen sulphide, which is, in turn, a product of sulphate-reducing bacteria. Many inflammatory bowel disease patients describe offensive flatus and it is generally the case that sulphur-containing gases are responsible. It is difficult to perform objective studies of flatus for obvious reasons [74] but data do exist, and Levine *et al.* [75] have examined gas production in sealed samples of faeces, demonstrating striking differences between control and colitic stools, the latter producing up to four times as much hydrogen sulphide (but no differences in other metabolites studied). Hydrogen sulphide is not only unpleasant, it is also toxic, with an effect on mice not dissimilar to equimolar amounts of cyanide. A review by Pitcher and Cummings explores this area [76] and suggests that excess luminal sulphide overwhelms a genetically determined capacity for mucosal detoxification, with consequent impaired butyrate oxidation and the beginnings of colitis. There is here an attractive set of potential links between this observation, the abnormalities in faecal mucinases described above, and the postulated links with (abnormal?) gut flora. The resident colonic bacteria are found predominantly to ferment residual dietary carbohydrate in the proximal colon, but a much greater proportion of peptides and amino acids on the left side. There is consequently a greater release of nitrogenous (and sulphur-containing) moieties more distally. As these are arguably more pathogenic than the methane produced more proximally from anaerobic metabolism of carbohydrate, this provides another possible explanation for the distal distribution of ulcerative colitis (J. Cummings, personal communication).

Specific organisms in Crohn's disease aetiology

Three specific organisms have been seriously proposed as the cause of Crohn's disease: *Mycobacterium paratuberculosis*, the measles virus and *Listeria*; groups of potential pathogens are also suggested and a number of additional groupings of potential pathogens. Each has its protagonists, and this is probably the area above all others that has led inflammatory bowel disease research workers to follow faith rather than science. This is unfortunate as it has led to relatively sterile debates that have probably combined to delay a fuller understanding of the pathogenesis of the diseases. The evidence in favour of the three candidate organisms is incomplete and in each case falls a long way short of fulfilling Koch's postulates. It may also be apposite to remember that bacterial overgrowth in the small bowel is responsible for malabsorption and diarrhoea and yet that the organisms concerned are normal gut flora, and that overgrowth of *C. dif-*

ficile (a relatively inconspicuous member of some individuals' normal flora) is responsible for a distressing and sometimes catastrophic colitis.

Mycobacterium paratuberculosis

Mycobacterium paratuberculosis is causatively associated with a granulomatous disease of cattle – Johne's disease – which shares a number of features with Crohn's disease. The organism is relatively ubiquitous in the human environment, and is both present in cows' milk and prone to survive pasteurization. The evidence for *M. paratuberculosis* in intestine from Crohn's disease patients is convincing, with only occasional detectable bacteria, but bacterial antigens or DNA found in around 65% of samples studied, compared to frequencies of well under 20% in most control tissues (including those from ulcerative colitis patients as well as from normal individuals) [77]. These observations are relatively consistent from centre to centre, but reports using modern technology which fail to demonstrate a different prevalence of detection of the organism in Crohn's disease from that in other patient groups are also to be found [78]. In distinction from Johne's disease, there is often no associated inflammatory response at the sites of these antigens, and there are concerns that polymerase chain reaction assay techniques may be responsible for some false positives. No series has been able to demonstrate anything near to a 100% association in well-documented Crohn's disease, and there is a frequency of detection of DNA even at the sites of granulomata of under 25% [79]. Neither Koch's postulates nor modifications thereof which take account of advances in molecular biology are satisfied [80]. There is no substantial body of epidemiological evidence favouring a higher frequency of Crohn's disease in those particularly closely exposed to *M. paratuberculosis*, indeed rather the opposite given the negative association with exposure to environmental organisms in farmers [81], and the comparative incidence of Crohn's disease in First and Third World populations. The question of antibiotic therapy in inflammatory bowel disease will be returned to (Chapter 3), but the general failure of antimycobacterial regimes to help in Crohn's disease, and the generally positive effects of corticosteroids, also argue against the case for continuing infection with *M. paratuberculosis*. A small number of centres around the world remain convinced that it is truly causative, but a scientific basis for this conclusion is lacking.

Measles

A number of human diseases have been linked to persistent infection with paramyxoviruses, of which subacute sclerosing panencephalitis is now very firmly associated with prior measles infection. Although, until the advent of immunization, acute measles infection was virtually the rule in childhood, preliminary epidemiological evidence and the observation of putative viral particles in tissues from Crohn's disease patients have prompted further exploration of measles as a causative agent of IBD. Clinical support is arguably lent by the well-known occurrence of oral aphthous ulcers (and vasculitis) in both acute measles and Crohn's disease. Measles antigens were detected in Crohn's disease tissues by use of a novel nucleoprotein antibody immunogold technique, supporting the view that the virus may persist in the intestine after acute infection [82]. Low levels of antigen were also found in tissues from a patient with ileocaecal tuberculosis, leaving open the possibility that persistently infected immune cells aggregate in foci of inflammation without necessarily having any causal association. It is also possible that the (immune) patient with intestinal disease who is re-exposed to measles is not able to prevent uptake of the virus into the inflamed tissues, though obviously able to mount an adequate immunological response to avoid a recurrence of acute measles. Comparable studies in other laboratories have so far failed to lend support to a specific involvement of measles virus, and Haga *et al.* were unable to demonstrate any evidence of genetic material from measles, mumps or rubella viruses in intestinal resections from patients with Crohn's or ulcerative colitis, or in controls without inflammatory bowel disease [83].

There are good epidemiological links between perinatal measles infection and subsequent development of Crohn's disease, with infants born during epidemics being almost 1.5 times more likely to develop Crohn's disease within 30 years than those born in non-epidemic periods [84]. The four (of 25 000) pregnancies complicated by clinically diagnosed measles in Uppsala between 1940 and 1949 prove especially striking. Of the offspring of these four women no fewer than three have required multiple resections for severe Crohn's disease [85]. Interestingly the fourth child, without Crohn's disease, was the only one of the four to have suffered clinical measles. However, the dramatic reductions in clinical measles infections in developed and developing countries have not been associated with a reduction in the incidence of Crohn's disease – rather the converse, a phenomenon perhaps even exaggerated by the administration of measles vaccination [86]. The proposed explanations put forward by the Royal Free group are largely based on the premise that the timing of exposure to measles virus or its antigens is crucial, and it is at least plausible that those who previously died of overwhelming measles infection and now survive (because of improved social circumstances or vaccination) are those who now go on to develop Crohn's disease. There are also important questions to be answered in respect of ulcerative colitis, which is also linked to measles by some of the Ekbom/Wakefield data, but without a comparable rationalizing hypothesis, and of linkage with influenza epidemics.

An interesting study from Guinea-Bissau may provide part of the explanation for the link between infection and inflammatory bowel disease [87]. The study was of adults, and hinges on documentation of

measles infections during an epidemic in their childhood; it is accordingly subject to some reservations. Nevertheless atopy (skin-prick positive)
proved almost twice as common in those who had been vaccinated and
avoided measles in 1979, compared to their unvaccinated compatriots
who developed measles (25.6% v. 12.8%). The difference remained significant when corrected for such factors as breast-feeding. If childhood
measles infection can in some way prevent development of atopy, then it
seems very reasonable to suppose that it might have other long-term
immunological effects. Equally, there is no reason that this response (or
responses) should be unique to measles amongst putative pathogens.

Listeriosis
Listeria is the latest specific micro-organism to be suggested as the cause of
Crohn's disease [88]. In something of a fishing expedition, intestinal tissues
and mesenteric lymph nodes were examined for a whole variety of micro-
organisms. Again there was overrepresentation of specific bacterial antigens
in Crohn's tissues, with 75% of 16 patients expressing listerial antigens, particularly at sites of ulceration and inflammation, in comparison to only 13%
of colitics and in no controls. *Listeria monocytogenes*, like *M. paratuberculosis*,
is ubiquitous in the environment, is known to invade intestinal M cells and
can produce an experimental ileo-colitis in which it is found to be an intracellular pathogen. The fact that the very same study records similar data for
E. coli and streptococci (57% and 44% positive, respectively) must be considered to weaken the case for an aetiological link, but rather to confirm that
the (already) abnormal intestine is excessively permeable to, or poor at eliminating, a range of microbial antigens. Greater significance might be drawn
from the French group's inability to demonstrate certain putative
pathogens such as the measles virus; corroborative data are required.

Enteropathic E. coli
A study of enteropathic *E. coli* lysates demonstrated that these organisms
have the potential to inhibit selectively the production of IL-2, IL-4, IL-5
and γ-interferon (γ-IFN), but not of several other cytokines, from peripheral blood mononuclear cells [89]. Transfection experiments confirm that
this behaviour of the bacteria is genetically determined, and while not necessarily transferable to the situation *in vivo*, indicates that bacteria have the
ability to provoke a more complex immune response, and one that could
have bearing on the expression of inflammatory bowel disease.

Normal gastrointestinal flora in pathogenesis of inflammatory bowel disease
It looks increasingly likely that the correct interpretation of the link
between micro-organisms and Crohn's disease is that disease is the result
of a dysregulated host immune response to ubiquitous normal intestinal
flora or to not especially damaging pathogens. Normal luminal bacteria

appear to have the potential to influence Crohn's disease, and the sites most commonly involved (terminal ileum, caecum and left colon) are also those at which concentrations of micro-organisms tend to be maximal. Many measures which reduce intestinal microflora (such as gut lavage, intestinal bypass, creation of ileostomy, exclusive elemental or parenteral nutrition, antibiotic regimes) may also produce therapeutic benefit (Chapters 3 and 4).

There is also evidence for a humoral immune response to intestinal organisms, with significant levels of circulating antibodies to a variety of antigens. Purified subcellular bacterial components such as lipopolysaccharide and peptidoglycan polysaccharide can produce intestinal inflammation (sometimes with an associated systemic reaction). A reproducible granulomatous enterocolitis can be provoked by intramural injection of streptococcal cell wall fragments into rat intestine. This persists to give chronic inflammation and is associated with mesenteric and lymph node disease in nearly half of the challenged animals [90].

Since the excitement in the late 1950s when cross-reaction between a circulating antibody and the colon was demonstrated in ulcerative colitis [91], and the subsequent demonstration of an *E. coli* antigen that is shared by colonic mucosa [92], there has been a quest for evidence of destructive autoimmunity. This has been relatively unproductive as these antibodies are not specific for inflammatory bowel disease, and are not themselves cytopathic. It seems probable that this is not an important mechanism in Crohn's disease, but there are newer, provisional, but potentially significant data in ulcerative colitis, albeit concentrated in work from a small number of interested centres.

Models of inflammatory bowel disease

The older animal models of inflammatory bowel disease are falling into disuse, and not only because of concerns about animal welfare. Many of them (for example those induced by acetic acid, immune complexes, trinitrobenzene sulphonic acid/ethanol, non-steroidal anti-inflammatories) induce a short-term, self-limiting disease which lacks the chronic self-perpetuating nature that defines spontaneous inflammatory bowel disease. The more current animal models and their particular attributes (including those from carrageenan, dextran sulphate sodium, peptidoglycan-polysaccharide, cyclosporin or lymphogranuloma venereum infection), and the mutant and transgenic animals such as the SCID (severe combined immunodeficiency) mouse, the HLA-B27-β_2-microglobulin transgenic rat, and mice mutant for IL-2, IL-10 or T-cell receptors, were recently reviewed by Elson and colleagues [93]. It is striking that bacteria, and perhaps especially *Bacteroides*, are involved in the expression of almost all of the spontaneous/mutant/immunological models, and even in non-steroidal-induced colitis are responsible for perpetuation of disease. The gene knock-out animal models express 'inflammatory bowel diseases' only when the animal is exposed to a normal laboratory environment, and disease is prevented by upbringing in a germ-free unit.

Few animals get a spontaneous disease at all like inflammatory bowel disease, but an endangered monkey, the cottontop tamarin, and a mouse strain (C3H/HeJBir which develops a spontaneous proximal colitis with perianal ulcers) are exceptions. The tamarin develops a spontaneous colitis, which has much in common with ulcerative colitis, including the propensity for colorectal carcinoma, and may be responsible for death; the disease only seems to affect animals held in captivity. The tamarin also expresses the abnormal 40 kDa protein which has been associated with ulcerative colitis (see below) [94].

Although very useful information continues to emerge from intelligent study of animal models and from application of cell culture technology, there are also two situations in which we have a situation approaching a human model for inflammatory bowel disease. Recurrence at the site of anastomoses in Crohn's disease, and so-called pouchitis in ulcerative colitis are sufficiently common in patients considered free of inflammatory bowel disease shortly beforehand that the patient with a new anastomosis or pouch can be considered a model system or to have 'pre-inflammation'.

The anastomotic recurrence as an aetiological model for Crohn's disease

Post-resection relapse in Crohn's disease affects up to 100% on endoscopic criteria by 3–5 years postoperatively, with up to 40% affected by symptomatic relapse over the same time period (Chapters 2 and 4). Relapse is much rarer if a terminal ileostomy is performed (<20%), but if continuity is then restored, relapse is frequent and usually occurs at, or just above, the anastomosis. It is odd that the recurrence typically affects the neoterminal ileum rather than the previously defunctioned bowel distal to the anastomosis, as might more obviously be suggested. Rutgeerts described five such patients who relapsed in this way, having been well prior to ileostomy closure, and suggests that reflux of the faecal stream is crucial to this phenomenon [95]. Other suggestions to explain the predominance of the neoterminal ileal site of recurrence include mechanical or neurovascular impediments imposed by the surgery itself, but why these influences should apply to the bowel in continuity and not to the arguably more pathological end ileostomy is more difficult to conceptualize. Some light may be shed in this area by a curious epidemiological observation. Meckel's diverticulum – a relic of vitelline duct embryology – is present in somewhere between 0.6 and 3.0% of Caucasian populations, depending on how the data are collected. In a study of 294 patients having their first resection for Crohn's disease we found a 5.8% prevalence of these diverticula [96]. Their presence was not associated with heterotopic, acid-secreting mucosa, and they are not obviously pathogenic in any conventional sense, but we have speculated that they may mark zones of local alteration in gastrointestinal permeability or immune reactivity, and they do, of course, lie in the high-risk area of distal ileum most affected by Crohn's disease. It is feasible that the surgical re-anastomosis within the peritoneum (as opposed to the ileostomy which is exteriorized) behaves in some degree like a Meckel's diverticulum and influences the expression of (recurrent) Crohn's disease in a comparable but exaggerated fashion.

The importance of the faecal stream has been further addressed in a study of patients with Crohn's disease undergoing faecal diversion or (different patients) having continuity restored, in comparison to those without Crohn's having the same procedures [97]. Faecal diversion, as expected, produced clinically and statistically significant improvement in the activity of Crohn's disease. This was associated with a fall in rectal mucosal glycoprotein synthesis and maintenance of the preoperative levels of rectal crypt cell production, and significant deterioration of the macro- and microscopic appearance of the rectum. However, in the control patients having faecal diversion (mostly for cancer, non-Crohn's-related fistula or incontinence), rectal crypt cell production rate fell and rectal mucosal glycoprotein synthesis was maintained postoperatively, with no deterioration in rectal appearance. Following restoration of continuity, mucosal glycoprotein synthesis and crypt cell proliferation then rose. In Crohn's disease mucosal synthesis and proliferation rose, but not significantly so, following restoration of continuity. These observations do not explain the pattern of recurrence, but indicate that the distal defunctioned bowel continues to behave abnormally even when global evidence of inflammation is absent or quiescent. They provide important clues as to why diversion colitis (Chapter 4) is over-represented in Crohn's disease, and further support for the view that the distal bowel is vulnerable to deprivation of luminal nutrients or trophic factors (short-chain fatty acids being particularly implicated).

The ileo-anal pouch as a model for ulcerative colitis
The rationale for, and clinical aspects of, creation of the ileo-anal pouch for patients with ulcerative colitis are discussed in Chapter 4, but its inflammatory complication – 'pouchitis' – deserves attention here as it represents a fascinating and unique disease model for ulcerative colitis itself. The pouch has, intentionally, a marked degree of luminal stasis, and consequently an altered exposure to bacterial flora, bile acids and other potential inflammatory mediators, which are relatively foreign to the small bowel from which it is formed. The pouch quite rapidly takes on a number of colonic features with colonic metaplasia of the mucosa (Chapter 4). All these elements are common to the pouch for colitis and that performed for familial adenomatous polyposis for which the surgical procedure is

identical. However, pouchitis occurs at some time in around 20% of patients who previously had ulcerative colitis, but hardly ever, if at all, in patients having the operation for familial polyposis. The histological (and endoscopic) features of pouchitis have much in common with ulcerative colitis, and earlier thoughts that pouchitis was the result of re-emergent (previously misdiagnosed) Crohn's disease have now been dismissed. The disproportionate coexistence of extra-intestinal manifestations of inflammatory bowel disease and pouchitis [98] suggests a systemic link and (as with the absence of pouchitis in polyposis patients) that the exposure of the ileum in the pouch to unfamiliar content is not an adequate explanation. It may be worth noting here the evidence for abnormalities of small intestinal permeability in a majority of patients with ulcerative colitis [99] – ulcerative colitis begins to appear a more diffuse intestinal or systemic disorder than is conventionally accepted. Study of unselected patients after pouch creation should help to determine the factors that lead to pouchitis and perhaps those that predispose to colitis in the first place.

Specific lymphocyte defects and tolerance

The problem in understanding inflammatory bowel disease might succinctly be described as the continuing failure to explain why a response of the bowel that would be appropriate for an acute infection (such as bacillary dysentery) persists and cannot be 'turned off'. This continued self-perpetuating inflammation has been attributed *inter alia* to defects in suppressor T-cell function, with consequent overactivation of CD4 cells. In testing this hypothesis, Chan and Mayer found that oral antigen administration (keyhole limpet haemocyanin) had the opposite effect in Crohn's disease patients [100]. When subsequent subcutaneous immunization with the antigen was performed, the Crohn's patients had an exaggerated T-cell response compared to normal controls and ulcerative colitis patients (but little difference from the colitics in antibody response). A recent paper from Mainz [101] points in a similar direction, finding selective tolerance to intestinal flora from autologous but not from heterologous intestine. Lamina propria lymphocytes taken from apparently healthy bowel of inflammatory bowel disease patients exhibited tolerance to bacterial preparations from the same intestine, as do those from the gut of healthy controls. However, exaggerated CD4 and CD8 expression, with resultant increased cytokine production, was demonstrable if bacteria from other than the host intestine were incubated with the lymphocytes. If lymphocytes from areas of active inflammatory bowel disease were employed, then both host and non-host bacterial preparations had this effect. It is not at all clear how this extraordinary recognition of 'pet' bacteria in the normal intestine is mediated. Further work is clearly warranted in this area, since it could begin to explain some of the influences of dietary variation, perhaps some of the geographical variation, as well as being of interest in its own right as the first descriptions of a functional defect in mucosal suppressor T cells in inflammatory bowel disease.

Immunoglobulins in inflammatory bowel disease

The principal immunoglobulin in the normal intestine is IgA, but in inflammatory bowel disease there is increased production of IgG (especially IgG1). The antigens provoking this change in antibody profile are becoming better understood, with recent evidence from the King's group suggesting, at least in Crohn's disease, that much of the exaggerated mucosal response is directed against non-pathogenic faecal bacteria [102]. The implied breakdown in tolerance to normal commensal gut flora is readily accounted for by a prior disruption of intestinal permeability – a point not lost on these authors who have long been interested in this field.

There is a 40 kDa colonic protein which is specifically recognized by tissue-bound IgG in samples from patients with ulcerative colitis, and circulating antibodies to this protein are found only in (a large majority of) patients with active ulcerative colitis [103]. It is suggested that an autoimmune response to this antigen leads to complement activation via IgG1 and thus to epithelial damage and continuing inflammation [104]. Interestingly, the protein is also expressed in certain of the epithelial tissues of the skin, eye, synovium and biliary tract but not at other sites [105, 106], raising the question as to its possible relevance to extra-intestinal manifestations of ulcerative colitis at these sites (Chapter 6). Although this could be important in respect of sclerosing cholangitis, which is much more often seen in ulcerative colitis, it does not fit so readily with the other extra-intestinal manifestations of inflammatory bowel disease which are seen as often in patients with Crohn's disease (Chapter 6).

Cytokines and pathogenesis

In inflammatory bowel disease, as in other inflammatory conditions, polypeptide cytokines are expressed by immunoreactive cells and play an important role in mediation of the disease process. They also contribute to the destructive effects on the target tissues. Most of the cytokines can be demonstrated in tissues and in the circulation at higher than normal levels in patients with inflammatory bowel disease (Table 1.1), and there is usually a positive correlation with disease activity. It is less certain that they have a primarily aetiological role, but they are strongly, if non-specifically, influenced by existing pharmacological measures, and their more targeted manipulation can be seen to have substantial therapeutic potential. This is not the place for a detailed review of the cytokines, not least since, in this rapidly changing field, new moieties are still being identified at regular intervals, and the preferred nomenclature is still somewhat in evolution. However, it may be helpful to recognize that they fall into broad functional groups, including those with (for example) predominantly pro-inflammatory effects (e.g. IL-1 or tumour necrosis factor-α (TNF-α)), those with a more regulatory role (e.g. IL-4 or IL-10), those which are predominantly chemokine (e.g. IL-8), or those with more specific roles in healing and repair (e.g. TGF-β).

Inflammatory bowel disease is associated with an enhanced activation of T cells [107] but the effect is much more pronounced in Crohn's disease than in ulcerative colitis. This is exemplified by the different response of lymphocytes of the lamina propria to IL-2. In Crohn's disease there is then enhanced cytotoxicity, whereas ulcerative colitis cells tend to be inhibited [108]. The distinct cytokine profiles of the Th1 and Th2 classes of CD4-positive T-helper cells (hence Th) may be a reflection of these differences. Th1 lymphocytes produce predominantly γ-IFN and IL-2 and are most involved with cell-mediated immunity, while Th2 cells, which secrete IL-4, -5, -10 and -13, are more associated with stimulation of the B cells and a brisk antibody response. This in turn suggests that differential cytokine expression may contribute to the differences in disease expression between ulcerative colitis and Crohn's disease.

One important reason for believing that cytokine abnormalities could have truly aetiological significance comes from the extreme case of genetically engineered animal models rendered deficient in one or other respect [93]. The IL-10 gene knock-out mouse, for example, gets progressive, patchy intestinal inflammation when reared in a normal, non-sterile environment, and has been considered to have a condition similar to Crohn's disease. The IL-2 knock-out mouse, on the other hand, develops a condition with many similarities to human ulcerative colitis, again only when raised in a normal, non-sterile environment. It is not, of course, suggested that diseased humans have cytokine defects of such profundity, but that lesser abnormalities of cytokine expression could have a predisposing influence on the development of inflammatory bowel disease – perhaps contributing to the dichotomy between the ulcerative colitis and Crohn's disease phenotypes. Such abnormalities could themselves be of genetic or acquired origin; continued study of mutant animals seems likely to be productive in the further understanding of inflammatory bowel disease pathogenesis.

Alteration in expression of TNF-α appears to occur early in the recurrence of Crohn's disease. In prospective endoscopic evaluation of postoperative patients [109] high and sustained levels were found, correlating to some extent with the severity of recurrence. Although this further legitimizes therapeutic manipulation of TNF-α (Chapter 3), it was felt that its influence was more likely in perpetuating than in initiating inflammation,

Table 1.1 Brief classification of cytokines

Cytokine	UC	CD	Effects
γ-IFN	N/d	i	Pro-inflammatory; activation of Th1 cells and macrophages increases release of IL-1
IL-1	i	i	Pro-inflammatory; activation of macrophages, T cells, polymorphs, mesenchymal cells and endothelial cells; increases release of IL-2
IL-2	N/d	i	Proliferation and activation of Th1 and cytotoxic lymphocytes; increases release of γ-IFN and IL-9
IL-3	d	d	Pro-inflammatory; stimulation of stem and mast cells
IL-4	d	d	Regulatory; activation of Th2 cells, suppression of Th1 cells
IL-5	?	?	Eosinophil and mast cell product; eosinophil differentiation
IL-6	i	i	Pro-inflammatory; stimulation of the acute-phase response
IL-7	?	?	Intestinal epithelial and goblet cell product; growth factor for intra-epithelial lymphocytes
IL-8	i	i	Chemokine; polymorph chemotaxis
IL-9	?	?	T-cell product; anti-apoptotic; responsive to IL-2
IL-10	i	N	Regulatory; down-regulation of Th1 cells and macrophages
IL-11	?	?	Marrow-derived growth factor for megakaryocytes and murine intestinal stem cells
IL-12	N	i	Pro-inflammatory and regulatory; stimulates Th1 and NK cells
IL-13	?	?	Monocyte down-regulation (especially of TNF-α)
IL-1RA	i	i	Regulatory; inhibits IL-1
TNF-α	N/i	N/i	Pro-inflammatory; activation of macrophages, polymorphs, mesenchymal and endothelial cells
TGF-β	N	N/i	Chemokine/healing/repair; monocyte chemotaxis, suppression of lymphocyte proliferation, increased collagen synthesis
IGF-1	?	i	Healing/repair; epithelial cell and fibroblast proliferation, increased collagen synthesis
GM-CSF	i	i	Product of many cell types; proliferation of granulocyte and monocyte precursors
EGF	?i	?i	Healing/repair; intestinal stem cell product in response to ulceration
MCP-1	i	i	Chemokine; macrophage chemotaxis

UC, ulcerative colitis; CD, Crohn's disease; i, increased; d, decreased; N, normal; IFN, interferon; IL, interleukin; TNF, tumour necrosis factor; TGF, transforming growth factor; IGF, insulin-like growth factor; GM-CSF, granulocyte/macrophage colony stimulating factor; EGF, epidermal growth factor; MCP, monocyte chemoattractant protein; NK, natural killer.

The data for the table have been pooled from many sources (including a summary given by R.B. Sartor at Digestive Diseases Week, San Francisco, 1996) and are intended to give only a general overview; it is recognized (for example) that expression in tissue and in circulation is not always the same for a given cytokine, and that the list will not be thought comprehensive by experts in the field.

given that there were changes in biopsy supernatant γ-interferon levels prior to the rise in TNF-α.

There are some further interesting human data specific to IL-2. Soluble IL-2 receptor levels are increased in active inflammatory bowel disease to the extent that it has been suggested as a useful marker of disease activity, by analogy with CRP or orosomucoid (Chapter 2). A recent paper examining the process of T-cell activation found these typical increases in IL-2 receptor but also an impairment of T-cell proliferation in Crohn's disease which could be normalized by exogenous IL-2 despite the apparent normality of endogenous IL-2 production [110]. Again, there may be therapeutic consequences of this observation.

IL-4 is considered to have a modulatory role, tending to influence the balance of Th1 and Th2 cells in an anti-inflammatory direction. It is deficient in lamina propria lymphocytes (mRNA and protein product) from patients with Crohn's disease and ulcerative colitis [111]. As IL-4 expression was most obviously impaired in cells from actively inflamed intestine, it is likely that it is not an initiating abnormality, but its manipulation is clearly another avenue open to therapeutic efforts.

IL-10 is an immunoregulatory cytokine of Th2 cells with predominantly inhibitory effects on other T cells and on antigen presentation, with down-regulation of class II histocompatibility antigens. The production and release of a variety of pro-inflammatory cytokines are suppressed by IL-10 both *in vitro* and *in vivo* [112]. Although IL-10 levels are well preserved or high in inflammatory bowel disease [113], there is evidence that the concentrations are inadequate to the demand and that supplementary therapeutic IL-10 may be beneficial (Chapter 3) .

γ-IFN appears capable of increasing antibody-dependent cellular cytotoxicity in ulcerative colitis [114], and may as such have a further role in pathogenesis in addition to its well-known effects on antigen presentation, and the possibility that some of the therapeutic influence of aminosalicylates may be by this route.

Reactive oxygen species and free radicals

Free radicals are responsible for tissue damage in most inflammatory conditions to a greater or lesser extent. The relationship of reactive oxygen moieties to secretory diarrhoea has recently been reviewed [115], some of these data being of potential relevance to the pathogenesis of inflammatory bowel disease. The diarrhoea in both Crohn's disease and ulcerative colitis has a secretory component, and it is reasonable to explore the possibility that oxygen radicals may contribute. *In vitro* studies of inflammatory cells from inflammatory bowel disease patients confirm that they are able to generate reactive oxygen metabolites in excess, and, to judge from tissue studies, it is likely that the same occurs *in vivo* [116, 117]. Rectal dialysate studies lead to a similar conclusion [118]. Together, the various strands of evidence have served to generate enthusiasm for therapeutic trials aimed at modifying free-radical expression, already with some success (Chapter 3).

Nitric oxide

Nitric oxide is produced to excess in biopsies from patients with active ulcerative colitis [119], and is liberated into the lumen at levels 100-fold greater than in controls [120]. Comparable changes are found in biopsies from patients with active Crohn's colitis, and prove amenable to therapy with steroids [121]. It is uncertain at which point in the inflammatory process this excess occurs, and whether it is an initiating or reactive process, but the latter is more likely. Increased expression of inducible nitric oxide synthase is, in any event, a non-specific feature of forms of gut injury as diverse as the creation of a surgical anastomosis and *Shigella* dysentery [122]. In this context it is interesting to find that inducible nitric oxide synthase is stimulated by TNF-α, affects the vascular endothelium, and that, in ischaemic cardiac disease, it probably contributes to the tendency to thromboembolism [123]. Non-specific though these manifestations are, they provide the potential for therapeutic endeavour (Chapter 3).

Enteric neurones in inflammatory bowel disease

The enteric neurones are probably abnormal in Crohn's disease, but it is difficult to establish whether the various changes observed are primary or epiphenomenal. Several lines of enquiry have suggested that there is abnormal innervation of the submucosa, muscularis mucosae and mucosa in ulcerative colitis. This is supported by immunohistochemical staining demonstrating increased numbers of mucosal nerve fibres and of the expression of neuropeptide Y and tyrosine hydroxylase [124]. A preliminary study describes a bizarre, but apparently reproducible, disturbance of the neuroendocrine system in ulcerative colitis [125]. In contrast to normal individuals and those with irritable bowel syndrome, repeated sigmoidoscopy causes a reduction in rectal sensitivity. Both of these studies have therapeutic potential and may contribute to our understanding of the frequency of defaecation that is so often apparently out of proportion to macroscopic evidence of inflammation (Chapter 2).

Evidence that substance P, a pro-inflammatory neurotransmitter, is overexpressed in both Crohn's disease and ulcerative colitis [126] can be assumed to be of some significance given improvement in animal models of colitis if specific inhibitors are administered, but study of substance P in isolation is as liable to mislead as study of a single cytokine. However,

GAP43, a marker of innervation in hypertrophic smooth muscle, is increased in Crohn's disease tissues, an observation that may be of more than passing significance as it is not elevated in experimental models of intestinal inflammation [127].

Platelet activating factor

Platelet activating factor may be of especial relevance given that it is found in high concentration in mucosal biopsies in both Crohn's disease and ulcerative colitis, that it has a pro-inflammatory effect on other cells, and that it is a potent stimulator of intestinal secretion. *In vitro* data indicate that it may be responsible for about half of the secretory response in cultured mucosal biopsies [128]. Whether this is quantitatively important in contributing to diarrhoea *in vivo* remains to be clarified.

Environmental factors

Non-steroidal anti-inflammatory drugs
Non-steroidal anti-inflammatory drugs (NSAIDs) may be implicated in the aetiology of some cases of inflammatory bowel disease. Labelled white cell scanning demonstrates small bowel ulceration (of a magnitude similar to that seen in Crohn's disease) in two-thirds of those receiving long-term NSAID therapy for arthritis [129], that can persist for more than a year after the drugs are discontinued, and may be associated with frank ileal disease on contrast radiography. A number of further studies in respect of the colon and reaching similar conclusions have recently been summarized [130]. The more common ill-effects include watery diarrhoea, and chronic blood loss with or without anaemia. These problems tend to be exaggerated in patients with inflammatory bowel disease – and prove a limiting factor in the use of NSAIDs in those with arthropathy (Chapter 6). Data from the Tayside Medicines Monitoring Unit support the many clinical anecdotes [131]. Although the study was limited to prescribed (and dispensed) non-steroidals, and to episodes of inflammatory bowel disease sufficient to warrant admission to hospital – both of which factors might be expected to diminish an apparent strength of association – they found that patients were more than 1.7 times as likely to have been taking the drugs than matched community controls. The possibility that non-steroidals might have been used for symptoms of inflammatory bowel disease or for associated arthropathy is not excluded and requires study of the patients themselves rather than the purely epidemiological approach taken by the Tayside group. Fresh data from the Channel Islands suggest that NSAIDs may be responsible for a high proportion of apparent new cases of inflammatory bowel disease and could logically be considered, at least

on epidemiological grounds, to account for most cases of acute self-limiting colitis [132]. There has probably been some ascertainment bias in the study but the striking preponderance of NSAID usage in patients is unlikely to be accounted for entirely on this basis.

Smoking and inflammatory bowel disease

Smoking proves one of the more intriguing environmental factors to be identified in inflammatory bowel disease (IBD), both from its potential relevance to disease expression, and from the clear differences found between its frequency in Crohn's and in ulcerative colitis. Studies from a number of different centres around the world have confirmed and extended the original observation from the South Wales group [133] that smoking is less common in ulcerative colitis than in healthy controls, with the highest frequency being found in ex-smokers [134]. Initial concern that this observation might be influenced by recall bias was effectively refuted by prospective data collection [135]. It is now generally agreed that, in contrast, smokers are over-represented amongst patients with Crohn's disease. The mechanisms for these differential effects remain speculative, but an altered production of arachidonic acid metabolites, disruption of mucus-producing capacity and alterations to the protective barrier function of the colon are probably important [136]. The predominant mucin in the normal colon is a glycoprotein known as MUC-2; this also predominates in ulcerative colitis [137]. The same group has gone on to study expression of MUC-2 at different phases of colitis and find that there are higher levels and evidence of greater synthesis in patients with quiescent disease, but lower levels and inhibited synthesis in (different) patients with active disease [138]. These observations need confirmation, but could have important implications.

In Crohn's disease there is increasingly good evidence that smokers, as well as being over-represented, form a group with a worse prognosis [139] and that continued smoking is associated with more frequent relapse [140]. This was recently re-addressed in two retrospective European studies. In the French study of 400 Crohn's patients followed for a mean of over 8 years, smokers constituted 55% of the total [141]. The sites of intestinal involvement were similar in smokers and non-smokers, and age at diagnosis was comparable. The need for surgery did not differ significantly, but there was a higher frequency of repeated surgery in heavy smokers (20% v. 11%) which did not quite reach statistical significance. However, there was a significantly greater cumulative use of systemic steroids and of other immunosuppressive therapy in smokers, an effect which was more pronounced for female smokers. At 10 years 52% of female smokers had required immunosuppression, compared to only 24% of non-smokers ($p < 0.001$). In the German study of 346 patients [142], there were 59 ex-smokers (who were not considered further), 144 smokers and 143 non-smokers. There were no important demographic differences between patients at the time of diagnosis, and the distribution of disease within the bowel was similar. Additional evidence for a higher cumulative recurrence rate (RR) in smokers was provided. Within 5 years of first surgery 43% of smokers had relapsed, compared to only 26% of non-smokers (RR, 3.1; CI, 1.7–5.8), apparently independently of the initial site of disease. The adverse effects again appeared to be more pronounced in women, and in those of both sexes having surgery early in the course of their disease, partly answering a question of bias introduced by the higher proportion of non-smokers who had had their disease for less than 5 years at the time of study (57% v. 47%). Many more surgical procedures had been required in the smokers – at least one operation in 73% v. 39% – and multiple episodes of surgery were 10.8 times more likely in smokers (CI, 5.3–22.1). The overall frequency of fistula and/or abscess formation also was higher, at 40% compared to only 13% in non-smokers. The differences between these two studies are ones of degree and emphasis only, and are probably fully explained by differing criteria for surgical as opposed to immunosuppressive intervention in the two countries concerned. The French GETAID investigators also demonstrated the benefit of lifelong non-smoking in a smaller but prospective study performed to examine the value of mesalazine after surgical resection [143], in which endoscopic recurrence by 12 weeks was significantly less in non-smokers (odds ratio, 0.2; $p < 0.002$).

The clinical significance of findings such as these is accordingly quite compelling, especially when one considers that the differences observed for relapse-free intervals equal or exceed those attainable with current options for maintenance therapy (Chapter 3). However, it remains unknown, and is probably untestable (a controlled trial of stopping smoking being the necessary tool) whether stopping smoking would remove the problem. It is possible that the 'smoking phenotype' marks a subgroup with poor prognosis Crohn's and that stopping smoking would therefore be irrelevant. Three modest pieces of evidence indicate that this would probably be an unnecessarily nihilistic conclusion. First, there is some evidence that stopping smoking after a diagnosis of Crohn's disease is made reduces the need for surgical intervention and improves duration of remission, stopping smoking being associated with a reduction of relapse rate by around 40% at 1 year [144]. Secondly, ex-smokers have an elevated frequency of ulcerative colitis (not of Crohn's disease); and thirdly there are a number of other clear-cut benefits to be obtained from stopping smoking. Patients, and especially women, with Crohn's disease who smoke should be advised to stop. Sadly, evidence to date suggests that few health-care professionals are addressing this issue adequately [145].

As an interesting aside, the Oxford group has explored the effects of smoking on the success or otherwise of pouch surgery (Chapter 4) for ulcerative colitis [146] and find that the link with non-smoking and colitis is carried on to influence the ileo-anal pouch. Amongst 72 non-smokers there were 46 episodes of pouchitis in 18 patients, compared to 14 episodes in four of the 12 ex-smokers, and only a single episode of pouchitis in one of 17 current smokers.

Appendicectomy and inflammatory bowel disease

Studies of other aspects of the epidemiology of inflammatory bowel disease suggested that previous appendicectomy was under-represented in patients with ulcerative colitis, with relative risks well under 0.5 [71]. In a study of 174 consecutive clinic attenders with ulcerative colitis (32% with pancolitis) only one had had a previous appendicectomy (0.6%) [147]. A control group attending an orthopaedic clinic had a slightly different sex ratio, and were a little older (40.9 v. 34.9 years), but had a very strikingly higher frequency of previous appendicectomy, at 25.4%. Scrutiny of the ages at appendicectomy and at onset of colitic symptoms indicates that the controls were appropriate, and suggests that appendicectomy is truly linked to a lower subsequent incidence of ulcerative colitis. The nature of the study makes it difficult to know whether acute appendicitis or laparotomy is the protective association, as the number of normal appendices removed is unknown. The clinical and epidemiological literature now includes several concordant studies, and apparently none that is contrary. It would be an unwarranted extrapolation to propose a direct causal relationship, but speculation that the absence of the appendix is of local immunological significance is supported by the not infrequent histological finding of inflammation in the appendix in otherwise more distal ulcerative colitis (the appendix skip lesion). An influence on permeability also is possible (see above).

A past history of appendicectomy has neither positive nor negative association with later development of Crohn's disease [71]. However, epithelioid granulomas in appendicectomy specimens are occasionally identified, with consequent concern that the patient – despite an absence of other features – has Crohn's disease. In a major epidemiopathological survey, six of 6051 appendicectomies performed in Copenhagen County had granulomas at contemporary histological examination [148]. Follow-up of these patients for a minimum of 9 years revealed no further gastrointestinal symptoms. Of 373 patients with an initial clinical diagnosis of Crohn's, there were three in whom the only evidence of disease was in the appendix. Follow-up of these patients to a median of 6 years revealed no recurrence and led the authors to suggest that isolated granulomatous disease of the appendix is not Crohn's disease. An earlier report [149] concluded that there was a 14% recurrence rate in such patients, but the nature of the report, culling incomplete information from many other sources makes this less secure. It is probably correct to consider isolated granulomatous disease of the appendix as a separate condition with a good prognosis (that incidentally protects against ulcerative colitis?).

Sex steroids in pathogenesis of inflammatory bowel disease
The combined oral contraceptive pill has been associated with an increased risk of Crohn's disease (and possibly of ulcerative colitis) [135, 150]. Whether this remains true for the lower hormone doses currently in use has not been fully addressed, but a link between hormonal status and inflammatory bowel disease expression is indicated. The frequent association that women with Crohn's find between their symptoms and certain phases of the menstrual cycle, and altered behaviour of inflammatory bowel disease in pregnancy (Chapter 5) lend clinical support to this assertion.

Environmental exposure to metals and granulomatous disease
Taking as our starting points the occasional hypersensitivity reaction to certain metals responsible for a cell-mediated granulomatous inflammation of the skin, and the observation that granular pigment containing aluminium, silica and titanium can be found in the intestine and mesenteric nodes of those with Crohn's disease, we gave intradermal injections of putative pathogenic metals to patients with granulomatous Crohn's and to normal controls [151]. Although foreign body granulomas could be elicited, there was no evidence to suggest that metal sensitivity is an important contributing cause of granulomatous Crohn's disease.

Diet as an aetiological factor
The response of some patients with Crohn's to dietary therapy (Chapter 3) has led to speculation that a 'trigger' exists at the point of contact of food/digests and the intestine wall, and that one or more dietary factors may be a contributing cause of inflammatory bowel disease. Although a question very frequently asked by patients, and one postulated reason for the increase in prevalence of Crohn's disease during the past half century, there is remarkably little evidence on which to base a scientific reply. There do not appear to be any clear causative associations between dietary factors and ulcerative colitis, other than in Japanese patients in whom consumption of a Western-type diet is positively associated with the disease [152]; clearly diet here is not an independent risk factor. In Crohn's disease there is an intermittent phase of excitement as a new problem food is proposed, whether this be refined sugar, cornflakes, margarine, or a less obviously dietary component such as toothpaste. Although there is some degree of consensus that carbohydrate consumption is higher in patients with Crohn's disease, even before the first symptoms of the disease [153] none of the ingested substances yet proposed has stood up to prolonged scrutiny as of major aetiological significance. The less dubious role of dietary amendment in Crohn's therapy is discussed later (Chapter 3).

REFERENCES

1. Ekbom A, Helmick C, Zack M, Adami HO. The epidemiology of inflammatory bowel disease: a large, population-based study in Sweden. *Gastroenterology* 1991; **100**: 350–358.

2. Trallori G, D'Albasio G, Palli D *et al*. Epidemiology of inflammatory bowel disease over a 10-year period in Florence (1978–1987). *Ital J Gastroenterol* 1991; **23**: 559–563.

3. Riegler G, Tartaglione M, Marmo R *et al*. Ulcerative colitis in old age: men more frequent than women? *Gastroenterology* 1996; **110**: A1002.

4. Srivastava ED, Mayberry JF, Morris TJ *et al*. Incidence of ulcerative colitis in Cardiff over 20 years: 1968–87. *Gut* 1992; **33**: 256–258.

5. Ranzi T, Bodini P, Zambelli A *et al*. Epidemiological aspects of inflammatory bowel disease in a north Italian population: a 4 year prospective study. *Eur J Gastroenterol Hepatol* 1996; **8**: 657–661.

6. Gower-Rousseau C, Salomez J-L, Dupas J-L *et al*. Incidence of inflammatory bowel disease in northern France (1988–1990). *Gut* 1994; **35**: 1433–1438.

7. Munkholm P, Langholz E, Nielsen OH *et al*. Incidence and prevalence of Crohn's disease in the county of Copenhagen, 1962–87: a six-fold increase in incidence. *Scand J Gastroenterol* 1992; **27**: 609–614.

8. Lee FI, Nguyen-Van-Tam JS. Prospective study of incidence of Crohn's disease in north-west England: no increase since the late 1970s. *Eur J Gastroenterol Hepatol* 1994; **6**: 27–31.

9. Cosgrove M, Al-Atia RF, Jenkins HR. The epidemiology of paediatric inflammatory bowel disease. *Arch Dis Child* 1996; **74**: 460–461.

10. Moum B, Bentsen B, Ekbom A *et al*. Incidence of inflammatory bowel disease in childhood. A prospective population based study of the IBSEN study group in south-eastern Norway 1990–93. *Gastroenterology* 1996; **110**: A974.

10a. Lennard-Jones JE, Shivananda S and the EC-IBD Study Group. Clinical uniformity of IBD at presentation and during the first year of disease in the north and south of Europe, *Eur J Gastroenterol Hepatol* 1997; **9**: 353–360.

11. Mayberry JF, Judd D, Smart H *et al*. Crohn's disease in Jewish people – an epidemiological study in south-east Wales. *Digestion* 1986; **35**: 237–240.

12. Fellows IW, Mayberry JF, Holmes GK. Crohn's disease in West Indians. *Am J Gastroenterol* 1988; **83**: 752–755.

13. Cave DR, Freedman LS. Seasonal variations in the clinical presentation of Crohn's disease and ulcerative colitis. *Int J Epidemiol* 1975; **4**: 317–320.

14. Tysk C, Järnerot G. Seasonal variation in exacerbations of ulcerative colitis. *Scand J Gastroenterol* 1993; **28**: 95–96.

15. Sonnenberg A, Jacobsen SJ, Wasserman IH. Periodicity of hospital admissions for inflammatory bowel disease. *Am J Gastroenterol* 1994; **889**: 847–851.
16. Moum B, Aadland E, Ekbom A, Vatn MH. Seasonal variations in the onset of ulcerative colitis. *Gut* 1996; **38**: 376–378.
17. Tysk C, Linberg E, Järnerot G, Flodrus-Myrhed B. Ulcerative colitis and Crohn's disease in an unselected population of monozygotic and dizygotic twins. A study of heritability and the influence of smoking. *Gut* 1988; **29**: 990–996.
18. Roth MP, Petersen GM, McElree C *et al.* Familial empiric risk estimates of inflammatory bowel disease in Ashkenazi Jews. *Gastroenterology* 1989; **96**: 1016–1020.
19. Orholm M, Iselius L, Sorensen TI *et al.* Investigation of inheritance of chronic inflammatory bowel diseases by complex segregation analysis. *Br Med J* 1993; **306**: 20–24.
20. Satsangi J, Welsh KI, Bunce M *et al.* Contribution of genes of the major histocompatibility complex to susceptibility and disease phenotype in inflammatory bowel disease. *Lancet* 1996; **347**: 1212–1217.
21. Polito JM II, Rees RC, Childs B *et al.* Preliminary evidence for genetic anticipation in Crohn's disease. *Lancet* 1996; **347**: 798–800.
22. Toyoda H, Wang SJ, Yang HY *et al.* Distinct associations of HLA class II genes with inflammatory bowel disease. *Gastroenterology* 1993; **104**: 741–748.
23. Masuda H, Nakamura Y, Tanaka T, Hayakawa S. Distinct relationship between HLA-DR genes and intractability of ulcerative colitis. *Am J Gastroenterol* 1994; **89**: 1957–1962.
24. Mathew CG, Easton DF, Lennard-Jones JE. HLA and inflammatory bowel disease. *Lancet* 1996; **348**: 68.
25. Gardiner KR, Crockard AD, Halliday MI, Rolands BJ. Class II major histocompatibility complex antigen expression of peripheral blood monocytes in patients with inflammatory bowel disease. *Gut* 1994; **35**: 511–516.
26. Reinshagen M, Loeliger C, Kuehnl P *et al.* HLA class II gene frequencies in Crohn's disease: a population based analysis in Germany. *Gut* 1996; **38**: 538–542.
27. Forcione DG, Sands B, Rustgi A *et al.* An increased risk of Crohn's disease in individuals who inherit the HLA class II DRB3*301 allele. *Gastroenterology* 1996; **110**: A908.
28. Danzé P-M, Colombel J-F, Jacquot S *et al.* Association of HLA class II genes with susceptibility to Crohn's disease. *Gut* 1996; **39**: 69–72.
29. Mansfield JC, Holden H, Tarlow JK *et al.* Novel genetic association between ulcerative colitis and the anti-inflammatory cytokine interleukin-1 receptor antagonist. *Gastroenterology* 1994; **106**: 637–642.
30. Satsangi J, Jewell DP. Are cytokine gene polymorphisms important

in the pathogenesis of inflammatory bowel disease? *Eur J Gastroenterol Hepatol* 1996; **8**: 97–99.

31. Tountas NA, Yang H, Coulter DL *et al*. Increased carriage of allele 2 of IL-1 receptor antagonist in Jewish populations: the strongest known genetic association in ulcerative colitis. *Gastroenterology* 1996; **110**: A1029.

32. Plévy SE, Targan SR, Yang H *et al*. Tumor necrosis factor microsatellites define a Crohn's disease-associated haplotype on chromosome 6. *Gastroenterology* 1996; **110**: 1053–1060.

33. Hugot J-P, Laurent-Puig P, Gower-Rousseau C *et al*. Mapping of a susceptibility locus for Crohn's disease on chromosome 16. *Nature* 1996; **379**: 821–823.

34. Satsangi J, Parkes M, Louis E *et al*. Two-stage genome-wide search in inflammatory bowel disease: strong evidence for susceptibility loci on chromosomes 3, 7 and 12. *Gut* 1996; **39**(suppl 1): A18.

35. Yacyshyn BR, Bowen-Yacyshyn MB. Intestinal and peripheral blood CD45RO+ expression on CD8+ T-cells and CD20+ B-cells corresponds with cellular apoptosis in patients with Crohn's disease and first degree relatives. *Gastroenterology* 1996; **110**: A1048.

36. Walmsley RS, Zhao M, Hamilton MI *et al*. Anti-neutrophil cytoplasm autoantibodies against bactericidal/permeability-increasing protein in inflammatory bowel disease. *Gastroenterology* 1996; **110**: A1041.

37. Satsangi J, Landers C, Welsh K *et al*. ANCA and HLA genes in North European patients with ulcerative colitis. *Gastroenterology* 1996; **110**: A1009.

38. Shanahan F, Duerr R, Rotter JI *et al*. Neutrophil autoantibodies in ulcerative colitis: familial aggregation and genetic heterogeneity. *Gastroenterology* 1992; **103**: 456–461.

39. Seibold F, Slametschka D, Gregor M, Weber P. Neutrophil autoantibodies: a genetic marker in primary sclerosing cholangitis and ulcerative colitis. *Gastroenterology* 1994; **107**: 532–536.

40. Vecchi M, Bianchi MB, Meucci G *et al*. Prevalence of p-ANCA in unaffected family members of Italian ulcerative colitis patients. *Gastroenterology* 1996; **110**: A1037.

41. Bansi DS, Lo S, Chapman RW, Fleming KA. Absence of antineutrophil cytoplasmic antibodies in relatives of UK patients with primary sclerosing cholangitis and ulcerative colitis. *Eur J Gastroenterol Hepatol* 1996; **8**: 111–116.

42. Lo SK, Fleming KA, Chapman RW. Prevalence of antineutrophil antibody in primary sclerosing cholangitis and ulcerative colitis using an alkaline phosphatase technique. *Gut* 1992; **33**: 1370–1375.

43. Estève M, Mallolas J, Klaasen J *et al*. Antineutrophil cytoplasmic antibodies in sera from colectomised ulcerative colitis patients and its relation to the presence of pouchitis. *Gut* 1996; **38**: 894–898.

44. Vasiliauskas EA, Plévy SE, Landers CJ *et al.* Perinuclear antineu-trophil cytoplasmic antibodies in patients with Crohn's disease define a clinical subgroup. *Gastroenterology* 1996; **110**: 1810–1819.
45. Teahon K, Somasundaram S, Smith T *et al.* Assessing the site of increased intestinal permeability in coeliac and inflammatory bowel disease. *Gut* 1996; **39**: 864–869.
46. Schmitz H, Barmeyer C, Fromm M *et al.* Diarrheal mechanism in ulcerative colitis: epithelial barrier defect and impaired ion transport. *Gastroenterology* 1996; **110**: A358.
47. Hollander D, Vadheim CM, Brettholz E *et al.* Increased intestinal per-meability in patients with Crohn's disease and their relatives. *Ann Intern Med* 1986; **105**: 883–885.
48. Hilsden RJ, Meddings JB, Sutherland LR. Intestinal permeability changes in response to acetylsalicylic acid in relatives of patients with Crohn's disease. *Gastroenterology* 1996; **110**: 1395–1403.
49. Yacyshyn BR, Meddings JB. CD45RO expression on circulating CD19+ B cells in Crohn's disease correlates with intestinal perme-ability. *Gastroenterology* 1995; **108**: 132–137.
50. Wyatt J, Vogelsang H, Hübl W *et al.* Intestinal permeability and the prediction of relapse in Crohn's disease. *Lancet* 1993; **341**: 1437–1439.
51. Frenette PS, Wagner DD. Adhesion molecules – Part 1. *N Engl J Med* 1996; **334**: 1526–1529.
52. Isberg RR. Discrimination between intracellular uptake and surface adhesion of bacterial pathogens. *Science* 1991; **252**: 934–938.
53. Koizumi M, King N, Lobb R *et al.* Expression of vascular adhesion molecules in inflammatory bowel disease. *Gastroenterology* 1992; **103**: 840–847.
54. Jones SC, Banks RE, Haidar A *et al.* Adhesion molecules in inflam-matory bowel disease. *Gut* 1995; **36**: 724–730.
55. Nielsen OH, Langholz E, Hendel J, Brynskov J. Circulating soluble intercellular adhesion molecule-1 (sICAM-1) in active inflammatory bowel disease. *Dig Dis Sci* 1994; **39**: 1918–1923.
56. Pooley N, Ghosh L, Sharon P. Up-regulation of E-selectin and inter-cellular adhesion molecule-1 differs between Crohn's disease and ulcerative colitis. *Dig Dis Sci* 1995; **40**: 219–225.
57. Schürmann GM, Bishop AE, Facer P *et al.* Increased expression of cell adhesion molecule P-selectin in active inflammatory bowel disease. *Gut* 1995; **36**: 411–418.
58. Mishra L, Mishra BB, Harris M *et al. In vitro* cell aggregation and cell adhesion molecules in Crohn's disease. *Gastroenterology* 1993; **104**: 772–779.
59. Fries W, Mazzon E, Martines D, Martin A. Small intestine tight junc-tions are altered in experimental colitis in the rat. *Gastroenterology* 1996; **110**: A909.

60. Sträter J, Wedding U, Barth TFE *et al*. Rapid onset of apoptosis *in vitro* follows disruption of β_1-integrin/matrix interactions in human colonic crypt cells. *Gastroenterology* 1996; **110**: 1776–1784.
61. Hermiston ML, Gordon JI. Inflammatory bowel disease and adenomas in mice expressing a dominant negative N-cadherin. *Science* 1995; **270**: 1203–1207.
62. Wakefield AJ, Sawyerr AM, Dhillon AP *et al*. Pathogenesis of Crohn's disease: multifocal gastrointestinal infarction. *Lancet* 1989; **ii**: 1057–1062.
63. Wakefield AJ, Sankey EA, Dhillon AP *et al*. Granulomatous vasculitis in Crohn's disease. *Gastroenterology* 1991; **100**: 1279–1287.
64. Sawyerr M, Pottinger BE, Savage CO *et al*. Serum immunoglobulin G reactive with endothelial cells in inflammatory bowel disease. *Dig Dis Sci* 1994; **39**: 1909–1917.
65. Collins CE, Rogers J, Hall C *et al*. Platelets aggregate and neutrophils sequester in the mesenteric microcirculation in Crohn's disease. *Gastroenterology* 1996; **110**: A886.
66. Hamilton MI, Dick R, Crawford L *et al*. Is proximal demarcation of ulcerative colitis determined by the territory of the inferior mesenteric artery? *Lancet* 1995; **345**: 688–690.
67. Pullan RD, Thomas GA, Rhodes M *et al*. Thickness of adherent mucus gel on colonic mucosa in humans and its relevance to colitis. *Gut* 1994; **35**: 353–359.
68. Poulson R, Chinery R, Sarraf C *et al*. Trefoil peptide gene expression in small intestinal Crohn's disease and dietary adaptation. *J Clin Gastroenterol* 1993; **17**: S78–91.
69. Finnie IA, Dwarakanath AD, Taylor BA, Rhodes JM. Colonic mucin synthesis is increased by sodium butyrate. *Gut* 1995; **36**: 93–99.
70. Dwarakanath AD, Campbell BJ, Tsai HH *et al*. Faecal mucinase activity assessed in inflammatory bowel disease using ^{14}C threonine labelled mucin substrate. *Gut* 1995; **37**: 58–62.
71. Gent AE, Hellier MD, Grace RH *et al*. Inflammatory bowel disease and domestic hygiene in infancy. *Lancet* 1994; **343**: 766–767.
72. Ferguson A. Ulcerative colitis: how can we test theories of immune dysregulation? *Eur J Gastroenterol Hepatol* 1996; **8**: 101–103.
73. Well CL, Van de Westerlo EMA, Jechorek RP *et al*. Bacteroides fragilis enterotoxin modulates epithelial permeability and bacterial internalization by HT-29 enterocytes. *Gastroenterology* 1996; **110**: 1429–1437.
74. Grimble G. Fibre, fermentation, flora and flatus. *Gut* 1989; **30**: 6–13.
75. Levine J, Ellis CJ, Furne JK *et al*. Sulfate reducing bacteria and ulcerative colitis. *Gastroenterology* 1996; **110**: A949.
76. Pitcher MCL, Cummings JH. Hydrogen sulphide: a bacterial toxin in ulcerative colitis? *Gut* 1996; **39**: 1–4.
77. Sanderson JD, Moss MT, Tizard MLV, Hermon-Taylor J.

Mycobacterium paratuberculosis DNA in Crohn's disease tissue. *Gut* 1992; **33**: 890–896.

78. Dumonceau J-M, Van Gossum A, Adler M, Portaels F. Identification of intestinal mycobacterial species in inflammatory and non-inflammatory bowel diseases. *Gastroenterology* 1996; **110**: A900.

79. Fidler HM, Thurrell W, Johnson NMcI *et al*. Specific detection of *Mycobacterium paratuberculosis* DNA associated with granulomatous tissue in Crohn's disease. *Gut* 1994; **35**: 506–510.

80. Travis SPL. Mycobacteria on trial: guilty or innocent in pathogenesis of Crohn's disease? *Eur J Gastroenterol Hepatol* 1995; **7**: 1173–1176.

81. Sonnenberg A. Occupational mortality of inflammatory bowel disease. *Digestion* 1990; **46**: 10–18.

82. Lewin J, Dhillon AP, Sim R *et al*. Persistent measles virus infection of the intestine: confirmation by immunogold electron microscopy. *Gut* 1995; **36**: 564–569.

83. Haga Y, Funakoshi O, Kuroe K *et al*. Absence of measles viral genomic sequence in intestinal tissues from Crohn's disease by nested polymerase chain reaction. *Gut* 1996; **38**: 211–215.

84. Ekbom A, Wakefield AJ, Zack M, Adami HO. Perinatal measles infection and subsequent Crohn's disease. *Lancet* 1994; **344**: 508–510.

85. Ekbom A, Daszak P, Kraaz W, Wakefield AJ. Crohn's disease after *in-utero* measles virus exposure. *Lancet* 1996; **348**: 515–517.

86. Thompson N, Montgomery S, Pounder RE, Wakefield AJ. Is measles vaccination a risk factor for Crohn's disease? *Lancet* 1995; **345**: 1071–1074.

87. Shaheen SO, Aaby P, Hall AJ *et al*. Measles and atopy in Guinea-Bissau. *Lancet* 1996; **347**: 1792–1796.

88. Liu Y, Van Kruiningen HJ, West AB *et al*. Immunocytochemical evidence of *Listeria*, *Escherichia coli*, and *Streptococcus* antigens in Crohn's disease. *Gastroenterology* 1995; **108**: 1396–1404.

89. Klapproth J-M, Donnenberg MS, Abraham JM *et al*. Products of enteropathic *Escherichia coli* inhibit lymphocyte activation and lymphokine production. *Infect Immun* 1995; **63**: 2248–2254.

90. Sartor RB, Cromartie WJ, Powell DW, Schwab JH. Granulomatous enterocolitis induced in rats by purified bacterial cell wall fragments. *Gastroenterology* 1985; **89**: 587–595.

91. Broberger O, Perlmann P. Autoantibodies in human ulcerative colitis. *J Exp Med* 1959; **110**: 657–674.

92. Perlmann P, Hammarstrom S, Lagercrantz R, Gustafsson BE. Antigen from colon of germfree rats and antibodies in human ulcerative colitis. *Ann NY Acad Sci* 1965; **124**: 377–394.

93. Elson CO, Sartor RB, Tennyson GS, Riddell RH. Experimental models of inflammatory bowel disease. *Gastroenterology* 1995; **109**: 1344–1367.

94. Das KM, Vecchi M, Squillante L *et al*. Mr 40,000 human colonic epithelial protein expression in colonic mucosa and presence of circulating anti-Mr 40,000 antibodies in cotton top tamarins with spontaneous colitis. *Gut* 1992; **33**: 48–54.

95. Rutgeerts P, Geboes K, Peeters M *et al*. Effect of faecal stream diversion on recurrence of Crohn's disease in the neoterminal ileum. *Lancet* 1991; **338**: 771–774.

96. Andreyev HJN, Owen RA, Thompson I, Forbes A. Association between Meckel's diverticulum and Crohn's disease: a retrospective review. *Gut* 1994; **35**: 788–790.

97. Winslet MC, Allan A, Poxon V *et al*. Faecal diversion for Crohn's colitis: a model to study the role of the faecal stream in the inflammatory process. *Gut* 1994; **35**: 236–242.

98. Lohmuller JL, Pemberton JH, Dozois RR *et al*. Pouchitis and extraintestinal manifestations of inflammatory bowel disease after ileal pouch-anal anastomosis. *Ann Surg* 1990; **211**: 622–629.

99. Oriishi T, Sata M, Toyonaga A *et al*. Evaluation of intestinal permeability in patients with inflammatory bowel disease using lactulose and measuring antibodies to lipid A. *Gut* 1995; **36**: 891–896.

100. Chan L, Mayer L. Antigen priming, not tolerance, with oral antigen administration in inflammatory bowel disease. *Gastroenterology* 1996; **110**: A881.

101. Duchmann R, Kaiser I, Hermann E *et al*. Tolerance exists towards resident intestinal flora but is broken in active inflammatory bowel disease. *Clin Exp Immunol* 1995; **102**: 448–455.

102. MacPherson A, Khoo UY, Forgacs I *et al*. Mucosal antibodies in inflammatory bowel disease are directed against intestinal bacteria. *Gut* 1996; **38**: 365–375.

103. Takahasi F, Shah HS, Wise LS, Das KM. Circulating antibodies against human colonic extract enriched with a 40kDa protein in patients with ulcerative colitis. *Gut* 1990; **31**: 1016–1020.

104. Halstensen TS, Das KM, Brandtzaeg P. Epithelial deposits of immunoglobulin G1 and activated complement colocalise with the M(r) 40kD putative autoantigen in ulcerative colitis. *Gut* 1993; **34**: 650–657.

105. Das KM, Vecchi M, Sakamaki S. A shared and unique epitope(s) on human colon, skin, and biliary epithelium detected by a monoclonal antibody. *Gastroenterology* 1990; **98**: 464–469.

106. Bhagat S, Das KM. A shared and unique peptide in the human colon, eye, and joint detected by a monoclonal antibody. *Gastroenterology* 1994; **107**: 103–108.

107. Raedler A, Schreiber S, Weerth A *et al*. Assessment of *in vivo* activated T cells in patients with Crohn's disease. *Hepato-Gastroenterol* 1990; **37**: 67–71.

108. Kusugami K, Youngman KR, West GA, Fiocchi C. Intestinal immune reactivity to interleukin 2 differs among Crohn's disease, ulcerative colitis and controls. *Gastroenterology* 1989; **97**: 1–9.

109. D'Haens G, Peeters M, Baert F *et al.* Increasing TNF-α and decreasing IFN-γ tissue concentrations in early recurrent Crohn's disease and correlation with endoscopic lesions. *Gastroenterology* 1996; **110**: A894.

110. Roman LI, Manzano L, De la Hera A *et al.* Expanded CD4+CD45RO+ phenotype and defective proliferative response in T lymphocytes from patients with Crohn's disease. *Gastroenterology* 1996; **110**: 1008–1019.

111. West GA, Matsuura T, Levine AD *et al.* Interleukin 4 in inflammatory bowel disease and mucosal immune reactivity. *Gastroenterology* 1996; **110**: 1683–1695.

112. Moore KW, O'Garra A, de Waal Malefyt R *et al.* Interleukin-10. *Ann Rev Immunol* 1993; **11**: 165-190.

113. Kucharzik T, Stoll R, Lugering N *et al.* Antiinflammatory cytokine interleukin-10 in patients with inflammatory bowel disease. *Gut* 1995; **37**(suppl 2): A65.

114. Hibi T, Ohara M, Watanabe M *et al.* Interleukin 2 and interferon-gamma augment anticolon antibody dependent cellular cytotoxicity in ulcerative colitis. *Gut* 1993; **34**: 788–793.

115. Gaginella TS, Kachur JF, Tamai H, Keshavarzian A. Reactive oxygen and nitrogen metabolites as mediators of secretory diarrhea. *Gastroenterology* 1995; **109**: 2019–2028.

116. Simmonds NJ, Allen RE, Stevens TRJ *et al.* Chemiluminescence assay of mucosal reactive oxygen metabolites in inflammatory bowel disease. *Gastroenterology* 1992; **103**: 186–196.

117. Keshavarzian A, Sedghi S, Kanofsky J *et al.* Excessive production of reactive oxygen metabolites by inflamed colon: analysis by chemiluminescence probe. *Gastroenterology* 1992; **103**: 177–185.

118. Roediger WEW, Lawson MJ, Nance SH, Radcliffe BC. Detectable colonic nitrite levels in inflammatory bowel disease – mucosal or bacterial malfunction? *Digestion* 1986; **35**: 199–204.

119. Middleton SJ, Shorthouse M, Hunter JO. Increased nitric oxide synthesis in ulcerative colitis. *Lancet* 1993; **341**: 465–466.

120. Lundberg JO, Hellström, Lundberg JM, Alving K. Greatly increased luminal nitric oxide in ulcerative colitis. *Lancet* 1994; **344**: 1673–1674.

121. Rachmilewitz D, Stamler JS, Bachwich D *et al.* Enhanced colonic nitric oxide generation and nitric oxide synthase activity in ulcerative colitis and Crohn's disease. *Gut* 1995; **36**: 718–723.

122. Mannick EE, Ribbons KA, X-J Zhang *et al.* Expression of inducible nitric oxide synthase is a general response to gut inflammation and is not disease or site specific. *Gastroenterology* 1996; **110**: A959.

123. Habib FM, Springall DR, Davies GJ *et al*. TNF and inducible nitric oxide synthase in dilated cardiomyopathy. *Lancet* 1996; **347**: 1151–1155.

124. Bjørck S, Dahlstrom A, Ahlman H. Topical treatment of ulcerative proctitis with lidocaine. *Scand J Gastroenterol* 1989; **24**: 1061–1072.

125. Chang L, Munakata J, An K *et al*. Evidence for the activation of endogenous pain modulation system in ulcerative colitis. *Gastroenterology* 1996; **110**: A645.

126. Mazumdar S, Das KM. Immunocytochemical localization of vasoactive intestinal peptide and substance P in the colon from normal subjects and patients with inflammatory bowel disease. *Am J Gastroenterol* 1992; **87**: 176–181.

127. Lamb DP, Blennerhassett MG. Inadequate remodelling of innervation in inflamed hypertrophic smooth muscle: contributing factor in Crohn's disease? *Gastroenterology* 1996; **110**: A701.

128. Wardle TD, Hall L, Turnberg LA. Platelet activating factor: release from colonic mucosa in patients with ulcerative colitis and its effect on colonic secretion. *Gut* 1996; **38**: 355–361.

129. Bjarnason I, Zanelli G, Smith T *et al*. Nonsteroidal antiinflammatory drug-induced intestinal inflammation in humans. *Gastroenterology* 1987; **93**: 480–489.

130. Davies NM. Toxicity of nonsteroidal anti-inflammatory drugs in the large intestine. *Dis Colon Rectum* 1995; **38**: 1311–1321.

131. Evans JMM, McMahon AD, Murray FE *et al*. Non-steroidal anti-inflammatory drugs are implicated in colitis: a record-linkage case-control study. *Gastroenterology* 1996; **110**: A905.

132. Gleeson MH, Hardman JV, Clinton C, Spencer D. Non-steroidal anti-inflammatory drugs salicylates and colitis – a strong association. *Gut* 1996; **39**(suppl 1): A17.

133. Harries AD, Baird A, Rhodes J. Non-smoking: a feature of ulcerative colitis. *Br Med J* 1982; **284**: 706.

134. Lindberg E, Tysk C, Andersson K, Järnerot G. Smoking and inflammatory bowel disease. A case control study. *Gut* 1988; **29**: 352–357.

135. Vessey M, Jewell D, Smith A *et al*. Chronic inflammatory bowel disease, cigarette smoking and use of oral contraceptives: findings in a large cohort study of women of childbearing age. *Br Med J* 1986; **292**: 1101–1103.

136. Cope G, Heatley R. Cigarette smoking and intestinal defences. *Gut* 1992; **32**: 721–723.

137. Tytgat KMAJ, Opddam FJM, Einerhand AWC *et al*. MUC2 is the prominent colonic mucin expressed in ulcerative colitis. *Gut* 1996; **38**: 554–563.

138. Van der Wal J-WG, Tytgat KMAJ, Einerhand AWC *et al*. MUC2 synthesis is lowered in active ulcerative colitis. *Gastroenterology* 1996; **110**: A1034.

139. Sutherland LR, Ramcharan S, Bryant H, Fick G. Effect of cigarette smoking on recurrence of Crohn's disease. *Gastroenterology* 1990; **98**: 1123–1128.
140. Holdstock G, Savage D, Harman M, Wright R. Should patients with inflammatory bowel disease smoke? *Br Med J* 1984; **288**: 362.
141. Cosnes J, Carbonnel F, Beaugerie L *et al*. Effects of cigarette smoking on the long-term course of Crohn's disease. *Gastroenterology* 1996; **110**: 424–431.
142. Breuer-Katschinski BD, Hollander N, Goebell H. Effect of smoking on the course of Crohn's disease. *Eur J Gastroenterol Hepatol* 1996; **8**: 225–228.
143. Florent C, Cortot A, Quandale P *et al*. Placebo-controlled clinical trial of mesalazine in the prevention of early endoscopic recurrences after resection for Crohn's disease. *Eur J Gastroenterol Hepatol* 1996; **8**: 229–233.
144. Duffy LC, Zielezny MA, Marshall JR *et al*. Cigarette smoking and risk of clinical relapse in patients with Crohn's disease. *Am J Prev Med* 1990; **6**: 161–166.
145. Shields PL, Low-Beer TS. Patients' awareness of adverse relation between Crohn's disease and their smoking: questionnaire survey. *Br Med J* 1996; **313**: 265–266.
146. Merrett MN, Mortensen N, Kettlewell M, Jewell DP. Smoking may prevent pouchitis in patients with restorative proctocolectomy for ulcerative colitis. *Gut* 1996; **38**: 362–364.
147. Rutgeerts P, D'Haens G, Hiele M *et al*. Appendectomy protects against ulcerative colitis. *Gastroenterology* 1994; **106**: 1251–1253.
148. Wettergren A, Munkholm P, Larsen LG *et al*. Granulomas of the appendix: is it Crohn's disease? *Scand J Gastroenterol* 1991; **26**: 961–964.
149. Timmcke AE. Granulomatous appendicitis: is it Crohn's disease? Report of a case and review of the literature. *Am J Gastroenterol* 1986; **81**: 283–287.
150. Lesko SM, Kaufman DW, Rosenberg L *et al*. Evidence for an increased risk of Crohn's disease in oral contraceptive users. *Gastroenterology* 1985; **89**: 1046–1049.
151. Lee JCW, Halpern S, Lowe DG *et al*. Absence of skin sensitivity to oxides of aluminium, silicon, titanium or zirconium in patients with Crohn's disease. *Gut* 1996; **39**: 231–233.
152. Epidemiology Group of the Research Committee of Inflammatory Bowel Disease in Japan. Dietary and other risk factors of ulcerative colitis. A case-control study in Japan. *J Clin Gastroenterol* 1994; **19**: 166–171.
153. Tragnone A, Valpiani D, Miglio F *et al*. Dietary habits as risk factors for inflammatory bowel disease. *Eur J Gastroenterol Hepatol* 1995; **7**: 47–51.

2

Clinical presentations

Inflammatory bowel disease is usually responsible for diarrhoea, and, when the colon is involved, the rectal passage of blood. Depending on severity and the particular site(s) affected there may also be weight loss, anorexia and fatigue, or other systemic features such as tachycardia and pyrexia. Features that point towards Crohn's disease or ulcerative colitis (Table 2.1) reflect, on the one hand, the relative frequency of recto-sigmoid involvement, and, on the other, the malabsorptive effects of small bowel involvement in Crohn's disease. The history alone will occasionally remove any significant differential diagnosis. A young adult Caucasian patient presenting with several months' diarrhoea, weight loss and right iliac fossa pain might well be considered to have Crohn's disease until proved otherwise. Equally, gastrointestinal infection must always be considered and especially so when the history is short.

The general examination will often contribute little, beyond confirming aspects of the history, but evidence of perianal disease is much more typical of Crohn's disease – affecting upwards of 15% of patients – than of ulcerative colitis. One recent study put the frequency of perianal fistula as high as 33%, but may have been biased towards those with more severe disease, as all had been in-patients for at least a month at some point [1]. However, it would be a mistake to consider that perianal disease is pathognomonic of Crohn's disease, since around 10% of all perianal disease associated with inflammatory bowel disease is in patients with ulcerative colitis. Severe perianal disease is nonetheless mainly confined to patients with Crohn's.

The various extra-intestinal features of inflammatory bowel disease (considered in detail in Chapter 6) are sometimes said to be more or less common in ulcerative colitis than in Crohn's disease. Factual support for such a view is difficult to find, but there is a strong association between involvement of the colon and extra-intestinal manifestations, and patients

Table 2.1   Clinical features which help to distinguish Crohn's disease from ulcerative colitis

	Crohn's disease	Ulcerative colitis
General		
diarrhoea	+++	+++
abdominal pain	+++	+
pyrexia	++	+
oral ulcers	+++	+
Reflecting recto-sigmoid site of disease		
rectal bleeding	+	+++
mucus/pus with stools	+	++
tenesmus	+	++
Reflecting small bowel involvement and malabsorption		
weight loss	+++	+
growth retardation	+++	+
Reflecting penetrating tissue damage		
abdominal mass	++	–
perianal disease	+++	+
fistula	++	–

+++: Very common; ++: Frequent; +: Seen but relatively uncommon; –: Most unusual.

with Crohn's disease rarely have these features if their disease is confined to the small bowel.

Up to a third of patients with predominantly distal colitis may, despite a clear history of diarrhoea, prove to be constipated to abdominal palpation; this is less common in Crohn's disease. One study has suggested that this proximal stasis is actually the cause of acute relapse in up to 10% of cases [2]. Distinction from functional bowel disorders may be obvious, but in more subtle cases, the presence of night-time symptoms sufficient to wake the patient from sleep is a strong pointer to an organic aetiology. Bleeding is generally a feature of ulcerative colitis and distal Crohn's disease, but catastrophic bleeding from the small bowel in Crohn's disease, or from more distal sites in both forms of inflammatory bowel disease, does rarely occur. Soulé and colleagues have reviewed 15 patients with Crohn's disease with isolated major gastrointestinal bleeding [3], and conclude that it is usually from a single major colonic lesion, and that bleeding correlates poorly with other evidence of disease activity, often presenting during periods of apparent remission.

A new observation suggests that there may also be differences in personality type between the two principal forms of inflammatory bowel disease [4]. Patients with Crohn's disease were found to be more extrovert and with a greater psychoticism score than those with ulcerative colitis, but with no differences in respect of neuroticism. While these features may be important, there must be some caution because prevalent cases were studied; the possibility that the course of the disease may have affected the prevailing personality state remains open (also relatively small numbers were studied, including only 27 with ulcerative colitis).

At sigmoidoscopy, the confluent erythema and ulceration of ulcerative colitis is, when typically exhibited, distinguishable from the more characteristic aphthoid ulceration, serpiginous ulcers and generally patchy distribution of Crohn's disease. In a patient with a history suggestive of inflammatory bowel disease and in whom the rectum appears normal, a Crohn's diagnosis is also supported. It is most unusual for ulcerative colitis to present with a normal-appearing rectum (and still less with a histologically normal rectum) unless topical therapy has already been utilized, but most authorities allow that this scenario very rarely occurs. Confluent proctitis is of course seen also in Crohn's disease.

Investigation will typically commence with the relatively routine laboratory tests such as full blood count and serum biochemistry. These will rarely contribute to the diagnostic process in patients with a typical history and examination but may be helpful in cases where these are atypical and in the differentiation from functional disorders, which are effectively excluded by an elevated platelet count, a low haemoglobin, or a low albumin, for example. Different blood tests to assess the magnitude of inflammation are favoured by different laboratories, for logistic and other reasons. There are no compelling arguments for a single choice, but the C-reactive protein (CRP) is less complex a phenomenon than the sedimentation rate and has been shown to have a close correlation with disease activity, while the sedimentation rate correlates only with colonic disease [5]. Orosomucoid, α_1-antitrypsin and other proteins of the acute phase reaction seem to offer no particular advantage [6] and disease activity, although good correlations exist between levels of various cytokines, and especially for circulating IL-2 receptor, they are no more specific [7]. It should be understood that correlation between the various options is incomplete and that there will inevitably be different false positives and false negatives depending on which test is selected. None of the inflammatory markers exhibits a correlation of better than 80% with a global assessment of disease activity.

The differential diagnosis of inflammatory bowel disease presenting with an acute colitis includes infection, non-steroidal drug-related, and acute, self-limiting colitis (which may itself be infective). The most likely organisms – *Shigella*, *Campylobacter*, *Escherichia coli* 0157, *Entamoeba*, and to a lesser extent (as bleeding is less frequent) *Salmonella*, *Aeromonas*, *Yersinia* and rota virus – are all fairly readily identified (or excluded) by conventional laboratory microbiological examination of the stools. More rigorous microbiological attention is required if the patient is immunodeficient. Pseudomembranous colitis from *Clostridium difficile* infection should be sought, by culture and by examination for its cytotoxin, especially if the patient has recently been exposed to antibiotics. It will be remembered also that the patient with inflammatory bowel disease may present acutely because of a secondary gastrointestinal infection. In the patient presenting for the first time, but in the absence of acute dysenteric symptoms, the differential diagnosis is rather wider and includes colorectal carcinoma, ischaemic colitis and radiation enteritis if there is rectal bleeding, and intestinal tuberculosis, irritable bowel syndrome and a variety of malabsorptive and other gastrointestinal conditions if diarrhoea is unaccompanied by bleeding. When the history does not provide obvious pointers it is then reasonable to proceed with investigation as for inflammatory bowel disease.

PATHOLOGY

The macroscopic pathology of inflammatory bowel disease correlates naturally with the clinical, radiological and endoscopic appearances, and simple examination of resected bowel rarely presents surprises. The key differences between Crohn's disease and ulcerative colitis are vested in their distribution longitudinally and transversely, Crohn's being potentially more extensive in both respects, and the serosal surface of the colon in ulcerative colitis often being nearly normal in appearance. However, it is not unusual for the colon of the fulminant colitic to appear in a much more parlous state than was anticipated preoperatively, with full thickness involvement, probably reflecting secondary ischaemia (also Chapter 4). In Crohn's disease there is characteristic 'fat wrapping' around a stiff, immobile, thickened bowel, and the surgeon may be seriously taxed by unexpected fistulous connections or widespread adherence of the bowel to adjacent structures. In all forms of aggressive disease the bowel may be alarmingly friable and difficult to anastomose safely.

The proximal limit of ulcerative colitis is often very strictly demarcated (hence the proposal that the extent of disease is determined by the underlying vasculature; Chapter 1); whether this is of vascular, mechanical or some other origin, the phenomenon itself remains striking. The colonic surface may be studded with inflammatory polyps or pseudopolyps. There appears to be considerable confusion in the use of these terms. The inflammatory polyp is a true polyp in the sense that it protrudes from the mucosal surface into the lumen on a stalk of variable breadth and length; these tend to occur at sites of past inflammation (and may be the only markers of previous extensive colitis in some patients in remission). Amazing architectural formations may develop, with long interlinked polyps and bridging. Pseudopolyps, on the other hand, are more of an artefact; although they may be described macroscopically and endoscopically, they are most likely to figure in radiological reports. Essentially they represent islands of normal or regenerative mucosa which appear elevated through the loss of the surrounding sloughed mucosa. Their presence will always coincide with active inflammation at the site implicated.

HISTOLOGY

In ulcerative colitis the histological changes are predominantly confined to the mucosa and submucosa. In active disease there will typically be an acute inflammatory reaction with a neutrophil infiltrate, crypt abscesses and goblet cells depleted of mucus (Plate 1); there may also be generalized oedema and vascular congestion. None of these features is pathognomonic of ulcerative colitis, although their occurrence together will be highly suggestive. With chronicity, architectural changes develop. There are then abnormal, irregular and excessively branched crypts, which will also typically be atrophied and shortened, and may no longer reach at least two-thirds of the distance from the luminal surface to the muscularis mucosa as is normal. These changes are more specific to ulcerative colitis, and help greatly in the pathological distinction from acute infective colitis or acute self-limited colitis [8].

Transmural involvement is the norm in established Crohn's disease and is associated with a predominantly lymphocytic infiltrate [9]. Crypt abscesses and neutrophil infiltrates occur in acute disease but are less prominent features than in ulcerative colitis. Goblet cells are less often drained of mucus. The mucosal architecture is generally better preserved than in ulcerative colitis. The most helpful specific features in Crohn's disease are granulomata which, when present, occur mainly in the submucosa and are non-caseating (Plate 2). The differential diagnosis for granulomatous colitis/ileitis includes not only tuberculosis, yersiniosis and sarcoid, but also the foreign body reaction which may confuse if typical inclusions are absent on polarized light microscopy. Pericryptal granulomata have been considered of lesser significance however, and most pathologists consider them evidence of crypt damage and therefore of non-specific nature. Fourteen patients with these lesions and with no other features (clinical or pathological) of Crohn's disease have now been followed for between 2 and 17 years, in comparison with eight patients with pericryptal inflammation and no granulomas [10]. Unequivocal evidence of Crohn's disease became apparent with follow-up in 10 of those with granulomas, but in only one without. It seems therefore that granulomas at any site should be considered important predictors of a final Crohn's diagnosis.

The aphthoid ulcers of early Crohn's typically occur over intestinal Peyer's patches and lymphoid aggregates, but whether they are necessarily the origin of the larger deep ulcers seen in more advanced disease is uncertain. Oral aphthous ulcers are definitely not peculiar to Crohn's disease, but those elsewhere in the gut, while not pathognomonic to inflammatory bowel disease, are sufficiently associated to make exploration of their pathogenesis of interest. It now seems probable, from a careful pathological study of lesions at various stages of their evolution, that (in the colon at least) aphthi originate in the follicle-associated epithelium in conjunction with an overexpression of HLA-DR antigens, and may reflect a role of this specialized epithelium as a portal for entry of potentially pathogenic agents [11].

INDETERMINATE COLITIS

Because of the absence of the differentiating markers of chronicity, the histopathologist is least likely to be able to make a firm distinction between ulcerative and Crohn's colitis in the colon removed at first presentation for fulminant disease. The term indeterminate colitis is applied to this group, and to any patient in whom there is chronic colitis in the absence of features – clinical, or from imaging as well as from histology – that amount to a diagnosis of ulcerative colitis or Crohn's disease. It can be seen therefore that the pathologist may record indeterminate colitis in a patient where there is no ileal histology but the barium follow-through shows obvious Crohn's disease. A diagnosis of indeterminate colitis then, to be meaningful, must carry with it the corollary that this is based on histology alone (in which case the clinician may be able to make a more or less certain assessment of whether it is Crohn's or ulcerative colitis) or that it is indeterminate colitis when all relevant disciplines have have completed their deliberations, in which case the diagnosis stands until new information becomes available (which in many cases it does not). Helpfully, Price has reviewed this area from the perspective of the histopathologist [12].

The difficulties of indeterminate colitis extend to the evaluation of the retained, defunctioned rectum prior to consideration of pouch surgery (Chapter 4). Unfortunately the histological characteristics of diversion colitis/proctitis share many of the features of Crohn's disease, and the pathologist may be unable to advise confidently as to whether the underlying diagnosis is ulcerative colitis, and that a pouch can sensibly be considered, or whether the clinician should be more wary.

Most patients categorized as having indeterminate colitis probably have ulcerative colitis, given that they will almost inevitably have continuous distal colorectal disease and disease limited to the mucosa, or presented with fulminant colitis. Accordingly, most of them retain this semi-diagnosis in the long term, as it is unusual for a feature so characteristic of ulcerative colitis to emerge that it outweighs the earlier uncertainty. A proportion (well under 25%) will nevertheless subsequently express features – especially small bowel involvement or obvious granulomata – that lead to a firm diagnosis of Crohn's disease. With this proviso, most patients with indeterminate colitis behave clinically much more like those with ulcerative colitis and should probably be managed accordingly [13]. From 46 patients in whom examination of a resected colon led the pathologist to call the colitis indeterminate, clinical features pointed to probable Crohn's disease in 19 and ulcerative colitis in 11. At a median of 10 years' follow-up, only five working diagnoses had been changed. One patient thought to have Crohn's was reclassified as ulcerative colitis, three with indeterminate colitis were subsequently considered more definitely ulcerative colitis, and only one patient with a single granuloma moved from the indeterminate to the Crohn's disease group (12 remained 'indeterminate' with no small bowel features). A cautious strategy nevertheless leads my patients with extensive and unresected indeterminate colitis both to enter surveillance for future development of neoplasia and away from pouch surgery (Chapters 4 and 8) .

IMAGING OF INFLAMMATORY BOWEL DISEASE

The traditional radiological methods of imaging the bowel have been increasingly challenged by newer modalities. Few would now argue that even the most carefully conducted double-contrast barium enema is superior to competent colonoscopy, but they remain complimentary investigations ([14], and see below). The alternatives to barium-based examination of the small intestine are less established. The principal competition comes at present from enteroscopy and from white cell scanning, but the potential value of abdominal magnetic resonance imaging, reconstructive 'three-dimensional' computed tomography and of newer methods of more specific isotopic imaging have not yet been exploited to the full. Angiography is rarely relevant in the context of inflammatory bowel disease.

Although controlled comparisons of colonoscopy and barium enema favour colonoscopy, which of course offers the advantage of permitting histological sampling, there remains a case for barium radiology. The potential value of the unprepared or 'instant' enema is discussed in the section on fulminant colitis (Chapter 4), and it retains a role in the early assessment of a new patient with colitic symptoms in whom the extent of the disease will have an immediate influence on management.

The plain abdominal radiograph is an undervalued and underused resource in many institutions caring for patients with inflammatory bowel disease. It will often be obvious from the supine film that the patient has faecal loading in the proximal colon which effectively excludes a diagnosis of total colitis. On the contrary, total colitis becomes an important possibility when there appears to be no faecal residue at any site (see also Chapter 4). Similarly neglected in many centres is the modest abdominal ultrasonographic scan. Quite apart from its role in detection and assessment of abscesses (Chapter 7), it will often be possible to identify a loop of thickened, inflamed bowel with proximal distension and fluid retention (see below).

Barium radiology

Contrast radiology is the longest-established imaging modality for diagnosis of inflammatory bowel disease. Barium sulphate is appropriately radiodense, is essentially inert and is not normally absorbed from the gut. However, extraluminal barium creates a vigorous and potentially fatal inflammatory reaction in the peritoneum with a high risk of subsequent devastating fibrosis. It behoves the clinician and radiologist to avoid barium where free perforation is a possibility, and to use instead a water-soluble contrast agent. Inferior definition is then to be expected, not least because many water-soluble media have a potent osmotic effect and tend to be diluted by resultant intestinal secretions.

The classical appearances of ulcerative colitis and Crohn's disease are well documented, and reference texts and atlases, such as those of Margulis and Burhenne, and Misiewicz *et al.* [15, 16], allow perusal of the variation in extent and severity and the more subtle aspects of radiological diagnosis. However, the key colonic and small bowel abnormalities may be summarized (Table 2.2).

Barium enema

The radiological distinction between ulcerative colitis and Crohn's colitis is based on the distribution, depth and presence/absence of complications, just as in the overall distinction of the two conditions. It is usually possible to draw a confident interpretation from the combination of the radiological signs and the clinical features. The double-contrast enema, using both air and barium, has almost completely superseded the single-contrast examination, but the unprepared ('instant') enema is still helpful in the rapid and non-invasive evaluation of acute colitis (see above and Chapter 4). In early/mild colitis the only abnormality may be a granularity of the mucosa, but in ulcerative colitis the changes will almost always

Table 2.2 Barium enema in diagnosis of inflammatory bowel disease

Feature	Crohn's disease	Ulcerative colitis	Other
Distal disease	+/−	++	+/−
Continuity	+/−	++	+/−
Asymmetry	++	−	+/−
Skip lesions	++	−	+/−
Deep perforating ulcers	+	−	+/−
Fistulae	++	−	+/−

be continuous from the rectum upwards. At a relatively early stage the retrorectal space becomes enlarged. It is probable that this reflects both thickening of the rectal wall and the beginnings of rectal shortening as the bowel becomes fibrotic. The so-called hose-pipe colon is less often seen with better medical therapy (or earlier surgery), but when present is strongly supportive of a diagnosis of chronic fibrotic ulcerative colitis.

Crohn's colitis may mimic ulcerative colitis but usually declares itself from deeper ulceration (the rosethorn ulcers), and a more patchy or asymmetrical distribution (with a strong tendency to affect the mesenteric border preferentially). In mild disease the halo appearance of aphthoid ulcers is characteristic (Figure 2.1). The presence of fistulous connections with other structures makes for a sure distinction from ulcerative colitis.

When polyps are demonstrated, the radiologist may be confident that 'bridging' seen between polyps (also referred to as filiform polyposis) is entirely the result of past inflammation, but otherwise will usually choose to defer to colonoscopic/histological assessment since it is not possible to make a clear distinction between the inflammatory polyp (common in inflammatory bowel disease and essentially harmless) and the adenoma

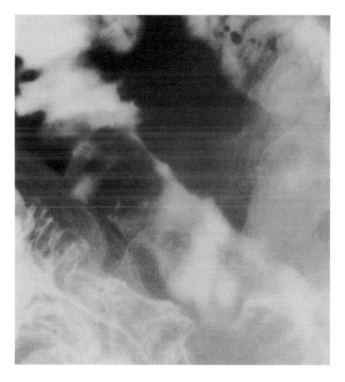

Figure 2.1 Barium follow-through in an early phase of Crohn's disease. The terminal ileum is seen in the centre of the image and bears several shallow aphthoid ulcers.

(which should be removed). Despite its limitations, the barium enema can sometimes provide information that cannot easily be obtained by other means. The proximal colon of a patient with a tight stricture can often be assessed adequately, and, perhaps more importantly, radiological recognition of abnormal distensibility and contour of the bowel may be the earliest sign of malignant transformation in the long-standing colitic (Chapter 8).

The radiological differential diagnosis for conditions other than inflammatory bowel disease includes ischaemia, which is patchy like Crohn's disease, but usually concentrated at vascular watershed zones such as at the splenic flexure. Infective colitides may be confused with inflammatory bowel disease (usually when the history is deficient), and there is a steady flow of accounts of mismanagement of acute amoebic colitis in which steroids have been given to treat an assumed diagnosis of inflammatory bowel disease. The classic cone-shaped caecum of more chronic amoebiasis is rarely seen in Western centres, and tends to yield a differential diagnosis of neoplasia rather than of inflammatory bowel disease when it appears. Pseudomembranous colitis poses more of a challenge as it may complicate underlying inflammatory bowel disease, but the radiological features of plaque formation and proximal distension may be helpful if the diagnosis has not been made as a result of clinical or endoscopic cues.

Barium studies of the small bowel

Barium studies of the small bowel are in a more secure position, clinical experience continuing to support their use in the investigation of patients with symptoms potentially attributable to the small bowel [17, 18]. There is still some debate in radiological circles as to the relative place of the traditional follow-through and the small bowel enema or enteroclysis, in which the barium is instilled through a nasal tube placed into the jejunum. My colleagues prefer the former for the reason that it tends to give relatively better visualization of the lower small bowel (very often the area of greater interest in inflammatory bowel disease) and because it generally remains possible to compress the contrast-filled bowel, which in turn helps to permit separation of superimposed intestinal loops [19]. The more distended bowel created in the adequately filled bowel at enteroclysis may be more difficult or painful to compress. The decision should rightly be that of the radiologist responsible for the examination, but the speedier completion of enteroclysis may be outweighed in the patient's eyes by the added discomfort of intubation. It may also be helpful to use pharmacological manipulation with anticholinergics (such as hyoscine or atropine) not only for their influence on intestinal motility but also because patients often find that the examination is then appreciably less uncomfortable (unpublished observations). A follow-through examination can be performed as a adjunct to assessment of the more proximal gastrointestinal tract (the meal and follow-through), but this is almost always second best for both parts of the examination as the ideal density and quantity of barium differs for the different purposes: it is not recommended.

It may be helpful, especially for comprehensive visualization of the terminal ileum, to introduce air into the colon (or to use an oral effervescent agent) to obtain partially double-contrast views. This is distinct from the retrograde examination of the small bowel obtained at barium enema when the ileocaecal valve is incompetent or absent, and which is not the investigation of choice if the ileum is the area of interest. Retrograde examinations are nevertheless valuable in patients with an ileostomy, and especially so when there is proximal stenosis or when the patient is unwilling or unable to retain oral barium.

The radiological features of small bowel Crohn's reflect its pathological nature and distribution. The early changes include granularity, aphthous ulcers and fold thickening, progressing with increasing severity to nodularity, including cobblestoning, frank focal ulceration, fissuring and stenosis. The asymmetry, typical of all aspects of Crohn's disease, is usually manifest as a disproportionate involvement of the mesenteric border of the gut. The classical 'string' sign (Figure 2.2), in which lengths of bowel

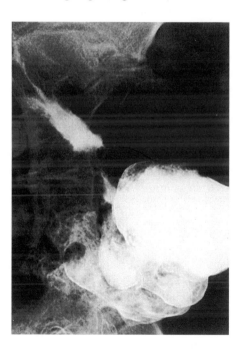

Figure 2.2 Barium follow-through in the same patient as in Figure 2.1, 12 months later when, despite 5-aminosalicylate (5-ASA) therapy, the disease has progressed, leading to stenosis of the terminal ileum which now almost exhibits the string sign; obstructive symptoms led to a surgical intervention.

appear narrowed and irregular, is as much the result of inflammation as of fibrous stricturing, and the separation of adjacent loops indicates that one is dealing with thickening of the bowel. In a dynamic examination it should be possible to make a distinction between motile but severely inflamed loops and those in which there is fixed stenotic scarring. This has clear therapeutic implications. 'Cobblestones' reflect the presence of deep and intersecting transverse and longitudinal ulcers and are rarely seen in other conditions. The presence of fistulae either between intestinal loops or from intestine to other structures is almost pathognomonic of Crohn's disease in developed countries.

Patients with extensive Crohn's disease may also exhibit the characteristic malabsorption pattern of barium dilution and flocculation; a modest diffuse dilatation (Figure 2.3) of the intestine may be seen. There tends to be a loss of the intestinal fold pattern in the proximal jejunum (and sometimes an increase more distally, although this is more a feature of non-Crohn's malabsorption). The special relevance of barium studies to short bowel syndrome is considered further in Chapter 7.

Intestinal tuberculosis poses special problems in the differential diagnosis at centres in developed countries because its relative rarity tends to lead to its neglect. The converse problem for patients with Crohn's disease in populations in which tuberculosis is more endemic is arguably less worrying given the therapeutic implications of a wrong diagnosis in one direction rather than the other. The radiologist may help by distinguishing the characteristic multiple transverse ulcers, the classic funnelled caecum, gross thickening of the intestinal wall and fixity of the terminal ileum, or from other manifestations of tuberculosis (not least of these being the chest radiograph – abnormal in about 50% of those with intestinal tuberculosis). A continued high index of suspicion in all population groups is needed if early infection is to be identified and late complications avoided. The differential diagnosis for terminal ileitis is often otherwise brief, but previous irradiation, Behçet's syndrome and yersinial infection deserve consideration. Intestinal lymphoid hyperplasia (idiopathic or related to a variety of acute and chronic infections) may be over-interpreted as Crohn's in young patients with gastrointestinal symptoms, but the experienced radiologist will usually be confident of the correct interpretation when associated ulceration is absent. At the opposite end of the age range, contrast examinations are increasingly performed in patients with intestinal ischaemia. Focal and segmental ischaemia can be difficult to distinguish from active Crohn's.

The clinician should regard a radiological verdict of Crohn's disease not as a diagnosis, but as a critical component to the formation of a global assessment. In practice there will very infrequently be disagreement with a confident conclusion arising from a small bowel series (Table 2.3).

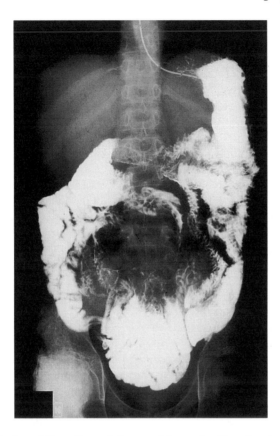

Figure 2.3 Barium follow-through in an adolescent with extensive small bowel Crohn's disease. The central loops of bowel are narrowed and their separation is indicative of their considerable thickening. The ulceration of the intestine is evident at several sites as is the degree of distal stenosis itself responsible for intestinal dilatation (most obvious in the left iliac fossa). The nasogastric tube was being used for primary nutritional therapy.

Fistulography

Fistulae are poorly demonstrated by endoscopic techniques and may be inadequately filled at intraluminal contrast studies for their full anatomy to be discerned. Although computed tomography (CT) and magnetic resonance (MR) scanning are proving helpful in the assessment of the patient with enterocutaneous fistulae (see below and Chapter 7), it is unlikely that the traditional 'fistulogram' will be superseded for some time. Introduction of water-soluble contrast directly into the cutaneous opening will usually permit adequate demonstration of the fistula track and the site of its origin from the bowel. The tendency of the contrast to spill back can be overcome by its introduction through a balloon-tipped catheter

Table 2.3   Small bowel series in diagnosis of inflammatory bowel disease

Feature	Crohn's disease	Tuberculosis	Other infection	Ischaemia
Terminal ileal	++	+	+	+/–
Enteric fistula	++	+	–	–
Strictures	++	++	+/–	++
Patchy distribution	++	+	–	++
Wall thickening	++	+++	+	+
Aphthous ulcers	++	+/–	+/–	–
Asymmetry	++	+	–	++
Cobblestones	++	–	–	–

which seals the skin opening; as relatively high pressure may be required, the caution of an experienced operator is advised to avoid damage and maintain the reputation of fistulography as a safe technique.

Endoscopy

Colonoscopy and ileoscopy

Endoscopic assessment of the intestine is most helpful in inflammatory bowel disease, but full colonoscopy is not always required: the high proportion of the needed information that can be obtained from simple sigmoidoscopy and biopsy is sometimes now underestimated. The characteristic appearances of confluent inflammation will permit the experienced endoscopist to diagnose ulcerative colitis with some confidence. Needless to say, this is substantially less reliable than the equivalent information from the pathologist, and no firm conclusion should be drawn without histological support. Colonoscopy comes into its own in ulcerative colitis (Plates 3 and 4) in determining the proximal extent of disease and in surveillance for neoplasia (Chapter 8). The upper limit of disease at colonoscopy tends to be somewhat more proximal than predicted by concurrent barium enema, and is often very well defined. In surveillance the endoscopist will be alert to focal areas of more abnormal mucosa and to mass lesions. The dysplasia-associated lesion or mass (DALM) has especial prognostic significance, but in the main the examination serves to permit the collection of a series of biopsies from around the colon (at least 10 biopsies for a reasonable chance of representative sampling) (Chapter 8).

Sigmoidoscopy is less helpful in Crohn's disease but it is always worth taking a mucosal biopsy even of normal-looking mucosa when the differential diagnosis includes Crohn's, as a single characteristic granuloma can lend substantial weight to the diagnostic process. Full colonoscopy (Plate 5) is proportionately more valuable in diagnosis than in ulcerative colitis given the potential for patchy disease expression and also because of the possibility of examining (and biopsying) the terminal ileum (Plate 6) in a majority of cases.

A number of centres have become interested in extending the sensitivity of colonoscopy by including infrared imaging which is thought to give additional information about the submucosal vascular pattern. Tamada *et al.* believe that this assists in the differential diagnosis between ulcerative colitis and Crohn's disease, only the former showing apparent rigidity and dilatation of terminal capillaries [20]. The technique currently requires a special endoscope but the principal is simple and could presumably be incorporated into regular instruments. There must be some scepticism that it may be wasted effort since histology will always be taken.

Other endoscopy
Upper gastrointestinal endoscopy is helpful in patients with proximal symptomatology (see below), and it is probable that enteroscopy will find a regular place in the diagnostic work-up of patients in whom the standard investigations are inconclusive or contradictory. One group already finds routine preoperative enteroscopy valuable in the full assessment of their patients with Crohn's disease [21]. At present enteroscopy by the 'push' technique will be preferred in inflammatory bowel disease practice because of the current inability to obtain biopsies from the sonde type of instrument.

Ultrasound

Modern ultrasound technology permits ready evaluation of the intestine at most sites in the abdomen, and radiologists (and gastroenterologists) are become more skilled at interpreting the findings. The presence of Crohn's-related abscesses or other complications may be obvious, but the thickness of the bowel wall, the presence of dilated fluid-filled loops and associated inflammatory masses or reactive fluid can also be determined. It therefore becomes possible to diagnose and to stage disease distribution and severity. Using a very simple single criterion to determine postoperative recurrence – namely the presence of a bowel thickness greater than 5 mm – ultrasonography proved nearly as reliable as full ileo-colonoscopy in one small, blinded study, and was possible in all patients, unlike the endoscopy, which was prevented by disease or its location in 13% [22]. Formal scoring systems are yet to be generally accepted, but one Japanese group has already proposed a complex activity index which takes into account the thickness of the bowel wall, and the ease with which the normal stratification of the intestine is discerned (i.e. mucosa v. submucosa v. muscularis) [23]. A good correlation with results of other imaging techniques is claimed, but the absence of a correlation with CRP levels suggests that it is not yet an activity index even if it is yielding useful non-invasive topography (see below).

Endoscopic ultrasound has not yet been widely adopted in inflammatory bowel disease, but it offers potentially useful information in assessment of complications such as pelvic fistulae, and may provide information additive to that of colonoscopy in (for example) a questioned neoplastic region in extensive colitis [24]. It is also proposed as a route to estimation of penetration and therefore of expected histology in inflammatory bowel disease in general [25]. It remains to be seen if this will prove of any clinical value.

CT scanning

CT scanning has mostly been used in the evaluation and management of complications of inflammatory bowel disease rather than in its initial diagnosis, but more modern scanners (and especially those with helical/spiral image capturing) permit detailed assessment of the entire alimentary tract. In Crohn's disease the thickening of the bowel loops and their approximate location are easily identified, and further information in respect of significant stenoses and fistulous connections is now beginning to be of comparable reliability to that of barium follow-through. CT appearances will differentiate reliably between ulcerative colitis and Crohn's colitis in most cases, and may occasionally avoid the need for colonoscopy [26]. Samples will still be needed for histology. A new feature, the 'comb' sign which results from vascular dilatation and tortuosity, and a wider spacing of the vasa recta, is proposed as a specific indicator of Crohn's disease [27]. Enhanced CT scans can be the best means of evaluating the retroperitoneum and iliopsoas region in patients with suspected abdominal sepsis, these areas often proving inaccessible to ultrasonography. Abscesses appear as relatively low-density spaces with enhancing walls, and can often be shown to contain gas (or previously administered contrast material). Evolving reconstructive techniques make it possible to create an image that apparently equates to the three-dimensional intraluminal view of the colon at colonoscopy. At present the resolution and pseudo-colour are greatly inferior to colonoscopy, but this may be just a question of time. However, it is unlikely that a therapeutic role, or means of obtaining biopsies, will easily supersede the endoscopic route to these. It is also probable that the high radiation dose of CT (Chapter 8) will accelerate the move towards magnetic resonance imaging in inflammatory bowel disease (see below).

Magnetic resonance imaging

MR scanning permits non-invasive three-dimensional imaging of the abdomen and pelvis, and the speedier image acquisition of modern equipment reduces earlier difficulties associated with artefact from intestinal movement. Already MR has outperformed the visual diagnosis made at colonoscopy in one small controlled study [28]. MR images are particularly helpful in the pelvis – a difficult area for most other forms of imaging – where unenhanced spin echo sequences can be invaluable in identifying and distinguishing inflammation/sepsis from surrounding normal tissues. Its application to patients with Crohn's disease has not been overlooked but financial constraints have so far restrained most UK practitioners from developing an adequate degree of familiarity with its strengths and weaknesses. In a representative review of initial experience of the technique in Crohn's, Kosa *et al.* describe a high sensitivity for clinically significant lesions, a relatively poor correlation with CRP levels, and the obtaining of otherwise unavailable information in respect of fistula anatomy [29]. It is probable that time will see faster (and less noisy) MR scanning, a wider selection of contrast agents, and that it will come to replace an increasing proportion of CT and barium examinations.

White cell scanning

Radiolabelled white cell scanning identifies areas of inflammation and may also be able to yield quantitative assessments. Given the limitations of clinical and biochemical means to distinguish inflammatory activity from the results of stenosis (see below), this is potentially valuable in inflammatory bowel disease. When autologous leucocytes are returned to the host circulation they migrate preferentially to areas of inflammation or, in the absence of inflammation, mainly to the bone marrow and spleen. Labelled neutrophils reinjected into patients with inflammatory bowel disease tend to localize to areas of bowel currently involved in the disease. Initial work with indium-111 permitted a distinction between patients with active and inactive disease, and the radioactivity of timed faecal collections led to a single 'excretion index' score. Indium has been superseded in most centres by labelling with technetium-99m which is cheaper, more readily available, has a shorter half-life, lower expected radiation exposure and gives images more quickly and of better resolution. The usual carrier, hexamethyl propylene amine oxime (HMPAO) is lipophyllic and easily able to enter white cells for labelling, but then becomes converted intracellularly to a hydrophilic form which cannot escape, leaving it and its associated technetium fixed within the cell. Crohn's disease activity and its predominant site(s) are reliably documented in most centres [30]. It is possible to quantify disease activity (not by stool collections, because of a normal degree of colonic excretion of the isotope), but there is still some difficulty in judging the accuracy and sensitivity of HMPAO scanning, not least because of the absence of a diagnostic gold standard.

The distinction between currently active Crohn's disease – amenable to steroid therapy or other non-surgical methods – and fibrostenotic disease – that can only be expected to respond to surgical resection or repair – is an important one. The radiologist may be able to make an informed judgement from barium images but will often acknowledge that a trial of therapy is a better indication of the predominant problem. White cell scanning has a definite role in this context – a normal scan in a symptomatic patient with known radiological abnormalities constitutes a strong indication for surgery. Unfortunately, the barium image is needed alongside the scan to obtain the full picture.

White cell scanning can be refined further by its combination with software developed for computed tomography to allow creation of single-photon-emission CT (SPECT) images, in which a three-dimensional reconstruction becomes possible. All of the variants of white cell scanning expose the patient to a great deal less ionizing radiation than barium imaging and X-ray CT, with typical doses in the region of that of a standard chest radiograph. Inflammatory bowel disease centres currently divide between those using a great deal of HMPAO scanning and those using it either not at all or for very selected cases. The St George's group in London encourages us to join the former camp [31] on the bases (*inter alia*) of quantitative reproducibility and low invasiveness, but I am not entirely persuaded for several reasons. Although a negative scan indicates that inflammatory bowel disease is probably absent, it does not exclude it (especially if the disease happens to be inactive at the time of the study), and I am not aware of published data that give the specificity of leucocyte scanning in patients relatively unlikely to have inflammatory bowel disease (such as the patient with atypical irritable bowel syndrome), but in whom one needs to have supportive negative investigations. If a scan is positive, histological support will usually still be sought, to discriminate idiopathic inflammatory bowel disease from other inflammatory conditions, and Crohn's from ulcerative colitis. Colonoscopy is not thereby necessarily avoided (and clearly not in respect of obtaining pancolonic biopsies in later surveillance work). As the quality of scans improves, it may be possible to define the topography of small bowel Crohn's sufficiently to reduce the need for barium radiology, but I am not sure that a scan will easily substitute for the detailed information on potential complications or in respect of the differential diagnosis that my radiological colleagues currently provide as a routine. There is an obvious role for white cell scanning in discriminating between fibrous and inflammatory strictures, and a good case for its use as an initial diagnostic method in children. It can sensibly be used to determine the extent of disease in a patient known from rectal histology to have inflammatory bowel disease (but who is not yet at risk of neoplasia). As an adjunct to Crohn's Disease Activity Index (CDAI) scores and biochemical assessments of disease activity, sequential scanning will also find use in clinical trials, but more conventional imaging is probably no further challenged at present.

E-selectin scanning

Arguably one of the most exciting of the newer imaging modalities is that under evaluation at the Royal Postgraduate Medical School in London [32]. The technique is derived from more conventional labelled white cell scintigraphy, but uses a labelled antibody to E-selectin, which is known to be overexpressed in endothelial cells at sites of inflammation. It has the advantage thereby of studying a more fixed entity that (unlike white cells) will not be shed at a variable rate into the bowel lumen, and is also applicable to the occasional neutropenic patient. Preliminary data indicate an accuracy comparable to that of HMPAO scanning and, with a planned switch to the more user-friendly technetium as the radioisotope employed, it could well take on a significant role.

CLINICAL VARIANTS OF INFLAMMATORY BOWEL DISEASE, DISEASE ACTIVITY AND PROGNOSIS

Oral and facial Crohn's disease

Oral aphthous ulcers are common in the general population but are definitely over-represented in groups of patients with inflammatory bowel disease – especially those with Crohn's disease. They are, however, not the only manifestations of inflammatory bowel disease in the mouth, focal oedema and polypoid papulous hyperplasia also being frequently identifiable [33]. Oral disease may be the first evidence of Crohn's disease and particularly so in the paediatric and adolescent age range. Topical steroid therapy (e.g. with hydrocortisone pellets) will lead to complete remission in at least 50% of cases but when this fails, intralesional injection of steroids, systemic steroids or azathioprine are reasonable options in response to facial distortion, disabling pain and inability to eat, even in the absence of disease activity at other sites. It is not unheard of for admission to be required for the administration of parenteral opiates for severe oral ulceration. Thalidomide may also have a role in treatment of these ulcers (Chapter 3). Orofacial granulomatosis is frequently the result of Crohn's disease, and particularly affects the lips and gums. It is unclear whether the orofacial granulomatosis syndrome, in which there are associated nerve palsies, is a separate condition, but a distinction from orofacial sarcoid is usually obvious from the presence of other gastrointestinal signs and the absence of pulmonary features.

Crohn's of the upper gastrointestinal tract

Gastroduodenal Crohn's is recognized but was thought generally unusual, with frequencies of well under 5% recorded in past literature. This may reflect its tendency to affect patients with more dramatic disease at other and more usual sites, thereby deflecting attention from both symptoms and from evidence on imaging even when relevant imaging has been performed. It has been my experience that most patients with Crohn's disease coming to upper gastrointestinal endoscopy have macroscopic changes in the stomach, but I had concluded that this was a result of the inevitable bias introduced by the selection of patients for this procedure. However, data from paediatric and adolescent series suggest a high frequency of upper gastrointestinal involvement in unselected cases [34], and Halme *et al.* [35] have now studied 62 consecutive patients with ileo-colic Crohn's disease and find a 42% frequency of histologically confirmed chronic gastritis. This was only associated with *Helicobacter pylori* in 9.7%; four of the 62 patients had gastric granulomas. The inflammatory changes were similar to those of Crohn's disease at other gastrointestinal sites, and there was a positive correlation between the severity of intestinal disease and the presence of gastritis. The corollary to this is that Crohn's disease accounts for a high proportion of *Helicobacter*-negative chronic gastritis. Oberhuber *et al.* describe similar features in their patients with Crohn's disease and suggest that a focal active gastritis found in the absence of *H. pylori* should prompt a search for Crohn's [36].

Functional symptoms in inflammatory bowel disease

It is not unusual for patients with well-established inflammatory bowel disease to present with symptoms that sound more functional, and in whom all investigations seeking evidence of current inflammation (such as raised platelet count or CRP) are normal. Symptomatic proximal constipation in those with distal colitis (see above) might also be included within this context. A group at the Mayo Clinic has tried to quantify the magnitude of functional disorder in patients with surgically treated ulcerative colitis [37]. Using a necessarily modified version of the Rome criteria for irritable bowel syndrome, they considered that 20.4% of their patients who had had a successful ileo-anal pouch for ulcerative colitis and in whom there was no evidence of pouchitis (Chapter 4) had irritable bowel syndrome. How this relates to the more complicated situation of separating the two conditions when the colitis is still active or potentially so is less clear. The possible impact of functional disorder should be remembered in patients with inflammatory bowel disease, and perhaps particularly so in Crohn's disease, in which active disease is less easily confirmed or refuted endoscopically. There are logical reasons for considering that such patients have superimposed irritable bowel syndrome, but that in this context this should be very much a diagnosis of exclusion. Management can then be along functional lines with avoidance of the more toxic options for therapy of inflammatory bowel disease.

Psychological problems in inflammatory bowel disease

The patient with inflammatory bowel disease has a chronic and often debilitating disease that can only (in the case of ulcerative colitis) be cured by radical surgery that itself leaves variable long-term sequelae. The symptoms of the disease are unpleasant, and are not considered ones for 'polite conversation'. It is inevitable therefore that psychological morbidity runs alongside the organic physical disease. No one now would seriously maintain that the inflammatory bowel diseases are caused by psychological disease, but there can be little doubt that psychological factors can be very important and presumably contribute to the functional symptoms described above. The unpredictability of inflammatory bowel disease is itself a major cause of anxiety and stress, especially when faecal incontinence is, or has ever been, a problem. Many patients limit their social lives dramatically and (to the physician's eyes) disproportionately because of these fears. The lay support groups have played an important role in reducing the social stigma of diarrhoea and urgency but the problem remains.

There is some evidence for excess neuroticism and obsessiveness in inflammatory bowel disease, but it is very difficult to distinguish the components of these observations that were present before the onset of the disease and which could have a partial causal role, from those that are reactive to the illness and its associated physical and psychological morbidity. The same difficulty applies to the analysis of formal psychological disorders such as depression and anxiety. Prospective studies do not exist, but the current great interest in family groups at high risk of inflammatory bowel disease will perhaps stimulate the collection of psychological data in individuals during the presymptomatic stages of disease.

Given time and a sympathetic ear, patients are remarkably candid about the influence of stress and emotional issues on their intestinal symptoms, and often appear to find such discussion therapeutically valuable in its own right. They may also be greatly helped by 'permission' to use moderately potent constipating agents such as loperamide to help them through times of predictable stress. This use of opioids is more prevalent among European than North American gastroenterologists for reasons that are unclear. There does not seem to be any risk attached to such a strategy so long as the patient knows to discontinue the drug if true constipation develops or if abdominal discomfort or pain indicative of developing obstruction begins.

In a tertiary referral practice, many inflammatory bowel disease patients have major psychological and emotional problems, and especially those who have been ill during adolescence and whose ability to manage their transition from childhood to adulthood has been seriously impaired by the illness (despite the best efforts of health-care workers and the best intentions of their parents). In this context the close involvement of counsellor, psychologist and psychiatrist is essential for comprehensive care, but even in the most straightforward case these issues should be addressed actively by the clinician. Faecal soiling and frank incontinence is rarely volunteered but is frequently experienced, and anxiety that it may be is almost universal in the patient with diarrhoea. The impact of this on (female) sexuality is alluded to elsewhere (see below and Chapter 5).

Patients with inflammatory bowel disease are not immune from other psychiatric diagnoses but these do not seem to be over- or under-represented relative to control populations, and their management can normally be conducted in a conventional fashion. Occasionally extensive small bowel Crohn's disease can lead to problems with absorption of psychoactive drugs, but in most respects therapy will be unaltered.

The acute pain associated with a specific complication or during a major relapse of inflammatory bowel disease rarely presents a management problem, but a substantial minority of patients with chronically active Crohn's disease have continual abdominal pain, which can prove intractable. The clinician's first role is, as far as possible, to confirm or refute the presence of a remediable physical cause of pain, but when pain remains idiopathic or is hugely out of proportion to the objective findings, management becomes a problem. There is a surprising paucity of reports in the literature on this difficult clinical problem, but the appropriate readiness of gastrointestinal physicians and nurses to resort to opiates in dealing with acute pain is probably a significant contributing cause to the emergence of opiate addiction in a high proportion of those who develop a chronic pain syndrome. One unit suggests that 5% of its entire inflammatory bowel disease population is drug dependent (excluding alcohol) [38]. The figure is clearly influenced by the prevalence of drug abuse in the general population to which patients belong, and it is unlikely that rates of this magnitude would be found other than in the most major cities in Europe. The problem is nevertheless real and probably reflects the gastroenterologist's uncertainty as to how to proceed and, once the problem is recognized, the reluctance of affected patients to accept help from pain clinics or drug-dependency centres. A high index of suspicion should be maintained and long-term use of opiates for pain control avoided whenever possible. Antidepressants may be valuable even in the absence of overt depression, as may alternatives such as carbamazepine and strategies based on hypnotherapy or acupuncture. However, there are no controlled data in respect of any of these in the context of inflammatory bowel disease. The early involvement of clinicians with skills complementary to those of the gastrointestinal team is always to be encouraged.

Inflammatory bowel disease that is not ulcerative colitis or Crohn's disease

Behçet's

Aphthous ulcers in the mouth in conjunction with arthropathy, uveitis or a variety of dermatological or neurological features will lead rapidly to a clinical diagnosis of the idiopathic condition, Behçet's disease, if aphthous ulcers are also found on the genitalia [39]. When there are no urogenital ulcers the differential diagnosis will usually include Crohn's disease, not least since around 50% of patients with Behçet's have gastrointestinal symptoms such as diarrhoea, vomiting and abdominal pain [40]. There are still no definitive tests for the diagnosis. The condition is very much more common in Middle Eastern and Asian populations [41]. Up to 1 in 1000 of the Japanese population may be affected, compared to less than 1 in 500 000 in North America.

Radiologically, the typical features of Behçet's are aphthous and geographical ulcers, with a patchy distribution not dissimilar from that of Crohn's disease [42]. The ulcers may be deep and punched-out, but do not often perforate nor lead to fistula formation. Intestinal lesions tend to be concentrated in the ileocaecal region and may be responsible for distortion and mass effects. Clinical remission is associated with parallel improvement in radiological signs. Histologically there is a non-specific chronic inflammatory process associated with the areas of ulceration. Treatment has usually included topical or systemic steroids, but a variety of alternative immunosuppressants have also been thought helpful. Controlled data do not yet exist.

Ulcerative jejunitis

Ulcerative jejunitis (or chronic non-granulomatous jejunitis) usually affects patients with coeliac disease, who lose or fail to achieve a response to gluten withdrawal [43]. Worsening malabsorptive symptoms, often associated with abdominal pain, lead to further investigation. The condition may also be present at the first presentation in some older patients in whom the differential diagnosis will usually be Crohn's disease. In either case, villous atrophy in combination with proximal small bowel ulceration is demonstrable. Radiological findings include prominence of the intestinal folds but the dilatation typical of untreated coeliac disease is not a feature [44]. It is probable that ulcerative jejunitis is a pre-neoplastic condition with a definite association with intestinal T-cell lymphoma, of which it may be a *forme fruste*. If very careful histological assessment reveals no malignancy, then the management will normally include a strict gluten-free diet and avoidance of potentially ulcerogenic drugs such as non-steroidals. This will sometimes suffice, but progression to frank lymphoma is nevertheless still seen. There are no prospective studies of therapy.

Lymphocytic and collagenous colitis

Definition of the microscopic colitides is problematic and there is consequent confusion clinically and in the literature. There should be first a
distinction between the microscopic forms of ulcerative colitis and
Crohn's disease where the endoscopist reports normal-looking mucosa
but the histologist is able to give a firm or suggestive report of one of the
two main forms of inflammatory bowel disease (usually ulcerative colitis). This is most obviously the case in proximal biopsies from colitics with
macroscopically distal disease. These patients have 'microscopic' colitis in
the sense of having no macroscopic evidence of disease, but equally clearly belong with those having other relatively mild forms of ulcerative colitis and Crohn's. If all patients with persistent but undiagnosed diarrhoea
are subjected to rectal biopsy (or better, colonoscopy and biopsy) other
conditions emerge. There are three relatively well-defined forms of 'specific' microscopic colitis – collagenous, lymphocytic and eosinophilic – of
roughly equal incidence. Eosinophilic cases probably have a different
aetiology and pathogenesis and are considered separately. However,
there seems to be a major degree of overlap between lymphocytic and
collagenous colitis (for example, at different sites in the colon or at different times). A recent case report from Central Middlesex Hospital illustrates this point particularly vividly, as there were unequivocal features
of collagenous colitis only 2 weeks before colectomy (itself a most unusual requirement), the operative specimen from which exhibited features
only of lymphocytic colitis [45]. There is also a substantial minority of
patients with definite histological abnormality which falls short of satisfying criteria laid down for collagenous or lymphocytic colitis. There are
minor histological abnormalities associated with a variety of gastrointestinal infections, but the presence of chronic symptoms and similar
biopsies taken over a period of several months suggest that there is a real
entity of non-specific microscopic colitis [46]. It should be noted also that
experienced endoscopists will often report a colonoscopy as 'not quite
normal' and a high proportion of these will turn out to be a (virtually)
microscopic colitis.

Collagenous colitis is the easiest to define, as it may be diagnosed from
a subepithelial collagen band of 10 μm or more in thickness (Plate 7), usually but not always with an associated chronic inflammatory infiltrate.
There is great variation in reported prevalence, but this may be a problem
of ascertainment since it is often necessary to have a histological assessment on multiple biopsies from a full colonoscopy to obtain positive samples. It has been argued that it should now be standard practice to obtain
such biopsies in all patients with chronic diarrhoea in whom a diagnosis
is otherwise lacking. Discussion indicates that those who have changed to
this practice find a uniform and sometimes striking increase in case detection, many patients having previously been considered to have irritable

bowel syndrome. As many as 95% [47] or as few as 65% [48] of cases may be identifiable from biopsies taken at flexible sigmoidoscopy.

Collagenous colitis is much more common in women (up to 20 to 1), typically in the sixth and seventh decades, and usually presents with chronic, almost watery, diarrhoea without bleeding [49]. It is associated with a number of other disease states, including coeliac disease, rheumatoid arthritis, seronegative arthritis and a variety of autoimmune and connective tissue diseases [50]. An autoimmune link is supported to a modest degree by higher levels of circulating IgM, and a higher frequency of autoantibodies to nuclear antigens but not of a wide range of other antibodies [51]. Laboratory abnormalities are otherwise present in a minority, and then reflect mild inflammatory activity. Treatment remains a problem and there are no controlled trials to guide us. Most patients will be exposed to 5-aminosalicylate (5-ASA) compounds, steroids, metronidazole and/or mepacrine, each of which has its protagonists. There are insufficient data to recommend one regime over another. The collected experience in 26 cases seen in New York [52] suggests that steroids and antibiotics are mostly unhelpful, but that a combination of 5-ASA and an antidiarrhoeal is effective in about half, with up to a quarter achieving a sustained complete remission.

Lymphocytic colitis is diagnosed from biopsies in which there is an excess of intra-epithelial lymphocytes, goblet cell depletion, sometimes with an increase in eosinophils, and in the absence of the characteristic architectural abnormalities of conventional inflammatory bowel disease. These features have been shown to be reproducibly recorded with only modest interobserver variation [53]. The similarity to another gastrointestinal condition in which inflammation is largely confined to the intra-epithelial site has not escaped attention, and there is a definite association between lymphocytic colitis and coeliac disease. The rectal gluten challenge test for coeliac disease produces changes that would otherwise point to a diagnosis of lymphocytic colitis [54]. Degranulation of mast cells is implicated in disease pathogenesis.

As with collagenous colitis, because it may be proximal or patchy in distribution, lymphocytic colitis is frequently missed if multiple colonoscopic biopsies are not performed. Patients frequently have symptoms for many months before a diagnosis is made. It too affects those in the sixth and seventh decades, but with a more equal sex distribution (females exceeding males at a ratio of about 1.3 to 1 [49]). Associations with other diseases are less obvious but similar to those of collagenous colitis, with coeliac disease predominating and with a number of autoantibody associations [50]. Therapeutic options are of unproven value and a regime of withdrawal of non-steroidals, 5-ASA drugs and/or steroids is used pragmatically. There do not appear to be any data on mast cell stabilizing agents.

Little is known about the natural or treated history of these 'lesser' forms of inflammatory bowel disease, so it is helpful to examine the preliminary retrospective data from the Cleveland Clinic [55]. The 25 patients with confirmed histological evidence for the conditions (of 38 seen during a 5-year period) had had symptoms (usually diarrhoea) for 0.5–120 months (mean 25 months) before diagnosis. Twenty-two were contacted for telephone review at a mean of 23 months from diagnosis. A variety of treatments had been employed, with fibre, opioids, 5-ASA drugs and steroids felt helpful by a majority in whom they had been used. At a mean of 47 months from diagnosis 17 patients were available for telephone review: no less than 14 were symptom-free and the remaining three were improved. It would be unwise to generalize from a single, relatively small series, but the data from St Mark's are very similar (unpublished observations), and the prognosis can probably be considered reasonable. Surgery is very rarely required. However, the value, if any, of the various therapies utilized must be seriously in question. Controlled trials involving multiple centres to recruit adequate numbers are needed.

Eosinophilic enteritis and colitis

Eosinophilic enteritis usually affects the upper gastrointestinal tract, but can be responsible for both ileal and, more rarely, colitic disease [56]. There is an association with other atopic conditions in at least a third of cases, and less often with a global hypereosinophilia syndrome (Churg–Strauss disease), most patients with gastrointestinal disease lacking a dramatic excess of eosinophils in the blood. The overall incidence is uncertain, the literature being comprised mainly of case reports. The clinical differential diagnosis is, depending on the principal site involved, often Crohn's disease. All ages can be affected. There may be non-specific thickening and ulceration visible at upper gastrointestinal endoscopy or colonoscopy, and the intestinal wall may be sufficiently thickened for this to be apparent radiologically as fold thickening or frank stenosis [57]. The diagnosis will usually be made from the characteristic eosinophilic infiltrate at histological assessment. There is nevertheless an overlap, with excess eosinophils in many biopsies from patients with collagenous colitis [58]. It is evident that parasitic infestation should be excluded before a diagnosis of eosinophilic enteritis is accepted, and as exposure to certain drugs may also lead to eosinophilic infiltrates a careful drug history also is required.

Eosinophilic enteritis at any site often proves to be steroid responsive but there are no controlled data to support this, nor detailed information in respect of other drugs, such as cromoglycate which has been advocated by several authors. In those patients with generalized hypereosinophilia, the gastrointestinal involvement is rarely the most pressing clinical issue, and management is appropriately devolved to others.

Inflammatory bowel disease of the HIV-infected patient
The special case of inflammatory bowel disease in patients infected with the HIV virus was highlighted by James, with the apparent remission of Crohn's disease on progression of HIV disease to fully established immunosuppression [59]. This scenario is absent as often as it is present in case reports, and Sharpstone *et al.* have now reviewed their eight cases with both diagnoses [60]. There were two patients with Crohn's disease and six with ulcerative colitis. The degree of inflammatory bowel disease activity did not appear to influence the gravity of immunosuppression, but there was some improvement in CD4 count after colectomy in four so-treated individuals. Equally, progressive immunosuppression as the viral disease advanced did not appear to be associated with improvement nor deterioration of the inflammatory bowel disease. The pertinent point is made that the colitic rectum places the patient at high risk for the viral infection, which may account for the relatively large number of patients with both diagnoses.

HIV enteritis exists but it is still unclear whether it is responsible for symptoms. It seems probable that in some patients it is the principal cause of malabsorption, but that this is relatively mild, and that the severely symptomatic patient will almost always have a second infecting organism such as a *Cryptosporidium* or *Microsporidium*. Cello's group suggests that there is also a non-specific colitis of HIV disease, which they identified in 15 of a group of 80 HIV-infected patients with diarrhoea in whom no infecting organism (or other diagnosis) could be elicited [61]. The condition was associated with relatively modest immunosuppression and was responsive to 5-ASA therapy in over half of those so treated. Is this in fact a *forme fruste* of idiopathic inflammatory bowel disease?

Diverticulosis and inflammatory bowel disease
Diverticulosis and inflammatory bowel disease are both relatively common, and as diverticulum formation increases with age it is not surprising that the conditions are seen together in the elderly. However, this seems to be more common in Crohn's disease than would be expected by chance alone, and Shepherd [62] suggests that there may be a subtype of Crohn's disease that is associated with diverticula, or indeed a new diagnosis – of diverticular colitis – indicating that the blind-ended diverticula may predispose to the adverse (bacterial?) effects of stasis. He analyses the difficulties in making a certain distinction between the two conditions, recognizing that some features considered typical (but never pathognomonic) of Crohn's may also occur in complicated diverticulosis in the absence of inflammatory bowel disease. I am sceptical of this proposal, in the absence of clear evidence, but agree that it deserves consideration, not least because of the link between appendicectomy and protection from ulcerative colitis (Chapter 1).

Clinical course and natural history of inflammatory bowel disease

The clinical course of inflammatory bowel disease is not easily predicted. With the proviso that concordance (for ulcerative colitis or Crohn's disease) is not complete, the disease does, however, tend to behave similarly in different members of an afflicted family (with an element of anticipation with succeeding generations; Chapter 1) [63]. There do not appear to be particular races or population groups in whom notably mild or severe disease can be expected. Ashkenazy Jews may be an exception to this general rule as they seem to have a predilection for unusually aggressive Crohn's disease. A recent questionnaire study organized by the Crohn's and Colitis Foundation of America [64] confirms a general tendency for Crohn's patients from poorer communities to fare less well, but with no independent effect from race.

In ulcerative colitis the initial extent of colonic involvement remains a good but fallible guide to its future course (as well as to the risk of neoplastic transformation; Chapter 8), but curiously the severity of individual severe acute relapses does not have an adverse impact on the frequency or severity of further relapses, nor on the need for surgery. If surgery is avoided despite systemic features such as fever and weight loss, the chance of subsequent 5-year remission is somewhat better than average. In an analysis of 1161 patients with ulcerative colitis, Langholz *et al.* provide additional detailed actuarial data for probability of relapse and remission [65]. At presentation, 44% had no macroscopic disease proximal to the sigmoid. At any one time about 50% of patients were in full remission, but 90% remained prone to intermittent relapses. Chronic disease activity in the first 2 years after diagnosis predicted continuing activity over the next 5 years to a high level of significance. Disease activity in a given year predicted a 70–80% risk of activity in the following year. The cumulative risk of colectomy in this (surgically orientated) centre was 24% at 10 years and 32% at 25 years. The rate of colectomy was 9% in the first year of diagnosis, 3% in each of the following 4 years and about 1% per year thereafter. One-quarter of those coming to surgery had disease limited to the rectum and sigmoid at the time of initial presentation, but their cumulative risk at 5 years was only 9%, compared to 35% in those with pancolitis at diagnosis. More than 90% of patients with colitis retained full working capacity at 10 years. In general, the likelihood that surgery will be necessary for non-fulminant ulcerative colitis is predicted by systemic signs, poor general condition, low serum albumin, mucopus in stools and more problematic diarrhoea [66].

There appear to be distinct subtypes of Crohn's disease, with, for example, some patients in whom perforating, fistulating disease is the norm, and others who never suffer these potentially very disabling complications. An intriguing study has taken the clinical phenotype back to the laboratory to help determine whether these are true, biologically determined subsets. Working on the premise that differential cytokine expression (or sensitivity) could account for the differences seen, Gilberts *et al.* [67] studied mRNA levels for a range of cytokine and related species. A bimodal distribution was found (only) for IL-1β and IL-1 receptor antagonist, with much higher levels of both of these in tissues from patients with non-perforating disease. These were not, perhaps, the expected results, given that levels of the mediators for fibrosis included did not distinguish between the two groups, but nevertheless support the hypothesis that underlying (genetic) differences play a significant role in determining the clinical manifestations of Crohn's disease.

Increasing age is probably linked to a diminishing severity and frequency of relapses of inflammatory bowel disease, but firm data are lacking. There was, however, definite ($p = 0.01$) advantage from increasing patient age in one dose-range study of a 5-ASA, 27% of the over-50s relapsing by 48 weeks compared to 53% of otherwise matched patients under 35 [68].

Frequency and significance of proximal extension of distal colitis
Ulcerative colitis is well established as a distal disease, the inflammation of which extends proximally, in continuity, but to a variable extent (see above). The proportion of the colon involved is clinically relevant because it has a bearing on both the severity of disease and the long-term risk of colitis-related colonic carcinoma (Chapter 8). Intensity and frequency of hospital follow-up is accordingly greatly influenced by the extent documented. However, the extent of the colitis may advance proximally after the initial diagnostic evaluation. The clinical importance of this is exemplified by no less than 12 colitis-related carcinomas recorded at St Mark's in patients who had documented distal disease and who were not therefore under special supervision, but who were found to have extensive colitis at the time of cancer surgery [69]. This proximal progression of colitis (and of ulcerative proctitis) is increasingly recognized. Several studies have reported extension up to the next colonic 'segment' (rectum to sigmoid; sigmoid to descending, etc.) in around 10% after 5 years, and the Birmingham group has recently reviewed both the literature and their own experience [70]. From 145 cases, followed for a median of over 10 years, disease had extended proximal to the sigmoid in 36% (at a median of 6 years). In 29% the progression was sufficient to make a diagnosis of macroscopic extensive colitis. Comparison between those with progression and those without presented no predictive cues. Actuarial analysis predicts progression proximal to the sigmoid in about 16% at 5 years (95% CI: 11–24%) and 31% at 10 years (23–40%). The frequency of progression to involve more proximal colon seems to be somewhat higher in those with disease initially confined to the rectum than in those with initial proctosigmoiditis.

The latest analysis from the County of Copenhagen [66] reflects a mammoth study based on 1161 patients with ulcerative colitis and, *inter alia*, examined disease progression in the subset of those with proctosigmoiditis. Similar methodology to that employed in Birmingham appears to have been used and a probability of progression of no less than 53% is recorded at 2 years. This group found that abdominal pain and continuing diarrhoea were associated independently with a greater tendency to disease progression. There was also evidence for regression (76.8% for extensive and 75.7% for pancolitis at 25 years).

Progression of initially distal disease does not necessarily seem to lead to more frequent or severe relapses that would warrant additional prophylactic therapy. However, the threshold for introducing systemic steroids (or other systemic agents) early in the course of a future relapse might reasonably be reduced. The substantial increase in colonic cancer risk in long-standing extensive colitis should not be ignored, as the St Mark's patients alluded to above demonstrate. It is therefore logical to re-evaluate the extent of colitis at intervals in patients with distal disease.

The foregoing provoke thoughts on the equivalent questions in Crohn's disease but there are few good data. Abstract data indicate a very high rate of progression indeed [71]. Almost half of a large group of patients with Crohn's colitis had total colitis at initial investigation, but between 32 and 60% of those without had progressed to pancolitis by 10 years, with the highest risk in those with predominantly left-sided colitis at presentation.

The constancy of the nature of disease at initial presentation and at subsequent relapse in Crohn's has been examined closely, not least by the Chicago group looking at the nature of postoperative recurrence. The generalities of postoperative recurrence and attempts directed at reducing its frequency are discussed in Chapters 3 and 4, but it is intriguing to examine the great similarity of the original disease and its later relapse. Not only does the general behaviour of the disease (fibrostenotic/fistulating) tend to run true, but so does the actual extent of bowel involved [72]. Remarkably, this implies that a patient from whom 20 cm of diseased terminal ileum is resected, tends to re-present with 20 cm of disease in the neoterminal ileum. This almost implausible scenario fits the experience at other centres but is unexplained.

Guides to disease activity

The most widely used and most frequently criticized scale of Crohn's disease activity is the Crohn's Disease Activity Index (CDAI) (Appendix A) [73]. This index is based on a series of self-reported symptoms during the week prior to its determination, coupled with additional scores for a number of clinical signs and complications. The most objective measures included are weight change and the haematocrit. It is precisely because of the subjectivity of the score that the CDAI is so much lambasted, given that patients with irritable bowel syndrome would frequently appear to have active Crohn's disease (CDAI >150) on the basis of a perceived severe illness. The same objection is raised to the Harvey–Bradshaw scale [74], although this is rather easier to compute and appears to give comparable information (Appendix A). Most authorities in the field have tried to improve this situation, whether by including additional laboratory markers (such as the platelet count or C-reactive protein) or by devising entirely independent measures of disease activity. Some of the more helpful of these will be discussed but it is important to recognize that we lack a gold standard either for diagnosis of Crohn's disease or its degree of activity. Comparisons of the different methods tend to be made against a global assessment made for all available information or against the CDAI: a new method may occasionally be better than either but appear deficient.

Best known of the more objective indices is the Dutch or Van Hees Index (Appendix A) [75]. Unsurprisingly, it correlates with other laboratory-based assessments and relatively poorly with clinical impressions or with the CDAI. However, the scale is based on nine parameters, each of which requires multiplication by a constant, before they are summated and a further constant subtracted; it is not a tool for the busy clinician!

A recent paper from Edinburgh tackles one potential solution to this problem [76]. This group pioneered the use of a lavage method of measuring, *inter alia*, intestinal protein loss, which they consider a very objective assessment of Crohn's disease activity. Other authors have been less convinced and have questioned the acceptability of the lavage technique to both patients and investigators. The recent study explored the CDAI, and the degree of protein-losing enteropathy, in conjunction with a global clinical assessment. Importantly, they included some subjects in whom active Crohn's disease was unlikely, some thought to have only (non-inflamed) fibrous strictures, and some in whom Crohn's was subsequently excluded. Patients in whom the clinical global judgement indicated active Crohn's disease (or ulcerative colitis for which the CDAI was, somewhat unconventionally, also used) had abnormal gut lavage protein levels (particularly IgG), but those with a high CDAI, thought falsely high because of prominent fibrous stricturing or predominant psychological symptoms, had normal gut lavage results. Unfortunately, in the continuing absence of a gold standard all one can conclude is that the lavage technique provides clinically plausible results. It is perhaps uncharitable to suggest that assessment of gut lavage by a more sceptical group might have led to different conclusions.

Increased blood flow in active Crohn's disease is readily and non-invasively demonstrable by Doppler flow characteristics, but reproducibility may be compromised by difficulties in localization of the area of interest.

Following on from Bolondi's pioneering work in this field [77], we have tried to standardize use of Doppler assessments. Measurements have been made at the origin of the superior mesenteric artery (SMA), which is easily defined and permits reproducibility [78]. Volume flow (normal < 500 ml/min) was significantly higher in subjects with Crohn's than in those with non-inflammatory conditions or normal diagnostic scans. The volume flows were not alone sufficiently discriminatory for diagnostic purposes, and comparison with contemporaneous CDAI, serum CRP and global clinical assessment in Crohn's patients revealed a strong but inexact correlation ($r = 0.7$; $p < 0.05$) for CDAI but not for CRP. The Doppler results are felt to provide additional, independent information, which may prove of practical value in devising new scoring systems for Crohn's disease.

Comparable scoring systems for defining the activity of ulcerative colitis have proved less controversial. Examples are given in Appendix A.

Quality of life in inflammatory bowel disease

It is obvious that inflammatory bowel disease has an adverse impact on the patient's quality of life, and yet this issue has not been well addressed by doctors. The medical profession's attention and interest is understandably focused on those aspects of the diseases that cause major morbidity and may even prove life-threatening. The creation and success of patient support groups (such as the National Association for Colitis and Crohn's Disease in Britain, or AMICI in Italy) has been partly in response to this perceived lack of attention. Many useful information leaflets and practical aids, such as the 'Can't wait' card (aiding urgent access to toilet facilities when away from home), have been produced, in addition to counselling services and more informal support. These groups have also taken steps to offset discrimination in the workplace and in respect of health and life insurance (see below). The profession has not been unsupportive of these initiatives, and Mayberry's group in particular has taken these and related issues in hand. Despite time lost from full-time education, young patients with Crohn's disease reach comparable [79] or higher [80] levels of academic success to their unaffected peers. Sadly this is not sufficient to preclude a somewhat higher frequency of subsequent unemployment and a desire of up to a third of these patients to wish to conceal their condition from actual or prospective employers [79], or indeed an inability to carry out the activities necessary for normal employment in 20% [80]. The similar proportion of women with Crohn's disease achieving marriage (81% v. 76% of age-matched controls) is probably also an acceptable surrogate for a marker of reasonable social functioning [81].

Internationally the lead in this area has been taken by Irvine and her colleagues who have devised and validated a disease-specific quality of life instrument known as the Inflammatory Bowel Disease Questionnaire (IBDQ) [82]. The IBDQ is complementary to so-called generic measures which are also applicable to the general population and to those with other diseases. Probably the most relevant in this context is the very extensively evaluated SF-36 questionnaire, a 36-item health status scale [83]. Few, if any, centres will apply these instruments routinely, but the wider recognition of the importance of quantification of quality of life is beneficial to patients in general and should be included in all future therapeutic trials. Unfortunately, copyright issues prevent the duplication here of these two scales, but both are readily available.

Sexuality
The relatively normal fertility of patients with inflammatory bowel disease is considered in Chapter 5, but it is important to recognize that fertility is only one component of sexual life, and that great morbidity can result from what may seem to be relatively minor defects in actual or perceived sexual functioning. Much has been written about the stigma of the gastrointestinal stoma, and all practitioners will aim to avoid stoma creation in the young patient if possible [84]; this has especial significance in Asian communities where it is not unusual for a young woman to be considered unmarriageable as a result of a stoma. Less attention has been focused on the concern that faecal incontinence will occur during intercourse; this is much more often a worry than an actuality, but the anxiety of the patient (particularly female) may be of such overwhelming intensity as to prevent the formation of any potentially sexual relationship. It is typical of the whole area of sexual functioning that this major concern of patients is one which is not conveyed to their medical attendants: the doctor should recognize this and introduce its discussion at an appropriate point in the consulting process. Fear of incontinence led to complete sexual abstinence in 14% of women with Crohn's disease in one study [85]. Achieving secure continence is more difficult, but pre-coital loperamide may suffice and will often provide the reassurance that is needed. Dyspareunia is likewise a problem that is often not mentioned in the inflammatory bowel disease clinic but should be enquired after in potentially sexually active women. Questionnaire data indicate a prevalence of dyspareunia as high as 38% compared to 18% in controls [86]. Painful intercourse in women with Crohn's disease is often the result of active inflammation and, when gynaecological causes are excluded, may itself be an indication for intestinal surgery if more intensive medical therapy is insufficient.

It is encouraging that reported frequency and enjoyment of sexual activity in inflammatory bowel disease patients seemed similar to that in controls but complacency should be tempered by the relatively low reply rates and the wide range of responses in both groups [86], especially since the same authors report six times the frequency of sexual abstinence in women with Crohn's compared to controls, when interviewed face-to-face (24% v. 4%) [85].

Causes of death in inflammatory bowel disease

Those aspects of morbidity and mortality specific to colorectal carcinoma are considered in Chapter 8, but in other respects the major inflammatory bowel diseases have generally been felt to have little effect on mortality. This may reflect a tendency for subjects from the relatively advantaged social classes to be affected by the diseases, and this is a major argument put forward by life assurance institutions when challenged as to why premiums for life cover are adversely loaded for inflammatory bowel disease patients. Their argument is that whatever the mortality data for ulcerative colitis or Crohn's disease relative to standard mortality data for the population, the company must quote on the basis of its average customer, who is from the upper echelons of society. Since it cannot be denied that inflammatory bowel disease sometimes kills, a financial consequence to the patient becomes inevitable.

There is surprisingly little in the literature on all-cause mortality from inflammatory bowel disease, or whether this is changing with time; past data have been somewhat contradictory. It is therefore helpful to analyse a new population study of nearly 3000 inflammatory bowel disease patients seen between 1955 and 1984 [87]. The criteria for case ascertainment and diagnosis would satisfy most clinical trials, and it is unlikely that better epidemiological data will emerge for this time period. It is probable that the great majority of cases of both ulcerative colitis and Crohn's disease to occur in the Stockholm area have been identified and included. Mortality data (n = 429) come from the national Death Register up to 1990, with causes of death codified according to the death certificate. In only 2.5% of patients was life-or-death follow-up to 1990 not available. Mortality from all causes and from specific causes was analysed by conventional relative survival statistics in comparison to the age- and sex-adjusted standard mortality data for Sweden. The relative survival for Crohn's disease was 93.7% at 15 years (95% CI: 91.8–95.7%) with no significant differences according to the site of the bowel involved. The standardized mortality ratio was 1.51. There was a slight worsening in prognosis in those diagnosed after 1970 (1.2% worse at 15 years) but this, too, failed to reach significance. In ulcerative colitis there was also a reduced life expectancy to the extent of 94.2% at 15 years (CI: 92.4–96.1%) which was most marked for those with extensive colitis (92.9%), but yet again this was not statistically different even from those with proctitis alone (96.4%). The standardized mortality ratio (SMR) was 1.37. As in Crohn's disease, the prognosis was less good in those diagnosed after 1970, which was attributed to an ageing population of new colitics (albeit with the mean age at diagnosis rising only from 30.8 to 36.4 across the study period).

The cause-specific mortality obviously includes patients dying from their inflammatory bowel disease (74 of the 429 deaths). When these are excluded, the SMRs remain elevated for both ulcerative colitis and Crohn's disease (1.20 and 1.14, respectively). The majority of these excesses occur within the purview of the gastroenterologist, as in addition to the threefold increase in colorectal carcinoma deaths in ulcerative colitis, there were increases in deaths from non-alcoholic liver disease in ulcerative colitis (SMR 4.8) (presumably from sclerosing cholangitis; see Chapter 6) and from other gastrointestinal disorders in both ulcerative colitis and Crohn's (SMRs 2.4–4.0).

There were also excess deaths from asthma, especially in ulcerative colitis (SMR 6.21; CI: 2.50–12.8) and increased deaths from other respiratory causes (SMRs 1.6–2.1) which was obviously not the result of a higher frequency of smokers (under-represented amongst colitics). In Crohn's disease there were very similar results, albeit with a more modestly increased SMR of 2.76 in asthmatics. The other major study of specified all-cause mortality (from Uppsala, also in Sweden) [88] also demonstrated increased mortality from respiratory causes, admittedly at a lower level (SMR 1.5; CI: 1.1–2.2); this should, accordingly, now be accepted as a true association – the explanation remains less certain.

Crohn's patients in Stockholm appeared relatively protected from death from colorectal carcinoma (SMR 0.30; CI: 0.01–1.66), and those from Uppsala were less likely to die from cerebrovascular disease (SMR 0.7; CI: 0.5–1.0). For no other major diagnostic grouping was substantially or statistically decreased risk found. There may be a tendency in each study for over-recording of inflammatory bowel disease as the cause of death, but this would have the effect of diminishing the likelihood of seeing excesses of other causes rather than the opposite observation as found.

The reasons for the worse prognosis with time in Stockholm are not fully explained and appear to conflict with published data for follow-up on patients in Uppsala and in other tertiary referral centres. However, an increased mortality in more recently diagnosed Crohn's patients was found in Leicestershire [89]. It is possible that the modest recent improvements in management are currently outweighed by an older affected population. As none of the statistics are robust, these data should be considered mainly as interesting observations, and not be permitted to influence clinical or health economic planning at this stage.

REFERENCES

1. Maeda K, Okada M, Yao T *et al.* Intestinal and extra-intestinal complications of Crohn's disease: predictors and cumulative probability of complications. *J Gastroenterol* 1994; **29**: 577–582.
2. Allison MC, Vallance R. Prevalence of proximal faecal stasis in active ulcerative colitis. *Gut* 1991; **32**: 179–182.

3. Soulé JC, Beaugerie L, Bouhmedi A, Bouhnik Y. Acute lower gastrointestinal hemorrhage of moderate severity in Crohn's disease. *Gastroenterology* 1996; **110**: A363.

4. Barrett SML, Standen PJ, Lee AS *et al*. Personality, smoking and inflammatory bowel disease. *Eur J Gastroenterol Hepatol* 1996; **8**: 651–655.

5. Sachar DB, Luppescu NE, Bodian C *et al*. Erythrocyte sedimentation as a measure of Crohn's disease activity: opposite trends in ileitis versus colitis. *J Clin Gastroenterol* 1990; **12**: 643–646.

6. Tromm A, Tromm CD, Huppe D *et al*. Evaluation of different laboratory tests and activity indices reflecting the inflammatory activity of Crohn's disease. *Scand J Gastroenterol* 1992; **27**: 771–778.

7. Schurmann G, Betzler M *et al*. Soluble interleukin-2-receptor, interleukin-6 and interleukin-1B in patients with Crohn's disease and ulcerative colitis: preoperative levels and postoperative changes of serum concentrations. *Digestion* 1992; **51**: 51–59.

8. Surawicz MC, Belic L. Rectal biopsy helps to distinguish acute self-limited colitis from idiopathic inflammatory bowel disease. *Gut* 1994; **24**: 519–524.

9. Price AB, Morson BC. Inflammatory bowel disease: the surgical pathology of Crohn's disease and ulcerative colitis. *Human Pathology* 1975; **6**: 7–29.

10. Lee FD, Maguire C, Obeidat W, Russell RI. The significance of cryptolytic lesions in inflammatory bowel disease. *Gastroenterology* 1996; **110**: A947.

11. Fujimura Y, Kamoi R, Iida M. Pathogenesis of aphthoid ulcers in Crohn's disease: correlative findings by magnifying colonoscopy, electron microscopy, and immunohistochemistry. *Gut* 1996; **38**: 724–732.

12. Price AB. Overlap in the spectrum of non-specific inflammatory bowel disease – colitis indeterminate. *J Clin Pathol* 1978; **31**: 567–577.

13. Wells AD, McMillan I, Price AB *et al*. Natural history of indeterminate colitis. *Br J Surg* 1991; **78**: 179–181.

14. Dijkstra J, Reeders JW, Tytgat GN. Idiopathic inflammatory bowel disease: endoscopic-radiologic correlation. *Radiology* 1995; **197**: 369–375.

15. Margulis AR, Burhenne HJ. *Practical alimentary tract radiology*. St Louis: Mosby, 1993.

16. Misiewicz JJ, Forbes A, Price AB (eds) *Atlas of clinical gastroenterology*, 2nd edn. London: Mosby, 1994.

17. Chernish SM, Maglinte DD, O'Connor K. Evaluation of the small intestine by enteroclysis for Crohn's disease. *Am J Gastroenterol* 1992; **87**: 696–701.

18. Lankisch PG, Gaetke T, Gerzmann J-F, Becher R. The impact of enteroclysis on the diagnosis of gastrointestinal symptoms: unexplained abdominal pain, gastrointestinal bleeding and chronic diarrhea. *Gastroenterology* 1996; **110**: A24.

19. Bartram CI. Barium radiology. *Scand J Gastroenterol* 1994; **203**(suppl): 20–23.

20. Tamada F, Honsako Y, Hirohata S *et al*. Usefulness of infrared video-endoscope for the diagnosis of ulcerative colitis. *Gastroenterology* 1996; **110**: A1025.

21. Smedh K, Olaison G, Nyström PO, Sjödahl R. Intraoperative enteroscopy in Crohn's disease. *Br J Surg* 1993; **80**: 897–900.

22. Andreoli A, Cerro P, Falasco G, Prantera C. Ultrasonographic evaluation in the diagnosis of post-surgical recurrence of Crohn's disease. *Gastroenterology* 1996; **110**: A854.

23. Futagami Y, Hata J, Haruma K *et al*. Development of an ultrasonographic activity index of Crohn's disease: comparison with endoscopy or barium studies. *Gastroenterology* 1996; **110**: A912.

24. Tio TL, Kallimanis GE. Endoscopic ultrasonography of perianorectal fistulas and abscesses. *Endoscopy* 1994; **26**: 813–815.

25. Shimizu S, Tada M, Kawai K. Value of endoscopic ultrasonography in the assessment of inflammatory bowel diseases. *Endoscopy* 1992; **24**(suppl 1): 354–358.

26. Philpotts LE, Heiken JP, Westcott MA, Gore RM. Colitis: use of CT findings in differential diagnosis. *Radiology* 1994; **190**: 445–449.

27. Meyers MA, McGuire PV. Spiral CT demonstration of hypervascularity in Crohn disease: 'vascular jejunization of the ileum' or the 'comb' sign. *Abdom Imaging* 1995; **20**: 327–332.

28. Shoenut JP, Semelka RC, Magro CM *et al*. Comparison of magnetic resonance imaging and endoscopy in distinguishing the type and severity of inflammatory bowel disease. *J Clin Gastroenterol* 1994; **19**: 31–35.

29. Kosa R, Hansmann HJ, Roeren T *et al*. Magnetic resonance imaging in Crohn's disease. *Gastroenterology* 1996; **110**: A941.

30. Lantto E, Jarvi K, Krekala I *et al*. Technetium-99m hexamethyl propylene amine oxime leukocytes in the assessment of disease activity in inflammatory bowel disease. *Eur J Nucl Med* 1992; **19**: 14–18.

31. Weldon MJ, Lowe C, Joseph AEA, Maxwell JD. Review article: quantitative leucocyte scanning in the assessment of inflammatory bowel disease activity and its response to therapy. *Aliment Pharmacol Ther* 1996; **10**: 123–132.

32. Bhatti MA, Chapman PT, Peters AM *et al*. Radioimmunoscintigraphy with 111-indium labelled monoclonal anti-E-selectin antibody and circulating soluble E-selectin in the evaluation of inflammatory bowel disease. *Gastroenterology* 1996; **110**: A864.

33. Plauth M, Jenss H, Meyle J. Oral manifestations of Crohn's disease. An analysis of 79 cases. *J Clin Gastroenterol* 1991; **13**: 29–37.

34. Mashako MNL, Cezard JP, Navarro J *et al*. Crohn's disease lesions in the upper gastrointestinal tract: correlation between clinical, radiological, endoscopic and histological features in adolescents and children. *J Ped Gastroenterol Nutr* 1989; **8**: 442–446

35. Halme L, Kärkkäinen P, Rautelin H *et al*. High frequency of *Helicobacter* negative gastritis in patients with Crohn's disease. *Gut* 1996; **38**: 379–383.

36. Oberhuber G, Puspok A, Oesterreicher Ch *et al*. Crohn's disease of the stomach is histologically characterised by focal active gastritis. *Gastroenterology* 1996; **110**: A982.

37. Nyam DCNK, Pemberton JH, Camilleri M, Sagar PM. Irritable bowel syndrome in patients with chronic ulcerative colitis: coexistence creates a clinical conundrum. *Gastroenterology* 1996; **110**: A725.

38. Kaplan MA, Korelitz BL. Narcotic dependence in inflammatory bowel disease. *J Clin Gastroenterol* 1988; **10**: 275–278.

39. Wechsler B, Davatchi F, Mizushima Y *et al*. Criteria for diagnosis of Behçet's disease. *Lancet* 1990; **335**: 1078–1080.

40. Kasahara Y, Tanaka S, Nishino M *et al*. Intestinal involvement in Behçet's disease. Review of 136 surgical case in the Japanese literature. *Dis Colon Rectum* 1981; **24**: 103–106

41. Jorizzo JL. Behçet's disease: an update based on the 1985 international conference in London. *Arch Dermatol* 1986; **122**: 556–558.

42. Kim JH, Choi BI, Han JK *et al*. Colitis in Behçet's disease: characteristics on double-contrast barium enema examination in 20 patients. *Abdom Imaging* 1994; **19**: 132–136.

43. Robertson DAF, Dixon MF, Scott BB *et al*. Small intestinal ulceration: diagnostic difficulties in relation to coeliac disease. *Gut* 1983; **24**: 565–568.

44. Lamont CM, Adams FG, Mills PR. Radiology in idiopathic chronic ulcerative enteritis. *Clin Radiol* 1982; **33**: 283–286.

45. Bowling T, Price AB, Al-Adnani M *et al*. Interchange between collagenous and lymphocytic colitis in severe disease with autoimmune association requiring colectomy: a case report. *Gut* 1996; **38**: 788–791.

46. Jawhari A, Sheaf M, Forbes A *et al*. Microscopic colitis: widening the definition. *Gastroenterology* 1995; **108**: A843.

47. Zins BJ, Tremaine WJ, Carpenter HA. Collagenous colitis: mucosal biopsies and association with fecal leukocytes. *Mayo Clin Proc* 1995; **70**: 430–433.

48. Offner FA, Jao R, Lewin KJ *et al*. Collagenous colitis: a histopathological analysis to define the optimal locations for diagnostic biopsies. *Gastroenterology* 1996; **110**: A983.

49. Giardello RM, Lazenby AJ, Bayless TM *et al.* Lymphocytic (microscopic) colitis. Clinicopathological study of 18 patients and comparison to collagenous colitis. *Dig Dis Sci* 1989; **34**: 1730–1738.
50. Zins BJ, Sandborn WJ, Tremaine WJ. Collagenous and lymphocytic colitis: subject review and therapeutic alternatives. *Am J Gastroenterol* 1995; **90**: 1394–1400.
51. Bohr J, Tysk C, Yang P *et al.* Autoantibodies and immunoglobulins in collagenous colitis. *Gut* 1996; **39**: 73–76.
52. Fiedler L, George J, Sachar D *et al.* Therapeutic outcomes in collagenous colitis. *Gastroenterology* 1996; **110**: A907.
53. Fasoli R, Talbot I, Reid M *et al.* Microscopic colitis: can it be qualitatively and quantitatively characterized? *Ital J Gastroenterol* 1992; **24**: 393–396.
54. Loft DE, Marsh MN, Sandle GI *et al.* Studies of intestinal lymphoid tissue. XII. Epithelial lymphocyte and mucosal responses to rectal gluten challenge in celiac sprue. *Gastroenterology* 1989; **97**: 29–37.
55. Bonner GF, Cheong DMO, Grewal ID *et al.* Short and long term follow-up of treatment for lymphocytic and collagenous colitis. *Gastroenterology* 1996; **110**: A869.
56. Naylor AR, Pollet JE. Eosinophilic colitis. *Dis Colon Rectum* 1985; **28**: 615–618.
57. Vitellas KM, Bennett WF, Bova JG *et al.* Radiographic manifestations of eosinophilic gastroenteritis. *Abdom Imaging* 1995; **20**: 406–413.
58. Lavy AM, Burgart LJ, Van Keulen VP *et al.* Eosinophil infiltration and major basic protein deposition are increased in colonic tissue from patients with collagenous colitis. *Gastroenterology* 1996; **110**: A950.
59. James SP. Remission of Crohn's disease after human immunodeficiency virus infection. *Gastroenterology* 1988; **95**: 1667–1669.
60. Sharpstone DR, Duggal A, Gazzard BG. Inflammatory bowel disease in individuals seropositive for the human immunodeficiency virus. *Eur J Gastroenterol Hepatol* 1996; **8**: 575–578.
61. Steuerwald MH, Kearney DJ, Scott MK *et al.* HIV-associated nonspecific colitis – prevalence, clinical presentation and response to 5-ASA compounds. *Gastroenterology* 1996; **110**: A1019.
62. Shepherd NA. Diverticular disease and chronic idiopathic inflammatory bowel disease: associations and masquerades. *Gut* 1996; **38**: 801–802.
63. Satsangi J, Grootscholten C, Holt H, Jewell DP. Clinical patterns of familial inflammatory bowel disease. *Gut* 1996; **38**: 738–741.
64. Straus WL, Eisen GM, Sandler RS *et al.* Race and Crohn's disease: clinical and therapeutic comparison of African–Americans and non-African Americans. Report of a multicenter survey. *Gastroenterology* 1996; **110**: A1021.

65. Langholz E, Munkholm P, Davidsen M, Binder V. Course of ulcerative colitis: analysis of changes in disease activity over years. *Gastroenterology* 1994; **107**: 3–11.

66. Langholz E, Munkholm P, Davidsen M *et al.* Changes in extent of ulcerative colitis. A study on the course and prognostic factors. *Scand J Gastroenterol* 1996; **31**: 260–266.

67. Gilberts ECAM, Greenstein AJ, Katsel P *et al.* Molecular evidence for two forms of Crohn's disease. *Proc Natl Acad Sci USA* 1994; **91**: 12721–12724.

68. Fockens P, Mulder CJJ, Tytgat GNJ *et al.* Comparison of the efficacy and safety of 1.5 vs 3.0g oral slow-release mesalazine (Pentasa) in the maintenance treatment of ulcerative colitis. *Eur J Gastroenterol Hepatol* 1995; **7**: 1025–1030.

69. Connell WR, Lennard-Jones JE, Williams CB *et al.* Factors influencing the outcome of endoscopic surveillance for cancer in ulcerative colitis. *Gastroenterology* 1994; **107**: 934–944.

70. Ayres RC, Gillen CD, Walmsley RS, Allan RN. Progression of ulcerative proctosigmoiditis incidence and factors influencing progression. *Eur J Gastroenterol Hepatol* 1996; **8**: 555–558.

71. Makowiec F, Schmidke C, Paczulla D *et al.* Progression of colonic involvement in Crohn's disease and the risk of surgery – a ten year follow-up study. *Gastroenterology* 1996; **108**: A869.

72. D'Haens GR, Gasparaitis AE, Hanauer SB. Duration of recurrent ileitis after ileocolonic resection correlates with presurgical extent of Crohn's disease. *Gut* 1995; **36**: 715–717.

73. Best WR, Becktel JM, Singleton JW, Kern F Jr. Development of a Crohn's disease activity index. National Cooperative Crohn's Disease Study. *Gastroenterology* 1976; **70**: 439–444.

74. Harvey RF, Bradshaw JM. A simple index of Crohn's disease activity. *Lancet* 1980; **i**: 514.

75. Goebell H, Wienbeck M, Shomerus H, Malchow H. Evaluation of the Crohn's disease activity index and the Dutch index for severity and activity of Crohn's disease. An analysis of the data from the European Cooperative Crohn's disease study. *Med Klin* 1990; **85**: 573–576.

76. Acciuffi S, Ghosh S, Ferguson A. Strengths and limitations of the Crohn's disease activity index, revealed by an objective gut lavage test of gastrointestinal protein loss. *Aliment Pharmacol Ther* 1996; **10**: 321–326.

77. Bolondi L, Gaiani S, Brignola C *et al.* Changes in splanchnic hemodynamics in inflammatory bowel disease: non-invasive assessment by Doppler ultrasound flowmetry. *Scand J Gastroenterol* 1992; **27**: 501–507.

78. Hare C, Hassan MT, Bartram CI, Forbes A. Superior mesenteric artery Doppler flow: a valuable indicator of disease activity in Crohn's disease. *Gastroenterology* 1996; **110**: A921.

79. Mayberry MK, Probert C, Srivastava E *et al.* Perceived discrimination in education and employment by people with Crohn's disease: a case control study of educational achievement and employment. *Gut* 1992; **33**: 312–314.

80. Duclos B, Planchon F, Jouin H *et al.* Socioprofessional consequences of Crohn's disease [original title in French]. *Gastroenterol Clin Biol* 1990; **14**: 966–972.

81. Mayberry JF, Weterman IT. European survey of fertility and pregnancy in women with Crohn's disease: a case control study by European collaborative group. *Gut* 1986; **27**: 821–825.

82. Irvine EJ, Feagon B, Rochon J *et al.* Quality of life: a valid and reliable measure of therapeutic efficacy in the treatment of inflammatory bowel disease. *Gastroenterology* 1994; **106**: 287–296.

83. Stewart AL, Hays RD, Ware JE Jr. The MOS short-form general health survey: reliability and validity in a patient population. *Med Care* 1988; **26**: 724–735.

84. Salter M. Sexuality and the stoma patient. In: Myers C, ed. *Stoma care nursing*. London: Arnold, 1996.

85. Moody G, Probert CS, Srivastava EM *et al.* Sexual dysfunction amongst women with Crohn's disease: a hidden problem. *Digestion* 1992; **52**: 179–183.

86. Moody GA, Mayberry JF. Perceived sexual dysfunction amongst patients with inflammatory bowel disease. *Digestion* 1993; **54**: 256–260.

87. Persson P-G, Bernell O, Leijonmarck C-E *et al.* Survival and cause-specific mortality in inflammatory bowel disease: a population-based study. *Gastroenterology* 1996; **110**: 1339–1345.

88. Ekbom A, Helmick CG, Zack M *et al.* Survival and causes of death in patients with inflammatory bowel disease: a population-based study. *Gastroenterology* 1992; **103**: 954–960.

89. Probert CSJ, Jayanthi V, Wicks ACB, Mayberry JF. Mortality from Crohn's disease in Leicestershire, 1972–89: an epidemiological community based study. *Gut* 1992; **33**: 1226–1228.

3

Medical therapy

INTRODUCTION

The medical management of inflammatory bowel disease is poised to enter an new era if the current promise shown by investigatory immunomodulatory regimes translates into confirmed effective therapy, but at present there are only a few firmly established routes to pharmacological success. Corticosteroids and the 5-aminosalicylate (5-ASA) drugs (sulphasalazine and its successors) still constitute the mainstays of therapy, with azathioprine/mercaptopurine an established second-line agent for resistant disease. Primary nutritional therapy has a place for some patients with Crohn's disease, and alternative immunosuppressants are finding their own niches.

This chapter will explore the current role of all of the above and, where possible, of the newer agents also. Fulminant ulcerative colitis is mainly considered in Chapter 4. The remitting and relapsing course of inflammatory bowel disease and the substantial rate of spontaneous improvement whatever therapeutic endeavours are employed, should be remembered, but the use of placebo arms in therapeutic trials is now ethically almost unacceptable given that we have effective (though admittedly insufficiently effective) established treatments. Historic placebo-controlled trials indicate that spontaneous clinical improvement and apparent full remission may reasonably be expected in around 30% and 11% of exacerbations of ulcerative colitis [1], and an apparent remission in about 30% of episodes of active Crohn's disease [2, 3].

CORTICOSTEROIDS

Corticosteroids – predominantly forms of prednisolone and hydrocortisone – remain a cornerstone in the medical management of patients with inflammatory bowel disease, providing rapid and effective relief of symptoms in acute exacerbations, though not always accompanied by full endoscopic remission. There is little difference between the response to hydrocortisone and to prednisolones when equivalent doses are compared (4 mg methylprednisolone; 5 mg prednisolone; 25 mg hydrocortisone), although there are some differences in their mineralocorticoid effects which can occasionally be important. Although intravenous therapy can be demonstrated to be more efficacious than oral administration in resistant cases, this is probably an effect of the more direct route, and usually also a higher dose, rather than because of a switch (say) from prednisolone to hydrocortisone.

The therapeutic effects of steroids are mediated by inhibition of several inflammatory pathways, including direct suppression of the 5-lipoxygenase-mediated metabolism of arachidonic acid, modulated transcription of glucocorticoid-sensitive proteins and suppression of mRNA for most of the interleukins [4]. More recent information suggests that a positive influence of steroids in stimulating apoptosis of lamina propria lymphocytes may also be an important contributor to the therapeutic response [5].

Typical regimes of systemic steroids for moderate to severe exacerbations of inflammatory bowel disease comprise oral prednisolone 0.5–1.0 mg/kg body weight, but with a suggested minimum of 30 mg daily. There are no good data to determine how long this dose should be maintained, and most gastroenterologists commence a fairly brisk reduction once response begins, in order to avoid unnecessary toxicity. I favour 7 days at the starting dose, reducing thereafter by 5 mg/week until weaning is complete, but as long as 4 weeks at 1 mg/kg has been advocated by others.

As steroids have been shown in all but one study (of Crohn's disease) [6] to be largely ineffective in maintaining remission, but contribute significantly to long-term morbidity via their side-effects, they should be withdrawn once the acute episode has settled. Growth suppression in children, osteoporosis, and suppression of the hypothalamic–pituitary axis have been of particular, though possibly overemphasized concern, especially with high doses and prolonged treatment (Chapter 5). Topical steroids also have the potential for toxicity when used for prolonged periods, as up to 80% of the applied dose may be absorbed systemically. More recent data suggest, however, that much of the apparent toxicity of steroids on bone mass (and growth) is actually a reflection of greater disease activity in patients treated with steroids, and that it is the active disease (and the need for steroids) that is the prime determinant of tissue damage [7] (see also Chapter 7). It is appropriate, none the less, that attention has centred on newer corticosteroids, which are poorly absorbed or extensively inactivated by the liver, and on new delivery systems which limit steroid absorption. Steroid sparing immunomodulatory drugs should continue to be considered in patients who remain apparently steroid dependent.

Topically active corticosteroids

Prednisolone metasulphobenzoate, which is available in enema form, is relatively poorly absorbed, yielding systemic levels significantly lower than those from a dose of prednisolone phosphate which achieves equivalent rectal tissue levels [8]. Therapeutic efficacy is similar, but measurable adrenal suppression can still be shown. It is fortuitous that the degree of systemic absorption is directly related to the degree of inflammation and therefore diminishes as the patient comes into remission [9]. Of the newer steroids, budesonide and beclomethasone are more rapidly metabolized in the liver and red blood cells. Budesonide, which is already widely used as a topical steroid in the treatment of asthma, has the additional benefit compared to prednisolone that it is poorly absorbed from the intestine and is highly protein-bound in circulation, permitting little 'free hormone' action. Trials of topical administration in an enema dose of 2 mg have demonstrated at least equal efficacy to hydrocortisone and prednisolone in the treatment of acute distal ulcerative colitis [10, 11]. There is low systemic bioavailability and less suppression of endogenous cortisol secretion than from prednisolone or hydrocortisone. Administration has been continued or repeated in uncontrolled longer-term follow-up studies and appears effective and well tolerated; even in this context there does not seem to be a special problem with adrenal suppression [12].

The new orally administered corticosteroids are also showing promise in Crohn's disease. Although trials using fluticasone propionate were disappointing, the results obtained with budesonide are more encouraging. The properties of this agent permit only about 10% of absorbed drug to reach the systemic circulation. To aid maximal delivery to the terminal ileum and colon it has been coated with Eudragit, an acrylic resin familiar to users of mesalazine, which dissolves at pH 6 (Eudragit-L), or pH 7 (Eudragit-S). There have been several trials of coated budesonide in the treatment of ileocaecal Crohn's disease. In the first, essentially a dose ranging study in active disease, doses between 3 and 15 mg daily were compared with placebo [13]. A 9 mg dose appeared optimal, there being no therapeutic gain, but appreciable increase in adrenal suppression, with 15 mg. In a European study, 9 mg budesonide daily was compared to a tapering dose of prednisolone (starting at 40 mg daily) [14]. The results indicate similar efficacy for the two agents. Adrenal toxicity from budesonide was certainly significantly less, but not absent, in this study, which was too short-term to provide information on other toxicological concerns. Abstract data from the German budesonide study group are very similar [15], a fourth study pointing to better clinical results with the new agent [16].

Oral budesonide has also been compared to prednisolone in the treatment of acute ulcerative colitis [17]. In a 9-week double-blind trial of 72 patients, 10 mg (of a different delayed-release form) of budesonide was compared with 40 mg prednisolone, the dose being gradually tapered in both cases. Plasma cortisol levels were not altered by budesonide, but were suppressed by prednisolone throughout the study period (albeit not significantly so at 9 weeks). Somewhat less impressive results were recorded with fluticasone [18].

Budesonide has also been assessed in the maintenance of remission in Crohn's disease. As a continuation of the therapeutic North American study into the remission phase, Greenberg *et al.* [19] have studied patients on 3 or 6 mg budesonide in comparison to placebo. They found value in delaying the onset of relapse with both doses in the medium term, but this benefit was lost by follow-up to 1 year. The European study [20] is a little more persuasive. Both 3 and 6 mg daily doses showed some benefit in comparison to a placebo group, and this was maintained for a useful interval with the 6 mg dose, which helped to achieve an 81% remission rate at 3 months compared to only 55% and 56% in the 3 mg and placebo groups, respectively ($p < 0.05$). By 12 months only 41%, 26% and 37% remained in remission, and all statistical advantage was again lost. As systemic side-effects were few, the authors conclude that this represents a worthwhile therapeutic advance. The 5-ASA preparations have been assessed in the same contexts (see below), and the scene is now set for formal comparison of the two types of therapy. While it is not suggested that any of the patients in these medium-term studies were steroid dependent (the comparisons were, after all, with placebo), it would be reasonable to draw from them further support for the use of budesonide in the steroid-dependent patient.

Data on the effects (or lack of them) of budesonide on bone metabolism and the longer-term risks of osteopenia are so far few, but there is evidence that osteoblast activity is less influenced than by apparently equipotent doses of prednisolone [21], which is clearly encouraging.

Further studies will no doubt clarify its most appropriate place in the overall management of inflammatory bowel disease.

AMINOSALICYLATES

Sulphasalazine has been used effectively in the treatment of ulcerative colitis since the early 1950s, when controlled trials demonstrated efficacy in treatment of acute colitis and maintenance of remission; reductions in annual relapse rates of up to threefold are typical (for example from 71 to 24% [22]). Early studies showed no benefit in Crohn's disease, but recent studies using newer formulations of 5-aminosalicylic acid (5-ASA), which has been shown to be the principal active ingredient of sulphasalazine, have shown more considerable promise. The mechanisms of action of 5-ASA in reducing intestinal inflammation in inflammatory bowel disease are not entirely clear, but include inhibition of 5-lipoxygenase metabolism and the production of interleukins and inflammatory leukotrienes; suppression of platelet activating factor, and of chemotaxis of neutrophils and monocytes, with normalization of intestinal permeability; reduction of epithelial HLA-DR expression; stimulation of cytoprotective prostaglandins; and scavenging of free radicals. All are documented (some only *in vitro*) and are potentially relevant [23]. However, a direct influence on colonic mucosal flora is probably not important [24].

Targeted delivery

Up to 15% of individuals are intolerant of the sulphapyridine moiety of sulphasalazine, but although (most of) its therapeutic benefit results from the 5-ASA (or mesalazine) molecule, oral administration of 5-ASA is ineffective because of proximal absorption and metabolism. Alternative formulations of 5-ASA have therefore been developed. In each case it proves possible to use larger equivalent doses than has usually been the case with sulphasalazine, as fewer patients develop upper gastrointestinal intolerance. There is also no problem with oligospermia with the newer agents. In 1996, five 5-ASA preparations were commercially available in Europe. Asacol® is 5-ASA coated with an acrylic-based resin (Eudragit-S) which dissolves rapidly above pH 7.0; this typically occurs in the region of the caecum and ascending colon. Eudragit-L dissolves at pH 6.0 and is used to coat Claversal® and Salofalk®, with which release in the ileum is to be expected. Pentasa® consists of microgranules of 5-ASA coated by a semipermeable ethyl cellulose membrane that releases 5-ASA steadily after tablet disintegration in the stomach, with enhanced release above pH 6.0; 5-ASA is made available throughout the small and large intestine. Olsalazine is a 5-ASA dimer, the two molecules linked by an azo bond, which is broken by the same azo-reductase of colonic bacterial flora that degrades sulphasalazine. The potential advantage for olsalazine shown over other 5-ASA preparations is limited by an osmotic diarrhoea provoked by the drug which affects up to 10% of patients, but may be minimized by taking the drug with food, and by commencing with a subtherapeutic dose and titrating up to the intended regime over a week or two [25]. Balsalazide (not available for general prescription in 1996 but expected soon) has a 5-azo bond linking 5-ASA to an inert carrier (4-aminobenzoyl-β-alanine), and is thus handled like sulphasalazine and olsalazine. The early publication record indicated comparable activity to other 5-ASAs and possibly a more favourable side-effect profile [26]. The most recent study, which compared balsalazide 6.75 g daily (equivalent to 2.34 g mesalazine) with Asacol® 2.4 g daily, has only been reported in abstract form [27]. Topical steroids were allowed in the study protocol, which confuses things a little, but it is highly probable that the higher proportion of clinical and sigmoidoscopic remissions obtained (88% v. 57%, and 62% v. 37%, respectively at 12 weeks) are of clinical as well as statistical significance ($p < 0.001$; $p < 0.05$). The responses obtained with balsalazide appeared also to be faster and associated with fewer side-effects.

It is evident, but surprisingly often neglected, that the 5-ASA preparations which depend on colonic bacteria for degradation of the azo bond cannot be effective in patients with colectomy and ileostomy. Too often sulphasalazine and olsalazine are still prescribed inappropriately and uselessly in this context.

Roles of 5-ASA in ulcerative colitis

Around 60% of patients with moderately active ulcerative colitis can be expected to respond to 5-ASA therapy alone. Meta-analysis [28] yields an odds ratio (OR) of 2.0 (CI, 1.50–2.72) for superiority of mesalazine over placebo in active disease, and of 1.15 (CI, 0.83–1.61) for superiority over sulphasalazine. No advantage relative to sulphasalazine was apparent in maintenance of remission (OR, 0.85; CI, 0.64–1.15). Long-term follow-up indicates, however, that overall benefit is better, and toxicity the same or less than for sulphasalazine [29] (see also p. 94). Olsalazine and mesalazine have been shown to be similarly efficacious in maintenance of remission, and in treating mildly to moderately severe active ulcerative colitis, only one fully presented maintenance study significantly favouring olsalazine [30]. In this study, in which it was compared to mesalazine as Asacol®, Courtney *et al.* demonstrated a lower relapse rate with olsalazine in left-sided ulcerative colitis (41.6% v. 70.4%), presumed due to relatively enhanced delivery of 5-ASA to the left side of the colon. However, this study has been criticized for its over-reliance on patient assessment and absence of sigmoidoscopic review. The relapse rate for mesalazine was also unexpectedly high, relapse rates of between 40% and 60% at 1 year being typical in other studies of 5-ASA. It is possible that olsalazine was favoured by the dosage schedule employed (1.0 g olsalazine v. 1.2 g Asacol®), given that the colonic concentration of 5-ASA after oral olsalazine is roughly double that after the same weight of mesalazine is given [31]. Kruis *et al.* have now performed a blinded comparison of olsalazine and pH-release mesalazine as Claversal®, in 172 patients with active colitis; 3 g daily doses of both drugs were used [32]. Their abstract indicates a somewhat higher frequency of adverse events from olsalazine, and little overall difference between the two agents, but again a strong suggestion that olsalazine has an advantage in those with predominantly left-sided disease (58% v. 30% attainment of remission).

Given continuing uncertainty as to the clinical relevance or otherwise of a dose response to 5-ASA and some concern about nephrotoxicity, the Dutch Pentasa Study Group [33] has recently reported on both the efficacy and safety of daily doses of 1.5 g and 3 g of 5-ASA in the maintenance of remission in ulcerative colitis. More than 150 patients with ulcerative colitis in remission were randomized to one of the two doses and monitored to 12 months or to earlier relapse on clinical, endoscopic and histological criteria. The higher dose of 5-ASA achieved a better 12-month remission rate on intention to treat – 67 v. 50%. This difference just failed to reach statistical significance. A dose-response effect was also strongly suggested by an American paper in which 4.8 g was more effective than 1.6 g in acute colitis, but some would argue that this lower dose was too low for therapeutic (as opposed to maintenance) use; no intermediate dose was used [34].

The appropriate duration of 5-ASA therapy in ulcerative colitis is debated, perhaps more by patients than by their doctors. There are strong suggestions that regular (and long-term) 5-ASA not only prolongs the relapse-free interval survival but also helps to reduce the risk of colonic neoplasia (Chapter 8). Patients in prolonged remission nevertheless usually seek to stop maintenance therapy (or simply stop it on their own initiative). Aside from the issue of cancer risk, which is still a little unclear, this becomes an increasingly reasonable proposition the longer the patient is from the last relapse. The Milan group suggests a 2-year remission as a cut-off point for discontinuing maintenance therapy in ulcerative colitis, the nuisance (and hypothetical hazard) of therapy then outweighing clear benefit [35].

5-ASA in Crohn's disease

Early studies failed to show worthwhile benefit from sulphasalazine in Crohn's disease, and studies of 5-ASA preparations have mostly been too small to avoid Type II error, but Prantera *et al.* [36] have now demonstrated significant value from Asacol® 2.4 g/day in the prevention of clinical relapse. Meta-analysis of the completed studies of 5-ASA therapy in maintenance of remission supports this conclusion [37]. Two recent randomized controlled trials add to a general consensus that the drug is effective also in preventing postoperative relapse. Caprilli *et al.* [38] showed that administration of Asacol® 2.4 g/day, beginning within 6 weeks of surgery, was effective in preventing postoperative recurrence, as judged endoscopically. There was a 39% reduction of all endoscopic recurrences and a 55% reduction of severe endoscopic recurrence at 2 years, with an accompanying reduction in symptomatic recurrence. Similar results come from a North American study of 163 patients [39], in which the clinical recurrence rate (symptomatic and endoscopic) of 31% on 3 g 5-ASA daily (as Rowasa® or Salofalk®) contrasted with 41% in placebo-treated patients. These findings are of clinical importance in view of the high rate of early postoperative endoscopic recurrence (29% at 6 months, 56% at 1 year and 85% at 2 years), and an evolution towards recurrent symptoms in around

90% of these patients by 3 years [40]. The generally positive view from studies using higher doses of 5-ASA is partially countered by a more recent trial from the French GETAID authors [41] in which Claversal®, 3 g daily, was compared with placebo in patients after macroscopically 'curative' resection. Over 100 individuals were evaluated, with apparently good matching between active and placebo groups. The drug was well tolerated, but although there was a small numerical advantage in respect of the endoscopic relapse rate at 12 weeks (50% in treated patients compared to 63% in those receiving placebo, or 58% v. 66% by intention to treat), this did not reach significance. It is implied, though not actually stated, that none of the GETAID patients had a symptomatic relapse during the study period. The very short follow-up period in this study and the uncertain relationship between endoscopic recurrence and clinical sequelae led me to consider this a part of the overall picture gently supporting the postoperative use of mesalazine. Longer follow-up of the various trial patients is required to determine whether the endoscopic advantages translate into prolonged decreases in morbidity. Although Singleton *et al.* [42] have shown substantial benefit from mesalazine in active Crohn's disease in a 16-week study, currently it appears that prevention rather than treatment of relapse is a better strategy in the postoperative management of patients with Crohn's disease [43].

A relatively large dose of 5-ASA seems to be required in Crohn's disease, there being a more obvious dose-response effect [37] than in ulcerative colitis (see above). At least 2 g daily, and perhaps as much as 4 g daily, may be necessary to yield therapeutic or prophylactic benefit in Crohn's.

Renal toxicity of 5-ASA

Increased usage of any drug, whether by increased numbers of recipients or by increased dose, raises anxieties about infrequent but important toxicity; 5-ASA is no exception. Since the late 1980s there has been concern that the upper gastrointestinal side-effects, reversible oligospermia, and occasional anaphylaxis from sulphasalazine, were being succeeded by renal toxicity from 5-ASA, sometimes responsible for endstage renal failure with the need for renal dialysis or transplantation [44, 45]. Debate continues as to the relative importance of idiosyncratic, dose-independent nephritis, which is described (though very rare) with sulphasalazine, and of dose-dependent renal toxicity in which direct renal exposure to 5-ASA is more likely to blame.

Although there is a substantial literature and much clinical experience supporting the renal safety of the pH-dependent delivery systems, the systemic availability of 5-ASA is higher [31], and renal failure is recorded more often with these agents [45]. This excess renal risk probably remains when corrected for the relative frequency of use of the different products, but is not of sufficient magnitude to warrant a major influence on choice of agent. Discussion with colleagues around the world suggests that the centres most concerned are those that have themselves seen and reported cases of renal failure.

Toxicity was actively sought throughout the Dutch Pentasa study [33] and a probable or definite drug-related adverse event affected seven patients (4%), with no difference in the toxicity profile for the two doses used, nor in the drop-out rate attributable to poor compliance. Pentasa® yields a high total circulatory 5-ASA concentration compared to other 5-ASA preparations, but relatively low free (non-acetylated) 5-ASA levels [31]. Two patients (1.3%) developed modest and reversible renal impairment (one with mesalazine-related interstitial nephritis).

Prescribers of other 5-ASA preparations, worried that they are responsible for excessive or avoidable renal toxicity, will be somewhat comforted to note that Pentasa® is also associated with renal problems quite frequently. However, if irreversible toxicity is the result of sustained high, or peak, concentrations of free 5-ASA, then the results for Pentasa® (or indeed those for the agents dependent on colonic bacteria for 5-ASA release) are not necessarily wisely extrapolated to all pharmaceutical formulations. The particular concern with pH-release systems is that there is the potential for release of a sufficiently large 'bolus' in the small intestine to overwhelm mucosal acetylation and thereby lead to a transient but high concentration 5-ASA challenge to the kidneys with each dose given.

The pharmacology of pH-release mechanisms has come under scrutiny following suggestions that the Eudragit-coated preparations behave in the stomach as if solids, and leave very late in the gastric emptying process. Accordingly, the tendency for insightful gastroenterologists to increase compliance by advocating twice rather than three times daily dosage develops a scientific rationale. Hussain and colleagues have taken this a step further by comparing the effects of Asacol® when normal volunteers were given 1.2 g as a single daily dose as compared to a more conventional 400 mg thrice daily [46]. Disposition of native 5-ASA and its acetylated form was similar regardless of the administration regime, but clearly there are objections to the use of healthy volunteers and examination of only a 7-day study period. There should perhaps be relatively greater concern when considering the larger daily doses customary in North America.

Whichever oral 5-ASA preparation is chosen, it must be remembered that it is likely to be employed in the very long term, and we must remain alert to the possibility of insidious nephrotoxicity developing after some years of treatment. As for phenacetin, there may be a rising incidence of late renal impairment with very prolonged use (10 years or more) for which data are not yet available. It is important that prescribers audit their practice carefully, taking account of the renal dysfunction that may complicate inflammatory bowel disease itself, quite independently of any drugs used in its therapy [47, 48]. Renal disease is discussed further in Chapter 6. Very occasionally mesalazine preparations are themselves the cause of exacerbation of colitis, the associated worsening of the underlying disease leading potentially to confusion until the correct interpretation is reached [49].

Topical 5-ASA derivatives in ulcerative colitis

The extent to which mesalazine enemas reach the less distal colon has been uncertain, with assumptions following from Farthing's paper of 1979 in respect of steroid preparations, suggesting that the splenic flexure will often be accessible in active disease [50]. Van Bodegraven *et al.* have re-explored this scintigraphically with a longitudinal examination of 31 patients with ulcerative colitis [51]. The patients received one of three dose/volume regimes of liquid mesalazine (Salofalk® or Pentasa®) labelled with technetium, and had a repeat labelled enema at 12 weeks. Disease activity was not found to influence the distribution, but there was a non-significant tendency for the enema to reach a little more proximally in the active phase of illness. Extent of distribution was determined mainly by the volume of the enema, the 30 ml enema remaining mainly confined to the sigmoid, 60 ml reaching the descending colon in 15%, and the 100 ml preparation reaching the descending colon in 25%. It is notable, and may be clinically important, that the enema was not imaged in the rectum in the great majority of patients (91–99%) whatever the phase of illness or volume of enema; it may be logical to use concurrent suppository therapy in these patients.

Topical mesalazine is firmly established as an effective agent in treatment of active proctitis and distal colitis, typically with a response rate in excess of 70% over 3–6 weeks. The results are at least comparable to those of topical steroids [52] and of oral 5-ASA [53]. One major study favours Asacol® foam over Predfoam® in acute active distal colitis [54]. This was a large (>300 patients) multicentre study conducted over 4 weeks and (by intention to treat) showed statistically significant advantage for the 5-ASA preparation, which fell short of conferring histological advantage. However premature it might be to alter prescribing habits on the basis of a single paper, the meta-analysis performed by Marshall and Irvine lends further support for topical 5-ASA in preference to topical steroids [55]. Where topical steroid foams are readily available, they may well remain many practitioners' first choice, given their undoubted efficacy, the wealth of clinical experience, and that the comparisons have been between relatively high doses of mesalazine (2 g daily) and more routine doses of prednisolone/hydrocortisone. In the UK there is also a substantial cost disincentive to the use of Asacol® foam instead of Predfoam® or Colifoam® (of the order of fivefold at 1996 prices). A useful case is also presented by Mulder *et al.* [56] who argue that in difficult cases it is not only logical but also effective to combine the two drug types. The editor of the journal concerned was evidently impressed by the importance of this observation, as the paper is accompanied by not only a leading article but also a review on the topic!

Topical 5-ASA has been compared with oral preparations in patients with distal ulcerative colitis, with comparable or better results [57], but it was difficult to be sure whether this was a dose-response effect given that the oral dose of 2.4 g daily was compared with Rowasa® enemas which contain 4 g mesalazine. Campieri *et al.* [58] have clarified this issue in a study of patients with ulcerative proctitis, comparing 2.4 g orally with 1.2 g daily by suppository (400 mg three times daily). Results strongly favoured the rectal route at 2 and 4 weeks for clinical effect and histological improvement. Topical 5-ASA has also been shown to achieve remission in some patients who have previously been resistant to oral 5-ASA or to topical steroids [9]. It is also effective in maintenance of remission, administered daily as a liquid enema, foam or suppository. Little is gained from dose escalation [59], and 1 g daily is not obviously inferior to 2 g or 4 g. When enemas are employed there is no difference in efficacy between foam and liquid preparation. However, patients tend to prefer the foam formulation and long-term compliance may therefore be improved should the drug be used for maintenance. Little 5-ASA is absorbed when it is administered rectally and it may therefore be inferred that the above results generally reflect topical effects. Although additional gain may be achieved from oral and topical therapy together [57, 60], the choice of route of administration may reasonably be left to the patient when the disease is entirely or predominantly distal.

No controlled data yet exist for the use of topical 5-ASAs in distal Crohn's disease, but personal experience suggests that some patients with otherwise resistant disease will respond.

Topical 4-ASA

Distal ulcerative colitis will also respond to topical 4-ASA (also known as para-aminosalicylic acid/PAS) with comparable results to topical prednisolone [61], and to topical 5-ASA [62]. Clinical experience suggests, as for 5-ASA, that although the overall proportion of responsive patients is virtually identical, the particular patients who respond may differ, making a switch to an alternative topical regime worthwhile in those who do not initially achieve remission.

IMMUNOSUPPRESSANT THERAPY

Immunosuppressant drugs are valuable in refractory inflammatory bowel disease, in which they help to achieve and maintain clinical remission, reduce steroid use and avoid surgery. However, their usefulness has been hampered by limited efficacy, lack of selectivity and significant toxicity. An increasing understanding of the mucosal immune response in inflammatory bowel disease should allow future agents to be targeted at particular, critical steps in immune activation. The central role of T-cell activation and involvement of associated pro-inflammatory cytokines in pathogenesis is increasingly established [63]. Trials of cyclosporin, which is mainly active against the CD4 cell, have therefore been conducted, and newer therapeutic approaches based on 'blocking' monoclonal antibodies, for example against tumour necrosis factor-α (TNF-α), are emerging.

Azathioprine and 6-mercaptopurine

Azathioprine and 6-mercaptopurine (6MP) are purine analogues that competitively inhibit the biosynthesis of purine nucleotides. Their mode of action is poorly understood but they are known to have selective suppressant effects on T cells. Once absorbed azathioprine is almost entirely metabolized to 6MP, by sulphydryl compounds such as glutathione. The 6MP is then metabolized by thiopurine methyltransferase (TMT) to 6-methylmercaptopurine (which may be immunoactive), by xanthine oxidase to the inactive 6-thiouric acid, or by a series of steps to active 6-thioguanine nucleotides. Congenital deficiency of TMT or inhibition of xanthine oxidase by allopurinol predisposes to accumulation of 6MP with the potential for severe bone marrow suppression [63]. Myelosuppression can occur in the normal population, especially when high doses are employed, but is more likely in heterozygotes for TMT deficiency, and is almost the rule in homozygotes who have almost undetectable concentrations of the enzyme.

Azathioprine and 6-mercaptopurine in Crohn's disease
Persuasive evidence for a role of azathioprine/6MP in the management of refractory Crohn's disease dates from Present's 1980 study in which induction of remission and reduction of steroid requirement were demonstrated [64]. In a 24-month placebo-controlled study of 83 patients (needing an initial mean daily prednisolone dose of 20 mg), 1.5 mg/kg of 6MP permitted full weaning from steroids in 55% with improvement in 75% of patients, whereas only 36% of the placebo group improved. Supportive data come from studies which have confirmed benefit in maintenance of remission [65, 66]. Whereas steroids and 5-ASA preparations appear to have no specific role in treatment of Crohn's-related enterocutaneous fistulae (Chapter 7), in an uncontrolled 6-month trial in 34 patients a 39% fistula closure rate was reported, with worthwhile improvement in a further 26%, mostly in patients who had not already been treated surgically for the fistulae [67]. The mean time to respond was over 3 months, as it was in the 1980 study; this delay adds to the continuing need for surgery in fistula patients.

Lémann *et al.* [68] have now studied azathioprine in patients after 'curative' resection for Crohn's disease. As this was a retrospective analysis with only historical controls, the interpretation should be somewhat guarded. The authors' view that the clinical recurrence rate (26% at 3 years) is better than with no maintenance therapy and of a similar order to that obtainable with 5-ASA seems reasonable, but whether controlled trial of a relatively hazardous agent is justified when a less toxic agent exists and may be of similar value must be considered carefully. A very large trial would be required to show differences between azathioprine and 5-ASA if Lémann's data are representative. It is probably no longer legitimate to initiate placebo-controlled trials in this context.

Azathioprine and 6-mercaptopurine in ulcerative colitis

Purine analogues have also been shown to be effective in induction and maintenance of remission in refractory ulcerative colitis, commencing with a study at St Mark's in 1982 in which 44 patients were randomized to azathioprine or placebo [69]. There was a clinical response and it was possible to achieve a significantly greater reduction in prednisolone dose by 3 months in the patients receiving azathioprine (mean prednisolone dose 6.7 mg v. 17.7 mg). Supportive data have come from other centres [70, 71], and there is a significantly greater relapse rate in patients in whom the drug is subsequently withdrawn [72].

Approximately two-thirds of patients selected for purine analogue therapy in the management of problematic inflammatory bowel disease will both tolerate and respond to it. The usual dose is 1.5 mg/kg of 6MP or 2.0 mg/kg of azathioprine. The onset of action is slow, as it depends on effects on newly differentiating cells, a phenomenon that necessitates treatment for at least 3 months before judging treatment a failure. It is perhaps unsurprising that this is not always readily accepted by the patient. Approximately 10% of patients are intolerant of azathioprine and 6MP, side-effects being mainly of a relatively trivial nature. Serious but idiosyncratic toxicities, including pancreatitis, hepatitis and hypersensitivity reactions, all of which recur on repeated administration, occur more rarely. Bone marrow suppression is dose related and reversible. It usually occurs in the first 6 months of treatment but can occur much later [73, 74] and therefore necessitates regular 4- to 6-weekly monitoring of the white blood cell count while therapy continues. In the St Mark's review, 5% of patients developed myelosuppression at some time [73]. In only five cases (<0.7%) were there associated clinical manifestations, but it is probable that at least one death from sepsis was azathioprine related. If myelosuppression develops, it may be possible to retain therapeutic efficacy safely by reduction of dosage. Indeed, it is proposed that efficacy is dependent on the development of some degree of leucopenia [75]. A prospective study to clarify this is said to be in progress, but for the time being the best data come from Berg *et al.* [76] who performed a retrospective study of 101 patients on 6-mercaptopurine. Of the 71 subjects who achieved complete remission on the drug, 65% were leucopenic (although the definition of this is not given in the abstract) at some time, compared to 43% of those in whom complete remission was not achieved. However, the two phenomena appeared unrelated as leucopenia followed the attainment of remission in 50%, and did not predict future remission.

As the benefits of azathioprine may be denied to some patients with florid disease because they cannot wait for its slow onset of action, Sandborn and colleagues have attempted to fast-track its effect by administering the drug intravenously at a very high dose [77]. Twelve patients with active Crohn's disease were given 50 mg of the drug by continuous infusion every hour for 36 hours having – crucially – first determined that each had adequate levels of red cell thiopurine methyltransferase to permit normal metabolism of the drug. Those with levels of enzyme activity in the low/homozygous range were excluded from consideration for intravenous therapy. The loading dose of 1800 mg was chosen to reflect an equivalent oral dose of around 4000 mg (or approximately 1 month's conventional therapy). Patients then continued with low-dose oral azathioprine (50 mg/kg). Toxicity was not obviously greater than for standard usage and the frequency of response (two-thirds) was comparable to that normally expected. When responses occurred they were indeed quicker, and always within 4 weeks of the infusion. Unfortunately, red cell thiopurine methyltransferase assays are not readily available, making this an unacceptably dangerous strategy for most centres. If controlled trial confirms the value of the new approach, additional laboratory support will also be needed.

Given continuing, and probably not entirely misplaced, concern about the long-term use of azathioprine, it behoves us to consider for how long therapy should be continued once remission is achieved. The data summarized above support its use for 12 months once the initial introductory phase is successfully negotiated. The data become less good thereafter, but the St Mark's data support use up to 24 months reasonably securely. Thereafter the data sets available refer to very small numbers. Bouhnik's study of 157 patients treated for more than 6 months is therefore helpful as well as interesting [78]. It reflects just over 40% of all their patients exposed to azathioprine or 6-mercaptopurine. The cumulative relapse rates at 1 and 5 years were 11% and 32% (compared to 38% and 75% in those who, having achieved remission on the drug, stopped it more than 6 months after its commencement). However, in those who stopped the drug more than 5 years after its initiation there was no apparent disadvantage. Although this may simply be a small number effect (12 continuing, five stopping) there were no relapses in those who stopped, compared to two in the 12 continuing, and for all other time brackets there was an obvious excess in those stopping, which failed to reach significance only in year 4, when 25% of those stopping relapsed compared to 17% of those continuing. Extrapolating a little from the French data, I now advocate a trial off azathioprine once 4 years of successful treatment have been completed.

The place (or otherwise) of azathioprine in pregnancy is considered in Chapter 5. Some concern in respect of the increased incidence of malignancy (particularly lymphomas) in transplant patients treated with azathioprine has not particularly been borne out in inflammatory bowel disease (Chapter 8).

An audit of azathioprine use was recently performed at St Mark's to determine whether it is practicable to use the drug safely outside the constraints and checks of a trial setting, and, as a secondary aim, to examine its efficacy in this same context. Clinical guidelines for its use had been established (Table 3.1) against which the audit sought to test compliance in regular clinical practice. All inflammatory bowel disease patients new to azathioprine in a 12-month period were followed (at this tertiary referral centre) for a further 12 months.

All patients commenced on azathioprine in 1993 were identified from case notes, the computerized inflammatory bowel disease database, and/or from pharmacy records. All 26 patients (11 Crohn's disease, 13 ulcerative colitis, two indeterminate colitis) had failed steroid withdrawal, with a period of at least 6 months on prednisolone, at a mean of more than 10 mg/day. Early surgery was not considered to be likely at the time of commencement of azathioprine. The results vindicated this view, with no patient proceeding to surgery in the first 4 months of azathioprine. All patients were correctly commenced on an initial 2 mg/kg dose, and hospital follow-up was uniformly organized at 2–3-month intervals. Haematological monitoring was impeccable (100%) for hospital visits, and a 6-weekly check (or better) was achieved in all patients during the first 6 months; thereafter most patients were checked less than 8-weekly. Nine adverse events were identified in seven patients (27% of subjects). In week 1, one patient developed an allergic reaction with bronchospasm: the drug was withdrawn. Another described hair loss and paraesthesia

Table 3.1 Guidelines for azathioprine use in inflammatory bowel disease

1	Established inflammatory bowel disease
2	Either failure to respond to steroid/5-ASA
	or failure to wean from steroids
	or need for systemic steroids > 4 months/year
3	Absence of need for early surgery
4	Prescription of 2 mg/kg
5	Regular clinical review
6	Full blood count every clinic visit
	and every 4–6 weeks
7	Dose reduction/stop if toxicity (total leucocytes < 3.5, or neutrophils < 1.5)

which resolved despite continuing azathioprine. After more than 6 months' treatment, one patient developed severe nausea which necessitated drug withdrawal, while two exhibited mild leucopenia requiring dose reduction. Benign macrocytosis unassociated with B_{12} or folate deficiency in three patients required no action. At 12 months, 17 patients were considered to have responded to azathioprine (prednisolone <5 mg/day for >4 months), three had been treated surgically, and six were on other medical therapy (including two of those withdrawn from azathioprine). We concluded that the guidelines were followed closely apart from the later haematological monitoring. The efficacy appeared encouragingly similar to that of trial data, and the safety profile appeared reasonable despite relatively poor monitoring. However, complacency was not felt justified given evidence of late toxicity both from the literature and current experience. It is noteworthy that this appears to be the first published audit on an inflammatory bowel disease-based topic.

Cyclosporin

Cyclosporin is a lipid-soluble fungal derivative with potent immunosuppressive effects, which acts primarily on T-cell function and proliferation, mainly by inhibition of interleukin-2 gene transcription. There is consequent loss of recruitment of cytotoxic cells and inhibition of cytotoxic lymphokines [79]. It has begun to be very much more widely used since the positive results reported for its use in fulminant ulcerative colitis [80].

Cyclosporin in Crohn's disease

Early uncontrolled open studies of cyclosporin in Crohn's disease and ulcerative colitis claimed impressive response rates within 5–10 days, followed then by a high late failure rate. There are currently four published, randomized, double-blind, placebo-controlled trials of oral cyclosporin in refractory Crohn's disease. Brynskov *et al.* [2] reported improvement in 50% of treated patients compared to only 32% in controls; although this was significant, only 19% of the responding patients retained their improvement to 6 months after tapering and discontinuing the drug. The subsequent study by Jewell *et al.* [81] was more disappointing even with continuing maintenance therapy. The Canadian Crohn's Relapse Prevention Trial Investigators [82] have since reported a multicentre double-blind placebo-controlled trial of low-dose cyclosporin in which a total of 305 patients were entered. Actively treated patients had a worse symptomatic outcome than the placebo group, and there was no reduction in requirement for other medication. Very similar conclusions come from the fourth study to report [83]. While it is possible that a better response might be obtained with higher doses, toxicity precludes this as a long-term measure (see below). A role may exist for the patient with fistulous disease

(Chapter 7), to judge from an uncontrolled study of 16 such patients [84]. All had failed on standard therapies, and were started on 4 mg/kg by continuous intravenous infusion. Fourteen patients showed some response, and seven fistulae closed. There was substantial toxicity, and a high relapse rate when parenteral therapy was discontinued. The authors concluded that intravenous cyclosporin was effective in fistulating Crohn's disease, but that its future role should be determined by controlled trial. This is probably an appropriate conclusion for the use of the drug in Crohn's in general, despite the occasional apparently dramatic anecdotal response. Its use is not currently justified outside formal clinical trials.

Cyclosporin in ulcerative colitis

The initial promising results from an open pilot study of intravenous cyclosporin in fulminant ulcerative colitis have subsequently been strongly supported by the same group. A dual-centre controlled trial was designed to include 40 patients failing to respond to 5 days of high-dose intravenous steroids [80]. Fulminant colitis was defined from the revised Oxford criteria [85] (see also Chapter 4). The patients were randomized to receive either intravenous cyclosporin 4 mg/kg as a continuous infusion together with continued high-dose steroids, or to continue conventional therapy alone. The study was stopped prematurely on statistical and ethical grounds after only 20 patients had been entered. Nine of 11 patients given cyclosporin responded as compared to none of the nine continuing conventional therapy alone. This improvement was maintained in 60% of patients at 6 months after discharge from hospital. Provisional data from Chicago indicate also that the quality of life in those treated successfully with cyclosporin was better than in those receiving surgery, but these seem flawed comparisons, as like is not compared with like. These results still require prospective verification from other centres, but indicate a place for the drug in selected patients with severe active or refractory ulcerative colitis. It should not need to be emphasized in the present context that all patients with severe colitis have a potentially life-threatening condition (Chapter 4). They are best managed jointly by physician and surgeon. The current practice at St Mark's mandates an agreement between all parties that cyclosporin is a short-term measure aiming to avoid surgery, but that this pharmacological intervention will not be permitted to delay surgery in the patient who continues to deteriorate or in whom there is no obvious response to medical therapy by a further 5–7 days (10–12 days in total). There is no place for cyclosporin in the management of patients with complications such as megacolon, perforation or major haemorrhage.

Monitoring cyclosporin and potential long-term use

To date there are no controlled data to determine whether cyclosporin has a role in maintenance or in the chronically active steroid-dependent patient. Most specialist centres are aiming to avoid such use, preferring to transfer patients who have responded to the drug in fulminant disease on to more established maintenance regimes – particularly azathioprine/6MP. However, cyclosporin enemas have been properly assessed in refractory ulcerative proctitis, and here prove no better than placebo [86].

Toxicity is relatively frequent even in short-term use and is mainly dose-related, there being a narrow therapeutic index. Reversible nephrotoxicity, hyperkalaemia, hyperuricaemia, hepatotoxicity, hypertension and seizures are not unusual even with careful use, and hypertrichosis, gingival hyperplasia, tremor and paraesthesiae are all common and of great concern to patients. The short-term control documented in six of seven patients in one small open study in Crohn's disease is heavily counterbalanced by the death of one of the six from opportunistic infection [87]. Caution in respect of possible coincidental cytomegalovirus infection is also appropriate [88]. The New York group has the most cumulative data for cyclosporin in inflammatory bowel disease [89], and reports 54 episodes of major toxicity in its first 111 patients. There were two deaths – one from septic shock and one from massive duodenal haemorrhage – and seven life-threatening infections. Fits occurred in three patients, attributed in part to low cholesterol levels. No less than 51% had paraesthesia, 43% hypertension and 42% hypomagnesaemia. The possible relevance of cyclosporin therapy to a subsequently increased risk of neoplasia is considered in Chapter 8.

Whole blood levels (not plasma) should be adjusted to 100–200 ng/ml in chronic low-dose oral therapy and to no more than 200–400 ng/ml in high-dose intravenous therapy, as measured by high performance liquid chromatography or monoclonal antibody radioimmunoassay. The intestinal absorption of the drug is affected by active intestinal disease and short bowel (and with cholestasis), and dietary factors such as grapefruit juice (but not other fruit juices) can significantly affect blood levels [90]. This may account in part for the poor results in most studies of Crohn's disease if insufficient active agent has been available.

Methotrexate

Methotrexate is a dihydrofolate reductase inhibitor which interferes with normal DNA synthesis. It has immunosuppressive and anti-inflammatory properties, and has accordingly been widely used in conditions such as psoriasis and rheumatoid arthritis, as well as in oncological practice. In 1989 Kozarek *et al.* [91] reported the results of an open trial of 12 weeks' methotrexate in patients with refractory Crohn's disease ($n = 14$) and ulcerative colitis ($n = 7$). There was an apparent short-term response in the majority of both groups of patients allowing significant reduction in steroid dosage, which was then sustained by maintenance therapy in two-thirds of the responders to 72 weeks. Previous failure to respond to aza-thioprine/6MP does not seem to preclude response to methotrexate. Controlled data have now been published by the North American Crohn's Study Group Investigators [92]. In a study which included 141 patients with active Crohn's disease, all were brought to a common daily dosage of 20 mg prednisolone, either by weaning down to this dose or by increasing a lower maintenance dose. A steroid weaning protocol was then followed for the study period. Half were randomized to receive intramuscular methotrexate 25 mg each week for 16 weeks (a relatively large dose by comparison with its use in other non-malignant conditions). The end-points comprised Crohn's activity and degree of weaning from steroids. Remission was achieved in 39.4% of those given methotrexate compared to only 19.1% in those given placebo (RR, 2.1; CI, 1.1–3.5), and with significantly greater reduction in final prednisolone dose. The overall rather poor results are accounted for by the prior severity of disease (all patients requiring prednisolone at a dose of at least 10 mg/day). Methotrexate was not associated with substantial toxicity in this relatively short-term study, although there was a deterioration in liver function parameters in 7%, and nausea led to withdrawal from the drug in 6% (total withdrawals 17% v. 2% in the placebo arm). A longer-term continuation of the study in the same group of patients, using 15 mg/week, is in progress to determine whether the apparent advantage from methotrexate is maintained without development of hepatic fibrosis, myelosuppression or other problems. Another positive North American placebo-controlled trial was reported in abstract form in 1992, but there must be doubt about its conclusions given the long delay to formal publication. Modigliani's group have been using methotrexate for longer than most, and continue to provide clinical data on its (uncontrolled) use in patients resistant to other forms of therapy [93]. A 72% success rate is claimed at 3 months but this falls to 42% at 12 months. Their protocol gives 25 mg intramuscularly each week for 3 months, and then switches to oral administration, reducing gradually to a minimum dose of 7.5 mg weekly. They report a continuing low incidence of important toxicity in these and in (a different?) 31 patients with Crohn's disease continuing the drug on an uncontrolled basis for longer periods (at least 7 months, median 19 months), only 16% of whom had to discontinue the drug [94].

Methotrexate has been less encouraging in ulcerative colitis than predicted from early data from the Canadian and French groups. A careful double-blind trial from Israel ($n = 67$) now demonstrates that a weekly oral dose of 12.5 mg in steroid resistant/dependent patients had no therapeutic effect over a 9-month study period [95]. It might be argued that the dose was inadequate, but it is unlikely that malabsorption was the reason for the poor result, as methotrexate is known to be absorbed in the proximal small bowel. There is therefore no current justification for the use of this drug in ulcerative colitis.

The traditional advice that a liver biopsy should be performed before methotrexate therapy is not warranted in inflammatory bowel disease patients with normal liver function, but regular estimation of hepatic biochemistry and coagulation status while on the drug is probably wise, with consideration given to liver biopsy once a total dose of 2 g has been given [96]. With the regimes currently being promoted this is not likely to occur much before 3 years of therapy (the Lémann regime rarely leads to more than 750 g being given even in the first year). The low but possible risk of malignancy complicating long-term methotrexate therapy is considered in Chapter 8.

Other immunosuppressants

Tacrolimus (previously FK506) is a macrolide with potent immunosuppressive activity. It has similar mechanisms of action to cyclosporin and has gained a major role in organ transplantation. Extrapolation from its use in patients undergoing small bowel transplant suggests that it may have a role in inflammatory bowel disease, and preliminary results suggest some benefit in chronic Crohn's fistulae and pyoderma gangrenosum [97].

K-76 is a fungal derivative of *Stachybotrys complementi*. It has been shown to have potentially beneficial immunomodulatory effects in inflammation, prompting a Japanese group to examine its effects in inflammatory bowel disease [98]. They report a good response as monotherapy in four of five patients. Seven of 21 patients with refractory disease unresponsive to steroids responded to the addition of K-76. Further assessment is clearly necessary.

ANTIBIOTICS IN CROHN'S DISEASE AND ULCERATIVE COLITIS

Antibiotics have a clear role in the management of certain of the complications of inflammatory bowel disease (Chapter 7). Their role in primary therapy is less certain. A number of broad-spectrum antibiotics have been evaluated in both ulcerative colitis and Crohn's disease. There is some evidence (mostly from small, uncontrolled studies) demonstrating efficacy for various agents, and rather better evidence for the use of metronidazole.

Metronidazole

Metronidazole is licensed as an antimicrobial with action against anaerobes and protozoa but it is probable that it also has independent anti-inflammatory actions. It is frequently used for management of perianal Crohn's disease given an expected benefit in two-thirds of recipients [99]. An earlier study in the UK was less enthusiastic; despite doubling the response rate at 2 weeks compared to placebo (from 35% to 67% or 71% depending on whether co-trimoxazole was also used), this effect was not sustained to 4 weeks [100]. Aside from its probable role in perianal Crohn's, some benefit from metronidazole given for a month or more at a dose of 10 mg/kg has also been demonstrated in ileo-colonic Crohn's disease (but not in disease affecting the small bowel alone) [3]. Finally, in a controlled trial of 60 patients undergoing terminal ileal resection given a 3-month course of metronidazole (20 mg/kg) or placebo starting within 1 week of surgery, there was a statistically significant reduction in clinically apparent postoperative recurrence at 1 year (4% v. 25%), but this was not maintained to 2 or 3 years [101]. Toxicity, particularly peripheral neuropathy, also remains a concern. In one study employing nerve conduction studies, 85% of treated patients had abnormalities, 46% were symptomatic, and in 11% the neuropathy was not reversible on discontinuing the drug [102].

Other antibiotics in ulcerative colitis

Burke *et al.* [103] reported long-term symptomatic and histological improvement in patients with refractory extensive colitis treated with a 1-week course of oral tobramycin. Some 90% of their patients were able to discontinue steroids, but relatively few subsequent trials have proved supportive. Amongst those that have, Malagelada's group have explored the use of co-amoxiclav in a Eudragit-coated delayed-release form [104]. When 3 g/750 mg was given daily to acute colitics, potentially beneficial changes were demonstrable in the cytokine content of rectal dialysates together with suggestive clinical differences of a magnitude to warrant formal clinical trial. Also a 6-month double-blind placebo-controlled trial of ciprofloxacin in 83 patients with moderate to severe ulcerative colitis, given in addition to conventional therapy, demonstrated a reduction in treatment failures from 56% in the placebo group to 21% in the ciprofloxacin group ($p = 0.03$) [105]. There was also an associated reduction in the need for colectomy from 40% to 16%. However, data from a blinded placebo-controlled trial performed in fulminant colitics showed no difference in response rate or need for surgery with ciprofloxacin 250 mg orally twice daily [106]. An effect may have been masked by concurrent high-dose steroids or overlooked because the antibiotic regime itself was inadequate (dose and/or route). There is as yet no mandate for routine use of antibiotics in ulcerative colitis, whether fulminant or not.

Other antibiotics in Crohn's disease

One early study [107] using a variety of broad-spectrum antibiotics given continuously for 6 months indicated symptomatic improvement in 93% of patients with Crohn's disease. Radiological improvement was seen in 57%, and 40% were able to discontinue steroids; it is unlikely that these impressive results were the direct consequence of antibiotics alone, given the inability of others to replicate this success. Ciprofloxacin, favoured in some centres [108], appears *in vitro* to have an anti-inflammatory effect on peripheral blood mononuclear cells, and potentially important non-antimicrobial effects, but as this effect is absent in biopsies from Crohn's disease patients, any therapeutic effect is most probably an antibiotic one [109]. Early uncontrolled data favouring clarithomycin in Crohn's also exist.

Antituberculous therapy for Crohn's disease

A variety of antimycobacterial regimes have been evaluated in the treatment of Crohn's disease (in part to test the hypothesis that *Mycobacterium paratuberculosis* is of aetiological relevance) [110] (Chapter 1). Although debate continues as to whether the result of inappropriate regimes or inappropriate logic, the early published results were disappointing. *Mycobacterium paratuberculosis* has much in common with the relatively non-aggressive opportunistic mycobacteria, and the therapeutic regimes developed for AIDS patients have now accordingly been applied in Crohn's disease. *In vitro* data support a combination of rifabutin with streptomycin, and an oddly constructed double-blind trial of 51 patients studied over 2 years (with 16 weeks of almost daily streptomycin injections), demonstrated improvements in those receiving streptomycin and rifabutin compared to those receiving streptomycin alone [111]. Remarkably, only 27% of the patients failed to complete the study. The magnitude of the apparent benefit from the two antibiotic regimes is difficult to judge as conventional therapies were continued and the overall response rates are within the range typical for Crohn's disease treated more conventionally. No pharmacologically 'clean' study yet demonstrates significant benefit. Trials using newer drugs and regimes continue.

NUTRITIONAL THERAPY IN INFLAMMATORY BOWEL DISEASE

A detailed account of nutrition in inflammatory bowel disease is beyond the scope of this volume, but some discussion of its therapeutic role is important. Nutritional intervention is crucial in malnourished patients, and most of all in children, where permanent growth retardation will result if it is neglected (see also Chapter 5). The patient with Crohn's of the small bowel is particularly at risk. This use of nutritional measures should be distinguished from primary nutritional therapy, in which a nutritional regime is used as the therapy (as opposed to providing nutritional support or treating malnutrition).

Primary nutritional therapy has not been shown to have any place in ulcerative colitis, although a number of lines of evidence suggest that modification of the colonic bacterial flora may be achieved by dietary manipulation, and that this in turn may have effects on disease expression (as is suggested, for example, by the data on antibiotic use (see above) or the effects of short-chain fatty acids or acetarsol (see below)). Also, many patients find that dietary modification has a major impact on their symptoms. It is difficult to give constructive advice that will be of general value, but it is worth recognizing this influence, and encouraging patients to make their own explorations into dietary manipulation. Reduction in consumption of milk products is more likely to be helpful than most other well-defined changes [112]. There is, however, an expanding literature indicating a role for dietary therapy in selected patients with Crohn's disease [113].

Dietary antigens have been thought to contribute to the pathogenesis of inflammatory bowel disease, and it was therefore logical to test exclusive parenteral nutrition encompassing 'bowel rest'. Early studies indicated a 65–95% response rate in patients with refractory Crohn's disease. However, it has been realized subsequently that elemental, 'pre-digested' and polymeric liquid formula diets can have similar efficacy to exclusive parenteral feeding in inducing remission [113]. It remains unclear whether nutritional repletion, relative bowel rest or other factors explain these improvements.

Much of the supportive literature for nutritional therapy comes from a small number of enthusiastic centres (reviewers including Silk [114], O'Morain [115], and Giaffer [116]), and analysis of results by strict 'intention to treat' has not always been volunteered. One is compelled to estimate a likely placebo response, as there are no placebo-controlled trials, so the 30% or so of Crohn's patients who will go into remission without specific intervention in most therapeutic settings should be kept in mind (see above). In the 10-year retrospective Northwick Park study published in 1990, nutritional therapy appeared to offer clear advantage, with remission being achieved in 96 of 113 acute Crohn's episodes (in patients with no previous surgery) [117]. Only 22% relapsed within 6 months, as did a further 9% per year thereafter. The Sheffield group examined enteral nutrition for those who had failed on high-dose steroids; there were only 16 patients, but 10 responded [118]. There are a number of other anecdotal reports and small series which reach similar conclusions.

Controlled (though inevitably unblinded) comparisons of nutritional therapy with steroid therapy permit a more objective view. O'Morain's landmark paper of 1984 found no difference between the two therapies in 21 Crohn's patients [119]. The same conclusion is reached by most of the other studies ($n = 16$ [120]; $n = 17$ [121]; $n = 95$ [122]; $n = 24$ [123]; $n = 32$ [124]; $n = 19$ [125]; $n = 42$ [126]). Only the Fourth European Crohn's study

[127], which included 55 patients, found a significant difference, and this was in favour of prednisolone.

If nutrition and steroids really are therapeutically equivalent, it would be appropriate always to choose the former on the basis of safety and freedom from toxicity, and particularly so in children given the concerns about steroid-related impaired growth, even if these latter concerns are somewhat misplaced (Chapter 5). It is therefore especially pertinent to examine the relative ease of use and the degree of compliance in routine use of these two options. The high drop-out rate for continuing enteral nutritional therapy, whether given orally or by overnight nasogastric intubation is therefore an important factor. As examples from two nutritionally orientated centres we find failure to complete maintenance studies in 33% and 55% of patients, even though the 42 and 78 patients, respectively, recruited had personal experience of the benefits of exclusive elemental feeding, having obtained their initial remissions in this way [128, 129]. It is also striking that despite the authors' enthusiasm for primary nutritional therapy, in the East Anglian study, of 228 eligible subjects only 136 were recruited (with a 57% response rate) [129]. The key to this issue thus lies in comparisons by intention to treat (Table 3.2).

These nine randomized studies (and 342 patients) are only broadly comparable, but more formal meta-analysis of primary nutritional therapy for Crohn's disease has now been performed. Griffiths *et al.* [113] included eight randomized controlled trials of steroid versus nutritional therapy ($n = 413$) and identified clinical remissions in 80.5% of those receiving steroids compared to 56.8% of those on nutritional therapy (odds ratio = 0.35; CI = 0.23–0.53). If remission was achieved, the relapse

Table 3.2 Examples of controlled comparisons of nutritional therapy with steroid therapy with response rates recorded by intention to treat

Author [reference]	Response rate		
	Steroids	TEN	Statistics
O'Morain [120]	70%	73%	NS
Saverymuttu [121][b]	100%	65%	$p < 0.05$
Sanderson [122]	?6/7	?7/8	NS
Malchow [123] [a]	73%	41%	$p < 0.05$
Lochs [128][a]	85%	53%	$p < 0.05$
Thomas [124]	?100%	?100%	NS
González-Huix [125]	88%	80%	NS
Seidman [126]	100%	60%	$p < 0.05$
Gorard [127]	85%	45%	$p < 0.05$
All nine studies	84.6%	58.9%	$p < 0.0005$

[a] Included sulphasalazine as well as steroids.
[b] Included antibiotics as well as total elemental nutrition.
TEN, total defined formula enteral nutrition.

rate at 12 months was the same for both therapies (65% and 67%). Nevertheless, meta-analysis does clearly support the view that nutritional therapy is more effective than placebo.

As it is possible that different nutritional regimes have different chances of inducing remission, the data have also been assessed according to the nature of the nutritional regime. Elemental nutrition does not appear to offer an advantage over semi-elemental or polymeric feeds; there is, in fact, a non-significant trend in the opposite direction, an odds ratio of 0.87 favouring non-elemental feeds (which may reflect better tolerability and better compliance). Current data do not permit an accurate assessment of the role of fat avoidance in successful Crohn's therapy but this is readdressed below.

If enteral nutrition is to be used in therapy, it would be helpful to know in advance which patients it is most likely to suit. Its value as a steroid-sparing manoeuvre is debatable (Chapter 5) but it is most likely to be considered when the patient, or the parents of a juvenile, are reluctant for steroids to be used. The literature suggests that those with colonic Crohn's are less likely to respond to nutritional therapy than those with predominantly ileal involvement, but there is little clarity in respect of the patient with extensive and proximal small bowel disease – who is equally in most need of non-surgical options if resection leading to short bowel syndrome is to be avoided. The issue is arguably a slightly artificial one as those with the most proximal disease are also those least likely to tolerate enteral regimes for the necessary time [130].

The greater commitment required of the patient for nutritional therapy coupled with a tendency for a slower induction of remission, lead most gastroenterologists to continue to favour systemic steroids as first-line treatment for acute relapses of Crohn's in the adult. There should be no doubt, however, that they can be effective in some patients who have failed on steroids, in those in whom steroids are strongly contra-indicated, and when steroids are refused by the patient. Whether there is a place for exclusion diets, with systematic slow reintroduction of foods once remission has been achieved – advocated as effective in maintenance of remission in inflammatory bowel disease [131] – remains ill-defined; these diets are difficult to implement even in patients brought to remission by nutritional therapy. The conclusions reached by the Northwick Park group seem to me appropriately pragmatic [128]. Although food sensitivities remain evident after nutritional treatment of Crohn's disease, they are very variable, are often transient and are ultimately of insufficient importance to warrant putting patients through the rigours of an elimination diet.

There is evidence that continued use of supplementary defined liquid enteral nutrition may help to maintain remission in Crohn's disease [132]. This comes from an uncontrolled study but one which may nevertheless be of practical value, since it has been difficult to give meaningful advice on whether nutritional therapy should be continued once remission is achieved, given that the patient will then wish to recommence eating (and our knowledge from the East Anglian study that continued food avoidance is not the long-term answer). Dietary supplements may be considered legitimate if not mandatory, and should certainly be encouraged in the patient who is still malnourished.

THE ROLE OF FATTY ACIDS AND EICOSANOIDS

Although controversial [113], it is possible that a component of the therapeutic response to nutritional therapy in Crohn's disease is from a reduced intestinal exposure to fat. Linoleic acid appears particularly disadvantageous [133], presumably because it is a key precursor of arachidonic acid and thus of inflammatory eicosanoids such as leukotriene B_4, thromboxane A_2 and prostaglandin E_2 (see also below). Other dietary methods of reducing eicosanoid synthesis have also been considered in both Crohn's disease and ulcerative colitis. Fish oils, which contain large amounts of eicosapentanoic acid, divert eicosanoid metabolism towards leukotriene B_5 and prostaglandin E_3, which are much less inflammatory than leukotriene B_4 and prostaglandin E_2 [134]. It is possible that useful inhibition of interleukins and TNF-α can be achieved, and in Crohn's disease there is also the possibility that inhibition of platelet aggregation may be helpful if microscopic multifocal infarction is indeed important (Chapter 1). It will also be noted that several of the standard therapeutic manoeuvres (5-ASA, azathioprine, cyclosporin) have significant, normalizing, influences on the eicosanoid content of colonic mucosa [135].

In a multicentre, double-blind, cross-over trial of eicosapentanoic acid in active ulcerative colitis, there was a significant reduction in rectal dialysate leukotriene B_4 levels, associated with clinical and histological improvement during the treatment period [136]. The Nottingham group also showed modest benefit from fish-oil supplementation in active colitis but no advantage in maintenance [137]. The most recent published study of fish-oil therapy was a more substantial two-centre Italian evaluation of a lipid concentrate in Crohn's disease maintenance [138]. The active agent included 40% eicosapentanoic acid and 20% docosahexanoic acid and provided 1.8 g of the former and 0.9 g of the latter each day for 12 months, in comparison to a mixed-acid triglyceride of fractionated fatty acids (60% caprylic, 40% capric acid). Compliance was surprisingly good, with only four of 39 patients ceasing active therapy because of side-effects (diarrhoea). At 1 year, and by intention to treat, 59% of the treated group remained in remission compared to only 26% of the control group ($p = 0.003$). Multivariate analysis indicated that the results could reasonably be attributed only to the specific therapeutic intervention. This response is equivalent to that predicted for 5-ASA regimes and now deserves comparative study.

Short-chain fatty acids are released from dietary fats by anaerobic bacteria and (particularly in the case of butyrate) are physiologically important colonocyte nutrients [139]. Good evidence now exists that their absence in the defunctioned colon is an important factor in the development of diversion colitis (Chapters 1 and 4), supported by a rapid response of some affected patients to short-chain fatty acid enemas [140]. Short-chain fatty acids are also depleted in ulcerative colitis, attributed (at least in part) to the effects of functionally abnormal anaerobic bacteria producing excess sulphur mercaptides [141] (Chapter 1), and have accordingly been used therapeutically in enema form. In a randomized trial in patients with acute distal colitis Senagore *et al.* [142] demonstrated a remission rate equivalent to that for topical steroids or mesalazine, with an overall 80% response rate. The attraction of using a natural agent with assumed low toxicity is offset by the current lack of availability of fatty acid preparations, the pharmaceutical difficulties resulting from their volatility and their unpleasant smell. In the face of these difficulties, and two similar trials with less promising results [143, 144], this is not a strategy that is currently recommended at St Mark's. Whether the apparent effect of short-chain fatty acids, in reducing the degree of proliferation in colitic rectal mucosa [145], has any bearing on risk of neoplasia such as to suggest a prophylactic therapeutic role, remains to be seen.

Similar mechanisms to those of the free fatty acids may also underlie the effect of topical arsenicals in the form of acetarsol – an agent of proven equivalence to topical steroids [146]. There is an appropriately high degree of caution in utilizing an arsenic-containing agent, but the short- and medium-term risks are low [147]. Uncertainty remains in respect of the long-term cancer risk, and the drug, which is not generally available, cannot be recommended.

Leukotriene (LT) B_4 (generated by the action of 5-lipoxygenase on arachidonic acid) has been shown to play a central role in the inflammatory cascade in inflammatory bowel disease, with elevated levels detected in the colonic mucosa of patients with active ulcerative colitis, but not in steroid-treated, quiescent disease [148, 149]. Several 5-lipoxygenase inhibitors now exist, including zileuton (A-64077), which inhibits 5-lipoxygenase without an effect on cyclo-oxygenase or phospholipase A, but with inhibition of LTB_4 production from neutrophils. Early results from zileuton suggested promise [150], comparable to the good results being recorded in respiratory disorders. Unfortunately, an 8-week, randomized, double-blind, controlled trial has shown poorer results than placebo in ulcerative colitis [151]. In maintenance of remission, zileuton is better than placebo, but no more effective than 5-ASA [152].

A leukotriene receptor antagonist appears effective in a rabbit immune colitis model, but human studies are still in their earliest stages [110]. Verapamil, a calcium-channel blocker, has been shown to reduce leukotriene B_4 release and accelerate healing in experimental colitis in the rat. This is probably because 5-lipoxygenase is calcium dependent; the use of calcium-channel blockers warrants study in man [153].

Prostaglandins in the normal gastrointestinal tract appear to have a protective role, contributing (for example) to microvascular integrity and mucus production. It is tempting to associate their inhibition with the general tendency of non-steroidal anti-inflammatory agents to worsen inflammatory bowel disease, and it was accordingly logical to explore therapeutic use of prostaglandin analogues. Unfortunately, misoprostol (one such agent) exacerbated proctitis (unpublished data). The undoubted efficacy of the 5-ASA drugs (which are after all a form of non-steroidal) contributes further paradox in this regard. Differing influence on expression of the two main classes of cyclo-oxygenase may provide the explanation. In the normal intestine, protective eicosanoids are synthesized by a constitutively expressed cyclo-oxygenase, but in inflammatory states an inducible cyclo-oxygenase (Cox-2) predominates, with uncoupling of oxidative phosphorylation and inhibition of prostaglandin synthesis [154]. There are preliminary data indicating that increased levels of mucosal inducible cyclo-oxygenase are associated with failure of steroid treatment in ulcerative colitis [155]. The interested reader is referred also to a recent review which considers the eicosanoids and their effects in the normal and diseased intestine in more detail [156].

THROMBOXANE SYNTHESIS INHIBITORS AND ANTAGONISTS

Thromboxanes are produced in excess in both ulcerative colitis and Crohn's disease [157–159]. They are produced by activated neutrophils, mononuclear cells and platelets. Increased mucosal permeability may be the trigger to their release, through allowing entry of bacterial antigens (such as lipopolysaccharides) which induce neutrophil activation. Ridogrel and picotamide both inhibit thromboxane A_2 synthesis and competitively block its receptors; ridogrel also blocks receptors for prostaglandin endoperoxide at higher dose. They may have a role in inflammatory bowel disease, given the demonstration of reduction of thromboxane A_2 and concomitant increase in thromboxane B_2 in incubated biopsy material from patients with both ulcerative colitis and Crohn's disease [159]. Picotamide also has important effects on platelet function and a fibrinolytic effect, and both agents stimulate production of prostacyclin. They are effective in experimental models of colitis, and preliminary studies in man are encouraging [158]. Unfortunately, work on picotamide is temporarily suspended for commercial reasons. Ridogrel is, however, being investigated actively in both major forms of inflammatory bowel disease. In a small comparative study in patients with ulcerative colitis, there were clinical and endoscopic improvements from oral ridogrel in a similar proportion to that from oral 5-ASA [160]. Concurrent colonic perfusion estimations confirmed that ridogrel had a more selective effect in reducing thromboxane B$_2$ (to 31% of basal) without the potentially adverse influence of the 5-ASA on prostaglandin levels. More recent abstract data on oral and rectal use of ridogrel in moderately active ulcerative colitis support a response rate comparable to oral mesalazine and rectal prednisolone, respectively [161, 162]. Sufficiently stringent trials are now under way.

TUMOUR NECROSIS FACTOR AND OTHER CYTOKINES

The pro-inflammatory cytokines are abnormally represented, contribute to the inflammatory response and may have an aetiological role in inflammatory bowel disease (Chapter 1) [163, 164]. Accordingly, a variety of means of their selective inhibition (by reduced synthesis, impaired release or by inhibited action) are under investigation. Preliminary reports of the use of monoclonal antibodies to anti-tumour necrosis factor-α (TNF-α) in refractory Crohn's disease yield particularly encouraging results.

A chimeric neutralizing antibody to TNF-α (cA2) was first used in an open study in 10 Crohn's patients with intractable disease [165]. One patient was unassessable because of an iatrogenic colonic perforation, but eight of the remainder had significant improvements in Crohn's Disease Activity Index (CDAI) and endoscopic healing by 4 weeks. The clinical responses had an average duration of 4 months. Concomitant histological improvements in Crohn's disease, but not in ulcerative colitis, were seen in another small study of the same antibody [166]. Two larger, multicentre trials of the cA2 antibody in Crohn's have also been presented [167, 168]. The McCabe study [167] gives additional safety information for single doses up to 20 mg/kg, and although a 90% response rate is quoted, this was an uncontrolled, open study. Targan's study, on the contrary, was a placebo-controlled trial of 108 patients with active Crohn's disease treated with 5, 10 or 20 mg/kg as a single dose and followed for 12 weeks [168]. The published abstract does give the response rate but these results were given at Digestive Diseases Week, San Francisco, May 1996. Taking a reduction in CDAI of at least 70 points as the primary end-point, there was a clear response to TNF-α antibody. There was remission in under 20% of the placebo group at all time points, whereas in each group treated with the antibody there was a response rate in excess of 50% at 2 and 4 weeks. By 12 weeks about one-third of all treated patients remained in remission. The response to further doses and incidence of neutralizing antibody formation is not yet known, but tachyphylaxis is expected.

The British multicentre TNF-α study, also in patients with active Crohn's disease (CDAI > 150), employed a different monoclonal antibody, CDP571, which is a cleverly engineered IgG4 designed to maximize its humanness and to reduce immunogenicity [169]. This was a relatively small study which fell short of a true placebo-controlled trial, but there was a significant response by standard criteria (CDAI, Harvey–Bradshaw, C-reactive protein (CRP)) at 2 weeks in patients receiving a single 5 mg/kg infusion of the antibody in comparison with the baseline values. Only a minority of treated patients achieved a full remission, and the effect did not appear to last as long as that quoted for cA2; by 4 weeks there was no longer any obvious difference from the entry criteria. Despite the humanized TNF antibody, seven of the treated patients developed antibodies directed against the therapeutic agent.

Both TNF-α antibodies have also been used to apparently good effect in small studies of ulcerative colitis, CDP571 in mild to moderate disease [170], and cA2 in severely ill, steroid-refractory patients [171].

TNF-α may be manipulated by means other than neutralizing antibodies. Thalidomide provides one such alternative route to benefit in inflammatory bowel disease. After reports indicating a useful therapeutic effect in a variety of inflammatory conditions, an impressive account of its value in two patients with HIV-related aphthae [172] has been critically discussed with reference to potential mechanisms [173]. Thalidomide is a specific inhibitor of TNF-α through enhanced degradation of TNF-α mRNA, which is probably how it exerts its activity in inflammatory conditions – immunomodulation without immunosuppression [174]. Only anecdotal data exist for thalidomide therapy in inflammatory bowel disease, especially in the management of intractable and painful oral ulcers in Crohn's disease, but formal trial is perhaps now warranted. Clearly the risk of phocomelia will always preclude its use in all but the very most carefully selected female patients.

It is also possible to inhibit TNF-α with oral pentoxifylline, but although an open study of 1.6 g daily in 16 steroid-dependent Crohn's patients confirms its suppressant effect on TNF-α secretion from *ex vivo* stimulated monocytes, no effect on any of the standard measures of disease activity (CDAI, CRP, endoscopic score) could be demonstrated [175]. If these results are correct, it suggests that the TNF-α antibody results stem from other mechanisms.

It is a reasonable hope that protocols to achieve better and prolonged neutralization of TNF-α will provide useful therapeutic advance. Whether the relatively clumsy use of antibodies to achieve this ambition will be the best route remains to be seen. Development of alternative 'small molecule' TNF-α receptor blockers that can be given orally is one possibility, the use of matrix metalloprotein inhibitors – which probably prevent initiation of the inflammatory cascade in a more general way – is another. That manipulation of a single (albeit important) cytokine has any meaningful impact on the clinical manifestations of inflammatory bowel disease is itself somewhat remarkable and should clearly be exploited, even if only as part of a package of targeted therapies.

Interleukin-10

The putatively inadequate IL-10 response in inflammatory bowel disease (Chapter 1) has led to hope that supplementary, therapeutic, IL-10 might be beneficial. Given in combination with zinc, IL-10 helps to prevent free radical damage in intestinal biopsies subjected to oxidative stress [176], and initial promise from an open study of topical IL-10 therapy in resistant distal colitis [177] has prompted further trials both in ulcerative colitis and Crohn's.

An extended, placebo-controlled phase II study has now been completed in 45 patients with steroid resistant Crohn's disease [178]. IL-10 was given daily for 7 days and the patients were followed for 4 weeks. Tolerance was good, and, combining the different doses used, there was an overall clinical response in 50% compared to 23% in the placebo group. Larger and more definitive trials in both ulcerative colitis and Crohn's disease are now in progress.

INTRAVENOUS IMMUNOGLOBULIN, T-CELL APHERESIS AND MONOCLONAL ANTIBODIES TO CD4 CELLS

Intravenous immunoglobulin has been used successfully in a number of autoimmune diseases. Given that inflammatory bowel disease may be mediated by an abnormal immune response to an unidentified infectious agent, a gut-associated antigen or an autoimmune disorder, assessment of immunoglobulin therapy has seemed reasonable. Preliminary open-label pilot studies in refractory inflammatory bowel disease are supportive [179], but the uncertain risks of transmission of viral infections (and considerable expense) mandate very careful assessment before sanctioning wider use in inflammatory bowel disease.

On similar grounds, T-cell apheresis and the use of anti-CD4 monoclonal antibodies have been proposed. T-cell apheresis using differential centrifugation has been assessed in patients with chronic resistant Crohn's disease in an open trial [180]. Interpretation of the results is complicated by the simultaneous administration of parenteral nutrition. However, long-term remission with steroid withdrawal in 64 of 72 patients is recorded. The French GETAID group have reported similarly good results from a controlled study of T-cell apheresis in 28 Crohn's patients recently brought to remission by steroids [181]. Steroid tapering and relapse rates were determined. The study group received lymphapheresis (nine procedures within 4–5 weeks) and all 12 achieved full weaning from steroids compared to only five of 12 controls (not significant). No adverse effects were seen, but there was a high rate of relapse in 18 months follow up after treatment (83% in the lymphapheresis group and 62% in the control group). A Japanese group has examined a similar technique in an open study of 30 patients with active ulcerative colitis [182]. The Plasauto 1000 apheresis unit equipped with a Cellsorba leucocyte removal filter was administered at 1 week intervals in 5 weeks of intensive therapy and at approximately 1 month intervals during 5 months of maintenance therapy; around 95% of all passaged white cells were removed. There were no side-effects, and clinical improvement was claimed for 24 patients. Heparin was thought unlikely to have contributed to the effect in the early studies and was not used in later patients (see below). Abnormalities of polymorphonuclear leucocyte function are well documented in inflammatory bowel disease [183] and the global effect on white cells of the Japanese device may explain its apparent effect. Only prolonged remission would justify the invasiveness and costs of such regimes, and it is unlikely that apheresis will ever have more than a peripheral place in inflammatory bowel disease management. It is further disappointing that, a year on, the same group have added only eight patients to their series with no other novel observations [184].

It may be hoped that similar or better results can be obtained from the use of monoclonal antibodies to CD4 cells. Humanized mouse antibodies have been synthesized to reduce the problems to be expected from the development of human anti-mouse antibodies. Initial studies using a chimeric anti-CD4 antibody in patients with active Crohn's disease yielded clinical remission in 10 of 12 patients (83%), with complete steroid withdrawal in two-thirds [185]. However, remissions were not long lasting, and the potential long-term ill-effects of iatrogenic CD4 cell suppression are a cause for concern. In a further study in severe Crohn's disease using a murine monoclonal antibody (B-F5) only four of 12 treated patients appeared to benefit, with sustained remission in only two of these [186].

REACTIVE OXYGEN METABOLITES

Oxygen free-radical production is increased in inflammatory bowel disease. Neutrophils and granulocytes, both in the peripheral circulation and in the intestinal mucosa, responsible for this, almost certainly thereby contribute to the inflammatory process [187] (Chapter 1). In animal models of colitis, inhibition of free-radical production reduces inflammation [188], and Millar *et al.* [189] indicate that this may prove useful in man also, an effect perhaps already in use as one of the mechanisms of action of 5-ASA.

Iron in its ferric state is known to contribute to the generation of reactive oxygen species, prompting a successful trial of chelation with desferrioxamine in pouchitis [190] (Chapter 4). This possibility has not yet been assessed in other forms of inflammatory bowel disease, but the addition of allopurinol (a xanthine oxidase inhibitor) or dimethyl sulphoxide (a hydroxyl radical scavenger) to sulphasalazine maintenance has been shown to improve symptoms and prolong remission in ulcerative colitis [191]. Emerit *et al.* [192] have also reported good long-term results in an open study of refractory Crohn's disease ($n = 34$) using copper zinc superoxide dismutase, an enzyme that accelerates the clearance of O_2^-. Again, controlled trials are awaited.

LOCAL ANAESTHETICS

Evidence for abnormal intestinal innervation [193] (Chapter 1) bolsters the same group's good results (all of 21 patients) from topical lignocaine therapy in distal colitis. There are other reasons for believing that local anaesthetic agents might be of therapeutic value in inflammatory bowel disease, as they can be shown to inhibit leucocyte migration to sites of inflammation [194], and may reduce platelet aggregation and cytokine production [195]. There are, however, still no controlled data for lignocaine use in colitis nor support from other centres, there being only a very modest clinical response in this author's patients given the same dose of topical gel. However, Arlander *et al.* suggest that ropivacaine, a new long-acting local anaesthetic, might usefully be employed [196]. A twice-daily 200 mg dose of ropivacaine gel was given to 12 patients with active distal ulcerative colitis without toxicity, and with indications that endoscopic and histological parameters improved usefully (as did clinical features despite the error in the published abstract that suggests the opposite). Formal comparisons of local anaesthetic agents with established drugs are indicated.

HEPARIN IN THERAPY FOR COLITIS

Heparin is best known as an anticoagulant but, like its endogenous equivalent, heparan, has important anti-inflammatory properties. The anticoagulant effects on thrombin themselves produce secondary inhibition of neutrophil activation and limit pathological increases in endothelial permeability. There is also inhibition of neutrophil elastase which reduces the ability of these cells to penetrate endothelium, associated with inactivation of a range of cytokines and binding of lactoferrin. In discussion of a fascinating case report, the Liverpool group [197] postulates that these effects of heparin contributed to its apparent therapeutic role in their patient (with pathergic arthropathy and pyoderma gangrenosum). It is suggested that margination of neutrophils – the degree to which the cells 'roll' along the endothelium – may be of key importance. This analysis lends scientific support for the impressive results from Eire [198] in which heparin, given for an incidental deep venous thrombosis, was apparently effective in problematic ulcerative colitis. This case and a further nine patients treated by full heparinization have now been reported. Nine of the 10 entered remission, rectal bleeding being the first symptom to resolve. Other centres, especially in Russia, are collecting similar data. Two further small series from Amiens record an apparent useful effect of therapeutic doses of heparin in a majority (7–10) of 13 patients with active Crohn's disease, and in five of six patients with extra-intestinal manifestations, indicating that the agent's actions may not necessarily be confined to ulcerative colitis [199, 200]. Controlled data for any of the uses of heparin in inflammatory bowel disease therapy are as yet lacking.

An apparent congenital absence of enterocyte heparan sulphate was associated with profound protein-losing enteropathy in the absence of conventional microscopic abnormalities in the small bowel biopsies of three infants [201]. Given the case for a therapeutic effect of heparin, it is tempting to speculate, first, whether acquired heparan deficiency is present in active ulcerative colitis, and secondly, if so, whether this could account for the hypoalbuminaemia seen in some colitics, and for the very occasional patient in whom a short bowel syndrome-like state develops and for whom parenteral nutrition becomes necessary.

NICOTINE

Intermittent smokers and those who restart after a period of abstinence often record improvement in ulcerative colitis symptomatology, suggesting that the act of smoking is of continuing direct relevance, and not a marker for other behaviour (or of a genetic predisposition – to both smoking and inflammatory bowel disease phenotype) (Chapter 1). In the absence of satisfactory explanations for these phenomena, it is suggested that nicotine may be an important mediator of the apparent beneficial effect in ulcerative colitis, perhaps acting via an effect on the neuromotor manifestations of acute inflammation. Nicotine has accordingly been assessed as a potential therapeutic agent.

A double-blind placebo-controlled trial of nicotine patches in active ulcerative colitis was reported in 1994 [202]. Encouraging results reached significance, but there were irregularities in the study which came in for some criticism, not least in an accompanying editorial [203]. A similar study has now been reported in abstract form from the Mayo Clinic [204] with comparable results (clinical responses in 39% compared to a mere 9% in the placebo group). These authors included histological assessment, which showed improvement at 4 weeks but of insufficient magnitude to reach significance. The Welsh group have followed up their original study with a maintenance study (see below), and now with a 6-week comparative study using a prednisolone-treated control group [205]. Sixty-one non-smoking patients with mildly to moderately active ulcerative colitis (about 50% of those seen) entered the study, and were randomized to treatment with either oral prednisolone or nicotine patches. Prednisolone was prescribed at 5 mg/day, rising over 9 days to a 15 mg daily dose that then remained static for the remainder of the study period. Nicotine-treated patients received an incremental dose administered by transdermal patch delivering 2.5 mg/day rising 'every 1 to 2 days' to 15 mg, and then to 25 mg daily if remission had not been achieved by 14 days. A reduced dose of nicotine was permitted if side-effects occurred. All other therapy was discontinued. Steroid-treated patients received dummy patches, while nicotine-treated patients had placebo capsules by mouth. Appropriate effort appears to have been taken to modify the dose/size of placebo patches similarly in the steroid-treated group to ensure maximal preservation of blinding. The rather unorthodox (and arguably suboptimal) steroid regime is defended on grounds of simplicity and homogeneity, but it seems a pity that a more conventional reducing course was not accommodated within the trial design. The steroid- and nicotine-treated groups proved well matched; the only differences of potential importance were a greater prior use of steroids in the prednisolone group, and somewhat higher global clinical and histological scores in the nicotine group at trial entry. Outcomes were recorded by intention to treat in respect of clinical, sigmoidoscopic and histological scores. There were fewer withdrawals in the steroid-treated group, and it seems probable that many of the withdrawals from the nicotine group were the result of (predictable) pharmacological effects of nicotine; 19 of 30 completed the trial protocol (compared to 24 of 31 with prednisolone). Lowered nicotine doses were required even amongst three of these, to minimize toxicity and retain compliance. Serum studies of nicotine and cotinine indicate that compliance was, however, as stated to the authors. The efficacy of continued blinding (of patients and investigators) is difficult to judge, but has probably not influenced the results of the study. In those who were able to complete the 6-week study period, there was a remission rate of only 32% with nicotine patches, compared to 58% of those completing 6 weeks in the steroid limb of the study. This difference does not reach significance, but when the data are analysed by intention to treat, prednisolone offers clear and significant advantage (e.g. 47% v. 21% for clinical remission; $p = 0.035$). For no criterion does nicotine score more favourably than prednisolone, and although there was clinical improvement with nicotine treatment, this was not accompanied by sigmoidoscopic improvement.

The authors recognize that the apparent effects of nicotine may be those of the placebo response, but it is reasonable to accept that this is unlikely to be the full explanation. Their previous study seemed to show additive benefit when nicotine was added to a 5-aminosalicylate (5-ASA), and, in the present study, a potential for deterioration from the withdrawal of prior 5-ASA therapy was not seen. It is also reasonable to propose that steroid responders and nicotine responders may be from different cohorts, and therefore that nicotine may have a place for the non-responder as well as for the patient who wishes strongly to avoid steroid treatment.

However, there is no case for nicotine in maintenance of remission of ulcerative colitis. In a careful study, again performed by the Welsh group, the results from nicotine appeared equivalent to those of placebo [206]. As there is unequivocal benefit from 5-ASA maintenance therapy, it is doubtful whether any further studies in this context could be considered legitimate.

The evidence in favour of smoking (as opposed to nicotine administration alone) is insufficient to warrant its recommendation to ulcerative colitis patients, given its other potentially fatal consequences. In Crohn's disease the gastroenterologist has a continuing and unequivocal mandate to direct its cessation.

CONCLUSION

The selective use of intravenous cyclosporin in acute severe colitis, of methotrexate in resistant Crohn's disease, and the 5-ASA derivatives for the maintenance of remission and prevention of postoperative recurrence in Crohn's are now becoming widely accepted. However, all currently available therapies have limited efficacy. Incomplete responses and the potential for short- and long-term toxicity leave a continuing need for pharmacological development. Although the portents are good, surgical intervention will continue to be necessary for a substantial minority of patients with inflammatory bowel disease for the foreseeable future.

REFERENCES

1. Ilnyckyj A, Shanahan F, Anton PA, Cheang M, Bernstein CN. The placebo response in ulcerative colitis. *Gastroenterology* 1996; **110**: A929.
2. Brynskov J, Freund L, Norby Rasmussen S *et al*. A placebo-controlled, double-blind, randomized trial of cyclosporine in active chronic Crohn's disease. *N Engl J Med* 1989; **321**: 845–850.
3. Sutherland L, Singleton J, Sessions J *et al*. Double blind, placebo controlled trial of metronidazole in Crohn's disease. *Gut* 1991; **32**: 1071–1075.
4. Fahey JV, Guyre PM, Munck A. Mechanisms of anti-inflammatory actions of glucocorticoids. In: Weissman G, ed. *Advances in Inflammation Research*, Vol 2. New York: Raven, 1981: 21–51.

5. Reich K, Lingnau F, Williams RM *et al*. Corticosteroids downregulate BCL-2 and induce apoptosis in CD4+ LPL in Crohn's disease. *Gastroenterology* 1996; **110**: A999.

6. Malchow H, Ewe K, Brandes JW *et al*. The European Cooperative Crohn's Disease Study: results of drug treatment. *Gastroenterology* 1984; **86**: 249–266.

7. Polk DB, Hattner JA, Kerner JA Jr. Improved growth and disease activity after intermittent administration of a defined formula diet in children with Crohn's disease. *J Parent Ent Nutr* 1992; **16**: 499–504.

8. McIntyre PB, Macrea FA, Berghouse L *et al*. Therapeutic benefits from a poorly absorbed prednisolone enema in distal colitis. *Gut* 1985; **26**: 822–824.

9. Anderson FH. The rectal approach to treatment in distal ulcerative colitis. *Lancet* 1995; **346**: 520–521.

10. Tarpila S, Turunen U, Sepäälä K *et al*. Budesonide enema in active haemorrhagic proctitis: a controlled trial against hydrocortisone foam enema. *Aliment Pharmacol Ther* 1994; **8**: 591–595.

11. Löfberg R, Thomsen OØ, Langholz E *et al*. Budesonide versus prednisolone retention enemas in active distal ulcerative colitis. *Aliment Pharmacol Ther* 1994; **8**: 623–629.

12. Pruitt, R, Katz S, Bayless T, Levine J. Repeated use of budesonide enema is safe and effective for the treatment of acute flares of distal ulcerative colitis. *Gastroenterology* 1996; **110**: A995.

13. Greenberg GR, Feagon BG, Martin F *et al*. Oral budesonide for active Crohn's disease. *N Engl J Med* 1994; **331**: 836–841.

14. Rutgeerts P, Löfberg R, Malchow H *et al*. A comparison of budesonide with prednisolone for active Crohn's disease. *N Engl J Med* 1994; **331**: 842–845.

15. Gross V, Andus T, Caesar I *et al*. Oral pH-modified release budesonide vs 6-methyl-prednisolone in active Crohn's disease. *Gut* 1995; 37(suppl 2): A104.

16. Campieri M, Ferguson A, Doe W *et al*. Oral budesonide competes favourably with prednisolone in active Crohn's disease. *Gut* 1995; 37(suppl 2): A64.

17. Löfberg R, Danielsson A, Suhr O *et al*. Oral budesonide versus prednisolone in patients with active extensive and left-sided ulcerative colitis. *Gastroenterology* 1996; **110**: 1713–1718.

18. Hawthorne AB, Record CO, Holdsworth CD *et al*. Double blind trial of oral fluticasonepropionate v prednisolone in the treatemnt of active ulcerative colitis. *Gut* 1993; **34**: 125–128.

19. Greenberg GR, Feagon BG, Martin F *et al*. Oral budesoninde as maintenance treatment for Crohn's disease: a placebo-controlled, dose ranging study. *Gastroenterology* 1996; **110**: 45–51.

20. Löfberg R, Rutgeerts P, Malchow H *et al*. Budesonide prolongs time to relapse in ileal and ileocaecal Crohn's disease. A placebo controlled one year study. *Gut* 1996; **39**: 82–86.
21. D'Haens G, Verstraete A, Baert F *et al*. Osteoblast function is suppressed by oral methylprednisolone but not by budesonide CIR in active ileocolonic Crohn's disease. *Gastroenterology* 1996; **110**: A894.
22. Misiewicz JJ, Lennard-Jones JE, Connell AM *et al*. Controlled trial of sulphasalazine in maintenance therapy for ulcerative colitis. *Lancet* 1965; **i**: 185–188.
23. Greenfield SM, Punchard NA, Teare JP, Thompson PH. Review article: the mode of action of aminosalicylates in inflammatory bowel disease. *Aliment Pharmacol Ther* 1993; **7**: 369–383.
24. Hartley MG, Hudson MJ, Swarbrick ET *et al*. Sulphasalazine treatment and the colorectal mucosa-associated flora in ulcerative colitis. *Aliment Pharmacol Ther* 1996; **10**: 157–163.
25. Järnerot G. Withdrawal rates because of diarrhea in Dipentum treated patients with ulcerative colitis are low when Dipentum is taken with food and dose-titrated. *Gastroenterology* 1996; **110**: A932.
26. McIntyre PB, Rodrigues CA, Lennard-Jones JE *et al*. Balsalazide in the maintenance treatment of patients with ulcerative colitis, a double-blind comparison with sulphasalazine. *Aliment Pharmacol Ther* 1988; **2**: 237–243.
27. Green JRB, Holdsworth CD, Lobo AJ *et al*. Balsalazide is more effective and better tolerated than mesalazine in acute ulcerative colitis. *Gut* 1996; **39**(suppl 1): A17.
28. Sutherland LR, May GR, Shaffer EA. Sulfasalazine revisited: a meta-analysis of 5-aminosalicylic acid in the treatment of ulcerative colitis. *Ann Intern Med* 1993; **118**: 540–549.
29. Abenhaim L, Sutherland LR, Field LG *et al*. Has the introduction of a new mesalamine containing compound altered the clinical course of ulcerative colitis patients? *Gastroenterology* 1996; **110**: A850.
30. Courtney M, Nunes D, Bergin C *et al*. Randomised comparison of olsalazine and mesalazine in prevention of relapses in ulcerative colitis. *Lancet* 1992; **339**: 1279–1281.
31. Laursen LS, Stokholm M, Bukhave K *et al*. Disposition of 5-aminosalicylic acid by olsalazine and three mesalazine preparations in patients with ulcerative colitis: comparison of intraluminal colonic concentrations, serum values, and urinary excretion. *Gut* 1990; **31**: 1271–1276.
32. Kruis W, Schreiber S, Theuer D *et al*. Comparison of an azo-bound amino-salicylate (olsalazine) vs a coated amino-salicylate (mesalamine) for active ulcerative colitis. *Gastroenterology* 1996; **110**: A942.

33. Fockens P, Mulder CJJ, Tytgat GNJ et al. Comparison of the efficacy and safety of 1.5 vs 3.0g oral slow-release mesalazine (Pentasa) in the maintenance treatment of ulcerative colitis. *Eur J Gastroenterol Hepatol* 1995; **7**: 1025–1030.

34. Schroeder KW, Tremaine WJ, Ilstrup DM. Coated oral 5-aminosalicylic acid therapy for mildly to moderately active ulcerative colitis. A randomized study. *N Engl J Med* 1987; **317**: 1625–1629.

35. Ardizzone S, Imbesi V, Molteni P et al. Is therapy always necessary for patients with ulcerative colitis in remission? *Gastroenterology* 1996; **110**: A856.

36. Prantera C, Pallone F, Brunetti G et al. Oral 5-aminosalicylic acid (Asacol) in the maintenance treatment of Crohn's disease. *Gastroenterology* 1992; **103**: 363–368.

37. Messori A, Brignola C, Trallori G et al. Effectiveness of 5-aminosalicylic acid for maintaining remission in patients with Crohn's disease: a meta-analysis. *Am J Gastroenterol* 1994; **89**: 692–698.

38. Caprilli R, Andreoli A, Capurso L et al. Oral mesalazine (5-aminosalicylic acid; Asacol) for the prevention of post-operative recurrence of Crohn's disease. *Aliment Pharmacol Ther* 1994; **8**: 35–43.

39. McLeod RS, Wolff BG, Steinhart AH et al. Prophylactic mesalamine treatment decreases postoperative recurrence of Crohn's disease. *Gastroenterology* 1995; **109**: 404–413.

40. Rutgeerts P, Heboes K, Vantrappen G et al. Predictability of the post-operative course of Crohn's disease. *Gastroenterology* 1990; **99**: 956–963.

41. Florent C, Cortot A, Quandale P et al. Placebo-controlled clinical trial of mesalazine in the prevention of early endoscopic recurrences after resection for Crohn's disease. *Eur J Gastroenterol Hepatol* 1996; **8**: 229–234.

42. Singleton JW, Hanauer SB, Gitnick GL et al. Mesalamine capsules for the treatment of active Crohn's disease: results of a 16-week trial. *Gastroenterology* 1993; **104**: 1293–1301.

43. Tremaine W. Maintenance of remission in Crohn's disease: Is 5-aminosalicylic acid the answer? *Gastroenterology* 1992; **103**: 694–704.

44. Anonymous. Nephrotoxicity associated with mesalazine. *Current Problems* (Committee on Safety of Medicines) 1990; **30**: 2.

45. Thuluvath PJ, Ninkovic M, Calam J, Anderson M. Mesalazine induced interstitial nephritis. *Gut* 1994; **35**: 1493–1496.

46. Hussain F, Ajjan R, Weir N, Trudgill N, Riley S. Single and divided dose delayed-release mesalazine: are traditional dosing regimens outmoded? *Gastroenterology* 1996; **110**: A928.

47. Asacol Study Group. Sensitive markers of renal dysfunction are elevated in chronic ulcerative colitis. *Gastroenterology* 1995; **108**: A919.

48. Bonnet J, Lemann M, Prunat A *et al*. Renal function in patients with inflammatory bowel disease on long-term mesalazine or olsalazine. *Gastroenterology* 1995; **108**: A786.

49. Sturgeon JB, Bhatia P, Hermens D, Miner PB Jr. Exacerbation of chronic ulcerative colitis with mesalamine. *Gastroenterology* 1995; **108**: 1889–1893.

50. Farthing MJG, Rutland MD, Clark ML. Retrograde spread of hydrocortisone containing foam given intrarectally in ulcerative colitis. *Br Med J* 1979; **287**: 822–824.

51. Van Bodegraven AA, Boer RO, Lourens J *et al*. Distribution of mesalazine enemas in active and quiescent ulcerative colitis. *Aliment Pharmacol Ther* 1996; **10**: 327–332.

52. Danish 5-ASA Group. Topical 5-aminosalicylic acid versus prednisolone in ulcerative proctosigmoiditis. A randomized, double-blind multicenter trial. *Dig Dis Sci* 1987; **32**: 598–602.

53. Rowasa Study Group. A double-blind comparison of oral versus rectal mesalamine versus combination therapy in the treatment of distal ulcerative colitis. *Gastroenterology* 1995; **108**: A909.

54. Lee FI, Jewell DP, Mani V *et al*. A randomised trial comparing mesalazine and prednisolone foam enemas in patients with acute distal ulcerative colitis. *Gut* 1996; **38**: 229–233.

55. Marshall JK, Irvine EJ. Rectal corticosteroids are not the best therapy for distal ulcerative colitis. *Gastroenterology* 1996; **110**: A957.

56. Mulder CJJ, Fockens P, Meijer JWR *et al*. Beclomethasone diproprionate (3mg) versus 5-aminosalicylic acid (2g) versus the combination of both (3mg/2g) as retention enemas in active ulcerative proctitis. *Eur J Gastroenterol Hepatol* 1996; **8**: 549–554.

57. Safdi M, DeMicco M, Sninsky C *et al*. A double-blind comparison of oral versus rectal mesalamine versus combination therapy in the treament of distal ulcerative colitis. *Gastroenterology* 1995; **108**: A909.

58. Campieri M, Gionchetti P, Rizzello F *et al*. A controlled trial comparing oral versus rectal mesalazine in the treatment of ulcerative proctitis. *Gastroenterology* 1996; **110**: A876.

59. Campieri M, Gionchetti P, Belluzi A *et al*. Optimum dosage of 5-aminosalicylic acid as rectal enemas in patients with active ulcerative colitis. *Gut* 1991; **32**: 929–931.

60. D'Albasio G, Pacini F, Camarri E *et al*. Combined therapy with 5-aminosalicylic acid tablets and enemas for maintaining remission in ulcerative colitis: results at 12 months. *Gastroenterology* 1995; **108**: A805.

61. O'Donnell LJ, Arvind AS, Hoang P *et al*. Double blind, controlled trial of 4-aminosalicylic acid and prednisolone enemas in distal ulcerative colitis. *Gut* 1992; **33**: 947–949.

62. Marteau P, Halphen M. Etude comparative ouverte randomisée de l'efficacité et de la tolérance de lavements de 2g d'acide 4-amino-salicylique (4-ASA) et de 1g d'acide 5-amino-salicylique (5-ASA) dans les formes basses de rectocolite hémorragique. *Gastroenterol Clin Biol* 1995; **19**: 31–35.

63. Kozarek RA. Review article: immunosuppressive therapy for inflammatory bowel disease. *Aliment Pharmacol Ther* 1993; **7**: 117–123.

64. Present DH, Korelitz BI, Wisch N *et al.* Treatment of Crohn's disease with 6-mercaptopurine. A long-term randomized double-blind study. *N Engl J Med* 1980; **402**: 981–987.

65. O'Donoghue DP, Dawson AM, Powell-Tuck J *et al.* Double blind withdrawal trial of azathioprine as maintenance treatment for Crohn's disease. *Lancet* 1978; **ii**: 955–957.

66. Markowitz J, Rosa J, Grancher K *et al.* Long term 6-mercaptopurine treatment in adolescents with Crohn's disease. *Gastroenterology* 1990; **99**: 1347–1351.

67. Korelitz BI, Present DH. Favorable effect of 6-mercaptopurine on fistulae of Crohn's disease. *Dig Dis Sci* 1985; **30**: 58–64.

68. Lémann M, Cuillerier E, Bouhnik Y *et al.* Azathioprine for prevention of Crohn's recurrence after ileal or colonic resection. *Gastroenterology* 1996; **110**: A948.

69. Kirk AP, Lennard-Jones JE. Controlled trial of azathioprine in chronic ulcerative colitis. *Br Med J* 1982; **284**: 1291–1292.

70. Present DH. 6-Mercaptopurine and other immunosuppressive agents in the treatment of Crohn's disease and ulcerative colitis. *Gastroenterol Clin N Am* 1989; **18**: 57–71.

71. Adler DJ, Korelitz BI. The therapeutic efficacy of 6-mercaptopurine in refractory ulcerative colitis. *Am J Gastroenterol* 1990; **85**: 717–722.

72. Hawthorne AB, Logan RFA, Hawkey CJ *et al.* Randomised controlled trial of azathioprine withdrawal in ulcerative colitis. *Br Med J* 1992; **305**: 20–22.

73. Connell WR, Kamm MA, Ritchie JK, Lennard-Jones JE. Bone marrow toxicity caused by azathioprine in inflammatory bowel disease: 27 years of experience. *Gut* 1993; **34**: 1081–1085.

74. Present DH, Meltzer ST, Krumholz MP *et al.* 6-Mercaptopurine in the management of inflammatory bowel disease: short- and long-term toxicity. *Ann Int Med* 1989; **111**: 641–649.

75. Colonna T, Korelitz BI. The role of leukopenia in the 6-mercaptopurine induced remission of refractory Crohn's disease. *Am J Gastroenterol* 1994; **89**: 362–366.

76. Berg PS, George J, Present DH *et al.* 6MP – is leukopenia required to induce remission in the treatment of ulcerative colitis? *Gastroenterology* 1996; **110**: A863.

77. Sandborn WJ, Van Os EC, Zins B *et al.* An intravenous loading dose of azathioprine decreases the time to response in patients with Crohn's disease. *Gastroenterology* 1995; **109**: 1808–1817.

78. Bouhnik Y, Lémann M, Mary J-Y *et al.* Long-term follow-up of patients with Crohn's disease treated with azathioprine or 6-mercaptopurine. *Lancet* 1996; **347**: 215–219.

79. Hodgson H. Cyclosporin in inflammatory bowel disease. *Aliment Pharmacol Ther* 1991; **5**: 343–350.

80. Lichtiger S, Present DH, Kornbluth A *et al.* Cyclosporine in severe ulcerative colitis refractory to steroid therapy. *N Engl J Med* 1994; **330**: 1841–1845.

81. Jewell DP, Lennard-Jones JE and the cyclosporin study group of Great Britain and Ireland. Oral cyclosporin for chronic active Crohn's disease. *Eur J Gastroenterol Hepatol* 1994; **6**: 499–505.

82. Feagan BG, McDonald JWD, Rochon J *et al.* Low-dose cyclosporine for the treatment of Crohn's disease. *N Engl J Med* 1994; **330**: 1846–1851.

83. Stange EF, Modigliani R, Pena AS *et al.* European trial of cyclosporine in chronic active Crohn's disease: a 12 month study. *Gastroenterology* 1995; **109**: 774–782.

84. Present DH, Lichtiger S. Efficacy of cyclosporine in treatment of fistula of Crohn's disease. *Dig Dis Sci* 1994; **39**: 374–380.

85. Chapman RW, Selby WS, Jewell DP. Controlled trial of intravenous metronidazole as an adjunct to corticosteroids in severe ulcerative colitis. *Gut* 1986; **27**: 1210–1212.

86. Sandborn WJ, Tremaine WJ, Schroeder KW *et al.* A placebo-controlled trial of cyclosporine enemas for mildly to moderately active left-sided ulcerative colitis. *Gastroenterology* 1994; **106**: 1429–1435.

87. Abreu-Martin MT, Vasiliauskas EA, Gaiennie J *et al.* Continuous infusion cyclosporine is effective for severe acute Crohn's disease ... but for how long? *Gastroenterology* 1996; **110**: A851.

88. Vega R, Bertrán X, Fernández-Bañares F *et al.* Cytomegalovirus infection in steroid resistant inflammatory bowel disease. *Gastroenterology* 1996; **110**: A1038.

89. Sternthal M, George J, Kornbluth A *et al.* Toxicity associated with the use of cyclosporin in patients with inflammatory bowel disease. *Gastroenterology* 1996; **110**: A1019.

90. Yee GC, Stanley DL, Pessa LJ. Effect of grapefruit juice on blood cyclosporin concentration. *Lancet* 1995; **345**: 955–956.

91. Kozarek R, Patterson D, Gelfand M *et al.* Methotrexate induces clinical and histologic remission in patients with refractory inflammatory bowel disease. *Ann Int Med* 1989; **110**: 353–356.

92. Feagan BG, Rochon J, Fedorak RN, Irvine EJ. Methotrexate for the treatment of Crohn's disease. *N Engl J Med* 1995; **332**: 292–297.

93. Lémann M, Chamiot-Prieur C, Mesnard B *et al.* Methotrexate for the treatment of refractory Crohn's disease. *Aliment Pharmacol Ther* 1996; **10**: 309–314.

94. Zenjari T, Lémann M, Mesnard B *et al.* Methotrexate in Crohn's disease: long-term efficacy and toxicity. *Gastroenterology* 1996; **110**: A1053.

95. Oren R, Arber N, Odes S *et al.* Methotrexate in chronic active ulcerative colitis: a double-blind, randomized, Israeli multicenter trial. *Gastroenterology* 1996; **110**: 1416–1421.

96. Whiting-O'Keefe QE, Fye KH, Sack KD. Methotrexate and histologic hepatic abnormalities: a meta-analysis. *Am J Med* 1991; **90**: 711–716.

97. Reynolds J, Trellis D, Abu-Elmagd K, Fung J. The rationale for FK506 in inflammatory bowel disease. *Can J Gastroenterol* 1993; **7**: 208–210.

98. Kitano A, Matsumoto T, Nakamura S *et al.* New treatment of ulcerative colitis with K-76. *Dis Colon Rectum* 1992; **35**: 560–567.

99. Sartor RB. Antimicrobial therapy of inflammatory bowel disease: Implications for pathogenesis and management. *Can J Gastroenterol* 1993; **7**: 132–138.

100. Ambrose NS, Allan RN, Keighley MR *et al.* Antibiotic therapy for treatment in relapse of intestinal Crohn's disease. A prospective randomized study. *Dis Colon Rectum* 1985; **28**: 81–85.

101. Rutgeerts P, Hiele M, Geboes K *et al.* Controlled trial of metronidazole treatment for prevention of Crohn's recurrence after ileal resection. *Gastroenterology* 1995; **108**: 1617–1621.

102. Duffy LF, Daum F, Fisher SE *et al.* Peripheral neuropathy in Crohn's disease patients treated with metronidazole. *Gastroenterology* 1985; **88**: 681–684.

103. Burke DA, Axon AT, Clayden SA *et al.* The efficacy of tobramycin in the treatment of ulcerative colitis. *Aliment Pharmacol Ther* 1990; **4**: 123–129.

104. Casellas F, Papo M, Guarner F *et al.* A trial of enteric coated amoxycillin–clavulinic acid in active ulcerative colitis. *Gastroenterology* 1996; **110**: A878.

105. Turunen U, Farkkila M, Hakala K *et al.* A double-blind, placebo controlled six-month ciprofloxacin treatment improves prognosis in ulcerative colitis. *Gastroenterology* 1994; **106**: A786.

106. Mantzaris GJ, Archavlis E, Christoforidis P. A prospective, randomized controlled trial of oral ciprofloxacin in acute ulcerative colitis. *Gastroenterology* 1996; **110**: A955.

107. Moss A, Carbone J, Kressel H. Radiologic and clinical assessment of broad-spectrum antibiotic therapy in Crohn's disease. *Am J Roentgenol* 1978; **131**: 787–790.

108. Peppercorn MA. Is there a role for antibiotics as primary therapy in Crohn's ileitis? *J Clin Gastroenterol* 1993; **17**: 235–237.

109. Reimund JM, Dumont S, Muller CD *et al.* Effect of ciprofloxacine upon cytokine production by peripheral blood mononuclear cells and intestinal biopsies in inflammatory bowel diseases. *Gastroenterology* 1996; **110**: A1000.

110. Lichtenstein G. Medical therapies for inflammatory bowel disease. *Current Opinion in Gastroenterology* 1993; **9**: 588–599.

111. Thayer WR, Reinert SE, Natarajan R, Szaro J. Rifabutin/streptomycin in the treatment of Crohn's disease. A double-blind controlled trial. *Gastroenterology* 1996; **110**: A1027.

112. Samuelsson SM, Ekbom A, Zack M *et al.* Risk factors for extensive ulcerative colitis and ulcerative proctitis: a population based case-control study. *Gut* 1991; **32**: 1526–1530.

113. Griffiths AM, Ohlsson A, Sherman PM, Sutherland LR. Meta-analysis of enteral nutrition as a primary treatment of active Crohn's disease. *Gastroenterology* 1995; **108**: 1056–1067.

114. Silk DB. Medical management of severe inflammatory disease of the rectum: nutritional aspects. *Baillières Clin Gastroenterol* 1992; **6**: 27–41.

115. O'Morain CA. Nutritional therapy in ambulatory patients. *Dig Dis Sci* 1987; **32**: 95S–99S.

116. Giaffer MH, Cann P, Holdsworth CD. Long-term effects of elemental and exclusion diets for Crohn's disease. *Aliment Pharmacol Ther* 1991; **5**: 115–125.

117. Teahon K, Bjarnason I, Pearson M, Levi AJ. Ten years' experience with an elemental diet in the management of Crohn's disease. *Gut* 1990; **31**: 1133–1137.

118. O'Brien CJ, Giaffer MH, Cann P, Holdsworth CD. Elemental diet in steroid-dependent and steroid-refractory Crohn's disease. *Am J Gastroenterol* 1991; **86**: 1614–1618.

119. O'Morain C, Segal AW, Levi AJ. Elemental diet as primary treatment of acute Crohn's disease: a controlled trial. *Br Med J* 1984; **288**: 1859–1862.

120. Saverymuttu S, Hodgson HJF, Chadwick VS. Controlled trial comparing prednisolone with an elemental diet plus non-absorbable antibiotics in active Crohn's disease. *Gut* 1985; **26**: 994–998.

121. Sanderson IR, Udeen S, Davies PSW *et al.* Remission inducuced by an elemental diet in small bowel Crohn's disease. *Arch Dis Child* 1987; **61**: 123–127.

122. Malchow H, Steinhardt HJ, Lorenz-Meyer H *et al.* Feasibility and effectiveness of a defined-formula diet regimen in treating active Crohn's disease. European Co-operative Crohn's disease Study III. *Scand J Gastroenterol* 1990; **25**: 235–244.

123. Thomas AG, Taylor F, Miller V. Dietary intake and nutritional treatment in childhood Crohn's disease. *J Pediatr Gastroenterol Nutr* 1993; **17**: 75–81.

124. González-Huix F, De León R, Fernández-Bañares F *et al*. Polymeric enteral diets as primary treatment of active Crohn's disease: a prospective steroid controlled trial. *Gut* 1993; **34**: 778–782.

125. Seidman EG, Griffiths AM, Jones A, Isserman R. Semielemental diet versus prednisone in the treatment of active Crohn's disease in children and adolescents. *Gastroenterology* 1993; **104**: A778.

126. Gorard DA, Hunt JB, Payne-James JJ *et al*. Initial response and subsequent course of Crohn's disease treated with elemental diet or prednisolone. *Gut* 1993; **34**: 1198–1202.

127. Lochs H, Steinhardt HJ, Klaus-Wentz XX *et al*. Comparison of enteral nutrition and drug treatment in active Crohn's disease. Results of European Co-operative Crohn's disease Study IV. *Gastroenterology* 1991; **101**: 881–888.

128. Pearson M, Teahon K, Levi AJ, Bjarnason I. Food intolerance and Crohn's disease. *Gut* 1993; **34**: 783–787.

129. Riordan AM, Hunter JO, Cowan RE *et al*. Treatment of active Crohn's disease by exclusion diet: East Anglian multicentre controlled trial. *Lancet* 1993; **342**: 1131–1134.

130. Davison SM, Johnson T, Chapman S *et al*. Disease localisation in elemental diet therapy for Crohn's disease: a study of response using 99mTc-HMPAO leukocyte scintigraphy. *Gastroenterology* 1996; **110**: A797.

131. Alun Jones V, Dickinson RJ, Workman E *et al*. Crohn's disease: maintenance of remission by diet. *Lancet* 1985; **ii**: 177–180.

132. Wilschanski M, Sherman P, Pencharz P *et al*. Supplementary enteral nutrition maintains remission in paediatric Crohn's disease. *Gut* 1996; **38**: 543–548.

133. Greenberg G. Nutritional support in inflammatory bowel disease: Current status and future directions. *Scand J Gastroenterol* 1992; **27**(suppl 192): 117–122.

134. Norday A. Is there a rational role for N-3 fatty acids (fish oil) in clinical medicine? *Drugs* 1991; **42**: 331.

135. Eliakim R, Karmeli F, Chorev M *et al*. Effect of drugs on colonic eicosanoid accumulation in active ulcerative colitis. *Scand J Gastroenterol* 1992; **27**: 968–972.

136. Stenson W, Cort D, Rodgers J *et al*. Dietary supplementation with fish oil in ulcerative colitis. *Ann Int Med* 1992; **87**: 609–614.

137. Hawthorne AB, Daneshmend TK, Hawkey CJ *et al*. Treatment of ulcerative colitis with fish oil supplementation: a prospective 12 month randomised controlled trial. *Gut* 1992; **33**: 922–928.

138. Belluzzi A, Brignola C, Campieri M *et al*. Effect of an enteric-coated fish-oil preparation on relapses in Crohn's disease. *N Engl J Med* 1996; **334**: 1557–1560.

139. Roediger WEW. The colonic eipithelium in ulcerative colitis: an energy deficiency disease? *Lancet* 1980; ii: 712–715.
140. Harig JM, Soergel KH, Komorowski RA, Wood CM. Treatment of diversion colitis with short chain fatty acid irrigation. *N Engl J Med* 1989; **320**: 23–28.
141. Pitcher MCL, Cummings JH. Hydrogen sulphide: a bacterial toxin in ulcerative colitis? *Gut* 1996; **39**: 1–4.
142. Senagore A, MacKeigan J, Scheider M, Ebrom S. Short chain fatty acid enemas: A cost effective alternative in the treatment of nonspecific proctosigmoiditis. *Dis Colon Rectum* 1992; **35**: 923–927.
143. Nightingale JMD, Rathbone BJ, West KP *et al.* Butyrate enemas are less effective than prednisolone enemas in treating distal or left sided ulcerative colitis. *Gut* 1995; **37**(suppl 2): A41.
144. Steinhart AH, Hiruki T, Brzezinski A, Baker JP. Treatment of left-sided ulcerative colitis with butyrate enemas: a controlled trial. *Aliment Pharmacol Ther* 1996; **10**: 729–736.
145. Scheppach W, Richter F, Boxberger F *et al.* Effect of short-chain fatty acids on mucosal hyperproliferation in ulcerative colitis. *Gastroenterology* 1996; **110**: A589.
146. Connell AM, Lennard-Jones JE, Misiewicz JJ *et al.* Comparison of acetarsol and prednisolone-21-phosphate suppositories in the treatment of idiopathic proctitis. *Lancet* 1965; i; 238–239.
147. Forbes A, Britton TC, House IM, Gazzard BG. Safety and efficacy of acetarsol suppositories in unresponsive proctitis. *Aliment Pharmacol Ther* 1989; **3**: 553–556.
148. Wardle TD, Hall L, Turnberg LA. Inter-relationships between inflammatory mediators released from colonic mucosa in ulcerative colitis and their effects on colonic secretion. *Gut* 1993; **34**: 503–508.
149. Hawthorne AB, Boughton-Smith NK, Whittle BJ, Hawkey CJ. Colorectal leukotriene B4 synthesis *in vitro* in inflammatory bowel disease: inhibition by the selective 5-lipoxygenase inhibitor BWA4C. *Gut* 1992; **33**: 513–517.
150. Collawn C, Rubin P, Perez N *et al.* Phase II study of the safety and efficacy of a 5-lipoxygenase inhibitor in patients with ulcerative colitis. *Am J Gastroenterol* 1992; **87**: 342–346.
151. Peppercorn M, Das K, Elson C *et al.* Zileuton, a 5-lipoxygenase inhibitor, in the treatment of active ulcerative colitis: a double blind placebo controlled trial. *Gastroenterology* 1994; **106**: A751.
152. Hawkey C, Gassull M, Lauritsen K *et al.* Efficacy of Zileuton, a 5-lipoxygenase inhibitor, in the maintenance of remission in patients with ulcerative colitis. *Gastroenterology* 1994; **106**: A697.
153. Gertner D, Rampton D, Stevens T, Lennard-Jones J. Verapamil inhibits *in-vitro* leucotriene B4 release by rectal mucosa in active ulcerative colitis. *Aliment Pharmacol Ther* 1992; **6**: 163–168.

154. Hayllar J, Bjarnason I. NSAIDs, Cox-2 inhibitors and the gut. *Lancet* 1995; **346**: 521–522.
155. McLaughlin J, Seth R, Cole AT *et al*. Increased inducible cyclooxygenase associated with treatment failure in ulcerative colitis. *Gastroenterology* 1996; **110**: A964.
156. Eberhart CE, Dubois RN. Eicosanoids and the gastrointestinal tract. *Gastroenterology* 1995; **109**: 285–301.
157. Hawkey C, Rampton D. Prostaglandins and the gastrointestinal mucosa: are they important in its function, disease or treatment? *Gastroenterology* 1985; **89**: 1462–1488.
158. Rampton D, Collins C. Review article: thromboxanes in inflammatory bowel disease-pathogenic and therapeutic implications. *Aliment Pharmacol Ther* 1993; **7**: 357–367.
159. Collins CE, Benson MJ, Burnham WR, Rampton DS. Picotamide inhibition of excess *in vitro* thromboxane B2 release by colorectal mucosa in inflammatory bowel disease. *Aliment Pharmacol Ther* 1996; **10**: 315–320.
160. Casellas F, Papo M, Guarner F *et al*. Effects of thromboxane synthase inhibition on *in vivo* release of inflammatory mediators in chronic ulcerative colitis. *Eur J Gastroenterol Hepatol* 1995; **7**: 221–226.
161. Skandalis N, Rotenberg A, Meuwissen S *et al*. Ridogrel for the treatment of mild to moderate ulcerative colitis. *Gastroenterology* 1996; **110**: A1016.
162. Van Outryve M, Huble F, Van Eeghem P, De Vos M. Comparison of ridogrel versus prednisolone both administered rectally, for the treatment of active ulcerative colitis. *Gastroenterology* 1996; **110**: A1035.
163. Beagley K, Elson C. Cells and cytokines in mucosal immunity and inflammation. *Gastroenterol Clin N Am* 1992; **21**: 347–366.
164. Murch S, Lamkin V, Savage M *et al*. Serum concentration of tumour necrosis factor in childhood chronic inflammatory bowel disease. *Gut* 1991; **32**: 913–917.
165. Van Dullemen HM, Van Deventer SJH, Hommes DW *et al*. Treatment of Crohn's disease with anti-tumor necrosis factor chimeric monoclonal antibody (cA2). *Gastroenterology* 1995; **109**: 129–135.
166. Baert F, D'Haens G, Geboes K *et al*. TNF-a antibody therapy causes a fast and dramatic decrease of histologic colonic inflammation in Crohn's disease but not in ulcerative colitis. *Gastroenterology* 1996; **110**: A859.
167. McCabe RP, Woody J, Van Deventer S *et al*. A multicenter trial of cA2 anti-TNF chimeric monoclonal antibody in patients with active Crohn's disease. *Gastroenterology* 1996; **110**: A962.

168. Targan SR, Rutgeerts P, Hanauer SB *et al*. A multicenter trial of anti-tumor necrosis factor antibody (cA2) for treatment of patients with active Crohn's disease. *Gastroenterology* 1996; **110**: A1026.

169. Stack W, Mann S, Roy A *et al*. The effects of CDP571, an engineered human IgG4 anti-TNFa antibody in Crohn's disease. *Gastroenterology* 1996; **110**: A1018.

170. Evans RC, Clark L, Heath P, Rhodes JM. Treatment of ulcerative colitis with an engineered human anti-TNFa antibody CDP571. *Gastroenterology* 1996; **110**: A905.

171. Sands BE, Podolsky DK, Tremaine WJ *et al*. Chimeric monoclonal anti-tumor necrosis factor antibody (cA2) in the treatment of severe, steroid-refractory ulcerative colitis. *Gastroenterology* 1996; **110**: A1008.

172. Ghigliotti G, Repetto T, Farris A *et al*. Thalidomide: Treatment of choice for aphthous ulcers in patients seropositive for human immunodeficiency virus. *J Am Acad Derm* 1993; **28**: 271–272.

173. Oldfield EC. Thalidomide for severe aphthous ulceration in patients with human immonodeficiency virus (HIV) infection. *Am J Gastroenterol* 1994; **89**: 2276–2279.

174. Moreria A, Sampaio E, Zmuidzinas A *et al*. Thalidomide exerts its inhibitory action on tumor necrosis factor alpha by enhancing mRNA degradation. *J Exptl Med* 1993; **177**: 1675–1680.

175. Bauditz J, Haemling J, Nikolaus S *et al*. Treatment of steroid dependent Crohn's disease with pentoxifylline. *Gastroenterology* 1996; **110**: A861.

176. Lih-Brody L, Collier K, Cerchia R *et al*. Zinc and rIL-10 prevents free radical mediated oxidant injury to the intestine. *Gastroenterology* 1996; **110**: A950.

177. Schreiber S, Koop I, Heinig T *et al*. Downregulation of IBD mononuclear phagocyte activation *in vitro* and *in vivo* by interleukin 10. *Gut* 1995; **37**(suppl 2): A112.

178. Van Deventer SJH, Elson CO, Fedorak RN *et al*. Safety, tolerance, pharmacokinetics and pharmacodynamics of recombinant interleukin-10 (SCH 52000) in patients with steroid refractory Crohn's disease. *Gastroenterology* 1996; **110**: A1034.

179. Levin S, Fischer S, Christie D *et al*. Intravenous immunoglobulin therapy for active extensive and medically refractory idiopathic ulcerative or Crohn's colitis. *Am J Gastroenterol* 1992; **87**: 91–100.

180. Bicks RO, Groshart KD. The current status of T-lymphocyte apheresis (TLA) treatment of Crohn's disease. *J Clin Gastroenterol* 1989; **11**: 136–138.

181. Lerebours E, Bussel A, Modigliani R *et al*. Treatment of Crohn's disease by lymphocyte apheresis: a randomized controlled trial. *Gastroenterology* 1994; **107**: 357–361.

182. Sawada K, Ohnishi K, KosakaT *et al.* Leukocytapheresis as new therapy for ulcerative colitis. *Gut* 1995; **37**(suppl 2): A153.

183. Kirk AP, Cason J, Fordham JN *et al.* Polymorphonuclear leukocyte function in ulcerative colitis and Crohn's disease. *Dig Dis Sci* 1983; **28**; 236–248.

184. Sawada K, Ohnishi K, Kosaka T *et al.* Leukocytapheresis as new therapy for ulcerative colitis. *Gastroenterology* 1996; **110**: A1010.

185. Emmrich J, Seyfarth M, Fleig W, Emmrich F. Treatment of inflammatory bowel disease with anti-CD4 monoclonal antibody. *Lancet* 1991; **338**: 570–571.

186. Canva-Delcambre V, Jacquot S, Robinet E *et al.* Treatment of severe Crohn's disease with anti-CD4 monoclonal antibody. *Aliment Pharmacol Ther* 1996; **10**: 721–727.

187. Verspaget H, Mulder T, Van der Sluys Veer A *et al.* Reactive oxygen metabolites and colitis: a disturbed balance between damage and protection: a selective review. *Scand J Gastroenterol* 1991; **26**: 44–51.

188. Kesharvarzian A, Haydeck J, Zabihi R *et al.* Agents capable of eliminating reactive oxygen species. Catalase, WR-2721, or Cu(II)2(2,5-DIPS)4 decrease experimental colitis. *Dig Dis Sci* 1992; **37**: 1866–1873.

189. Millar AD, Blake DR, Rampton DS. An open trial of antioxidant nutrient therapy in active ulcerative colitis. *Gut* 1994; **35**(suppl 5): S29.40.

190. Levin K, Pemberton J, Phillips S *et al.* Role of oxygen free radicals in the aetiology of pouchitis. *Dis Colon Rectum* 1992; **35**: 452–456.

191. Salim A. Role of oxygen derived free radical scavengers in the management of recurrent attacks of ulcerative colitis: a new approach. *J Lab Clinical Med* 1992; **119**: 710–717.

192. Emerit J, Pelletier S, Likforman J *et al.* Phase II trial of copper zinc superoxide dismutase in the treatment of Crohn's disease. *Free Radical Research Communications* 1991; **12–13**: 563–569.

193. Bjørck S, Dahlstrom A, Ahlman H. Topical treatment of ulcerative proctitis with lidocaine. *Scand J Gastroenterol* 1989; **24**: 1061–1072.

194. MacGregor RR, Thorner RE, Wright DM. Lidocaine inhibits granulocyte adherence and prevents granulocyte delivery to inflammatory sites. *Blood* 1980; **56**: 203–209.

195. Feinstein MB, Fiekers J, Fraser C. An analysis of the mechanism of local anesthetic inhibition of platelet aggregation and secretion. *J Pharmacol Exp Ther* 1976; **197**: 215–228.

196. Arlander E, Öst A, Ståhlberg, Löfberg R. Ropivacaine gel in distal ulcerative colitis and proctitis – a pharmacokinetic and exploratory clinical study. *Aliment Pharmacol Ther* 1996; **10**: 73–81.

197. Dwarakanath AD, Yu LG, Brookes C *et al.* 'Sticky' neutrophils pathergic arthritis and response to heparin in pyoderma gangrenosum complicating ulcerative colitis. *Gut* 1995; **37**: 585–588.

198. Gaffney PR, Doyle CT, Gaffney A *et al.* Paradoxical response to heparin in 10 patients with ulcerative colitis. *Am J Gastroenterol* 1995; **90**: 220–223.
199. Dupas JL, Brazier F, Yzet T *et al.* Treatment of active Crohn's disease with heparin. *Gastroenterology* 1996; **110**: A900.
200. Brazier F, Yzet T, Duchmann JC *et al.* Effect of heparin treatment on extra-intestinal manifestations associated with inflammatory bowel disease. *Gastroenterology* 1996; **110**: A872.
201. Murch SH, Winyard PJD, Koletzko S *et al.* Congenital enterocyte heparan sulphate deficiency with massive albumin loss, secretory diarrhoea, and malnutrition. *Lancet* 1996; **347**: 1299–1301.
202. Pullan, RD, Rhodes J, Ganesh S *et al.* Transdermal nicotine for active ulcerative colitis. *N Engl J Med* 1994; **330**: 811–815.
203. Hanauer SB. Nicotine for colitis – the smoke has not yet cleared. *N Engl J Med* 1994; **330**: 856–857.
204. Sandborn WJ, Tremaine W, Offord KP *et al.* A randomized, double-blind, placebo-controlled trial of transdermal nicotine for mildly to moderately active ulcerative colitis. *Gastroenterology* 1996; **110**: A1008.
205. Thomas GAO, Rhodes J, Ragunath K *et al.* Transdermal nicotine compared with oral prednisolone therapy for active ulcerative colitis. *Eur J Gastroenterol Hepatol* 1996; **8**: 769–776.
206. Thomas GAO, Rhodes J, Mani V *et al.* Transdermal nicotine as maintenance therapy for ulcerative colitis. *N Engl J Med* 1995; **332**: 988–992.

4

Problematic ulcerative colitis, and surgery for inflammatory bowel disease

ACUTE SEVERE OR FULMINANT COLITIS

Acute severe or fulminant colitis remains an important clinical problem and is still responsible for major morbidity and occasional mortality. In many respects the medical management is simple, but the necessity for and timing of surgery remain difficult to judge. Much of this section is therefore taken up with consideration of prognostic indicators early in the clinical course, and the related indications for timely surgical intervention. Fulminant colitis was defined in the 1950s by Truelove and Witts from the combination of frequent bloody diarrhoea with evidence of systemic illness. No better definition has emerged than in the form of minor modifications of the original description, such as that of the present Oxford group [1] (Table 4.1).

Most patients with very active disease have many of the signs of systemic disease, and any patient with a complication of aggressive colitis (such as toxic megacolon) would be considered to have fulminant colitis, even in the unlikely event of their absence.

The mortality of fulminant colitis has fallen substantially since the middle of the twentieth century, from around 50% before the introduction of

Table 4.1 Definition of fulminant colitis

In a patient with established ulcerative colitis, the presence of:
  more than 5 bloody stools per 24 hours
  and at least one of:
      fever (>37°C)
      tachycardia (>90/min)
      ESR >30 mm/h
      haemoglobin <100 g/l
      albumin <35 g/l

ESR, erythrocyte sedimentation rate.

steroids in the early 1950s, to around 1.5% in most centres now. However, this reduction has not been the result of single critical changes in practice, as even steroids brought the mortality down only to around 30% in the early 1960s. The improvement almost certainly reflects earlier diagnosis, better medical and perioperative care (including safer anaesthesia), but possibly most importantly the greater sharing of management between physicians and surgeons. Unfortunately this co-operation appears to function least well in centres with the least experience of life-threatening colitis. Any patient sick enough to warrant admission for ulcerative colitis really also warrants referral to both medical and surgical gastroenterologists. This practice makes joint planning easier and eliminates the surgeons' concerns that some patients are referred too late, as well as the physicians' frustrations when having managed the patient actively for some days and reached the conclusion that surgery is inevitable, that the surgeon chooses to observe for a further period while becoming familiar with the patient.

There is rarely a substantial differential diagnosis when the patient is already known to have ulcerative colitis, but the occasional patient with Crohn's disease presents in this way, and the largest group of patients with a final diagnosis of indeterminate colitis are those in whom an initial fulminant presentation led to early resection. However, in the known colitic as well as in the new case, it is essential to exclude infective causes, and perhaps especially, superimposed *Clostridium difficile* infection (Chapter 2).

The immediate management of fulminant colitis includes bed-rest and intravenous steroids, with parenteral fluids and blood if necessary. There are few data favouring a particular steroid, although ACTH may offer minor advantage if the patient has not previously been exposed to steroid therapy. It may not even be necessary to give the steroid parenterally as (for example) in Denmark similar results are obtained from high-dose oral therapy. A daily regime based on prednisolone or methylprednisolone 1 mg/kg, or hydrocortisone 4 mg/kg, is appropriate whichever route is chosen. Some centres consider that the addition of topical steroids is also helpful. Response to steroid therapy can be anticipated in about two-thirds of these patients [2]. There is no evidence that the routine addition of antibiotics is helpful, and one recent study demonstrated a small deleterious difference between treated and untreated groups from the development of antibiotic-related pseudomembranous colitis. There is no place for nutritional intervention as specific therapy (although it will clearly be an important part of adjunctive management and especially so in the malnourished patient). Bowel rest does not appear to offer any advantage, with evidence that normal eating produces similar results to fasting, with or without parenteral nutrition [3].

Urgent surgery is almost always indicated in fulminant colitis if complications arise. It is mandatory in the event of perforation and virtually so in massive haemorrhage (which can be considered to be the case in any patient requiring a transfusion of more than 6 units, or daily administration of blood). Surgery should naturally follow full resuscitative measures and should be performed by an experienced colorectal surgeon.

Toxic megacolon complicates no more than 10% of cases with fulminant colitis, but typically is the major indication for surgery in around 25% of the most urgent cases. The condition is readily defined from the diameter of the colon or caecum on a plain abdominal radiograph (Figure 4.1). It is usually easiest to identify in the transverse colon, where a diameter in excess of 5.5 cm is considered diagnostic in the context of acute colitis. The predominance of this site simply reflects the colonic anatomy, as this is generally the least dependent part of the colon when the patient lies supine and is therefore gas-filled and most easily visualized. A caecal diameter of more than 9 cm has identical significance. Many gastroenterologists and most surgeons consider megacolon to be an absolute indication for colectomy. This is a safe but perhaps unnecessarily aggressive strategy. It is probably reasonable to permit 24 hours of medical therapy in a patient who presents untreated with megacolon, but megacolon developing during therapy or persisting for more than 24 hours despite therapy should lead to colectomy. In this context the value of rolling the patient or encouraging the taking up of certain postures may be valuable (as also in the patient distressed by air insufflation at colonoscopy). The British technique [4] (Figure 4.2) places the patient in the knee–elbow position, while the North American method implies more rolling of the patient (to the prone position every few hours), often combined with the use of a rectal tube to help in deflation of the distal bowel [5]. Both techniques are reported to resolve megacolon without subsequent need for surgery. All forms of medical therapy for megacolon may, however, be considered to be temporizing manoeuvres, as around 50% of patients so treated come to colectomy within a year. Equally, some of these are able to have elective surgery with its obvious advantages relative to emergency resection.

It should be remembered that evidence even for such serious complications as perforation and frank faecal peritonitis can be masked by the high doses of steroids being used. A low threshold for surgical intervention should be maintained.

Predictors for failure of medical therapy once the major complications have been sought and excluded, reflect evidence of disease severity and involvement of the full thickness of the colon. A detailed review of patients presenting to St Mark's Hospital with fulminant colitis identified a number of criteria for poor outcome (Table 4.2). Much more recent data from Oxford [6] led to similar conclusions, shared by Meyers *et al.* in 1987, the latter group finding a short history, extensive colitis, anaemia and high erythrocyte sedimentation rate (ESR) also to be helpful [7]. The new

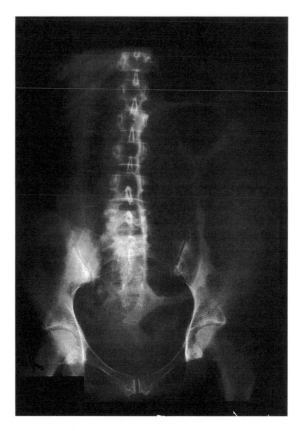

Figure 4.1 Toxic megacolon clearly demonstrated on plain abdominal film. This case was of interest because megacolon developed in the absence of pancolitis, and the well-preserved pattern of taeniae in the right colon even in the presence of distal dilatation testifies to this. There was no response to brief intensive medical therapy; surgery confirmed the severity of the condition but also its persistent limited extent.

Oxford data were derived from study of the 49 patients seen there on 51 occasions over an 18-month period in which cyclosporin was available but not uniformly used (14/51 cases) (Chapter 3). Outcomes were defined as: complete response (<4 stools with no blood by day 7); partial response (>3 stools or blood on day 7 but colectomy not performed that admission); or colectomy. As is typical in studies of fulminant colitis, 29% required colectomy during the acute admission. The stool frequency and the C-reactive protein (CRP) on days 1 to 5 were associated with the final outcomes, such that on day 3, 85% of patients with more than eight stools on that day, or between three and eight stools and a CRP greater than 45, would require colectomy. The authors comment appropriately that these patients should be identified and managed carefully, but there is an ele-

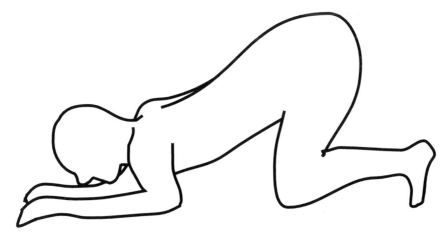

Figure 4.2 The knee–elbow position as advocated for relief of megacolon; when achieved the recto-sigmoid becomes the most superior part of the gastrointestinal tract, facilitating spontaneous passage of flatus.

ment of circular reasoning. Although surgery clearly will not have been decided upon because of continuing bloody diarrhoea and a high CRP alone, this combination is a very powerful one, as it includes a verifiable and distressing symptom, and one of the more objective markers of disease. It is most unlikely, therefore, that they were uninfluenced in their decisions about surgery by the very markers that they now propose as predictors. Of possibly greater value is the observation that the partial responders at 7 days had a 60% chance of continuing symptoms, an 82% risk of needing continuing immunosuppression, and a 40% chance of colectomy during the follow-up period (median 12 months).

The CRP is arguably more informative than the sedimentation rate in inflammatory bowel disease, and elevated levels have similar adverse significance. The failure of the CRP to fall with medical therapy is particularly important. As corticosteroids suppress all the acute-phase proteins even in the absence of reduced inflammation at the site of most interest, their failure to decrease the CRP indicates progressive and uncontrolled disease [10].

Severe diarrhoea is accompanied by a loss of sodium and hydrogen ions, and an abnormally acid stool. This can lead in turn to a systemic metabolic alkalosis. Given that most sick patients develop a metabolic acidosis, the presence of alkalosis should be taken seriously, and Caprilli *et al.* [11] consider this a useful adverse prognostic feature.

In addition to toxic megacolon itself, there are at least two other key abnormalities discernible from the plain film. The presence of mucosal islands along the length of the colon indicates a virtually complete loss of the mucosal surface, the beginnings of full-thickness damage to the bowel and a very high risk of later perforation if colectomy is not undertaken

Table 4.2   Adverse prognostic factors in fulminant colitis

Criterion	Failure rate
>8 stools/day	33%
Pulse rate >100/min	36%
Maximum temperature >38°C	56%
Serum albumin <30 g/l	42%
Presence of mucosal islands on plain abdominal radiograph	75%
Small bowel dilatation	73%

From refs [8, 9]

(Table 4.2). The islands – raised areas protruding into the lumen – are, in fact, the last remaining regions of relatively preserved mucosa. Similarly, the presence of (three or more) dilated loops of small bowel is predictive of a poorer outcome (Table 4.2), and indeed of the development of toxic megacolon itself [9, 12], the Oxford group finding this sign in 73% of those who subsequently required surgery, compared to only 43% in those responding to medical therapy. When there were five or more distended loops, all patients required surgery. Again, there is some difficulty in interpretation given that the earlier data of Lennard-Jones *et al.* [8] had predicted these outcomes and presumably had some bearing on the decision to elect for surgical intervention.

Almer *et al.* [13] have, in effect, expanded on the plain abdominal film with their study of 'air enema radiography' in 35 (of 49) patients with acute severe colitis who went on to surgery, and in whom they felt that the plain film was not adequate. Air was 'gently insufflated' under fluoroscopic control, with patients on their left sides, aiming to reach the caecum. A 'sufficient volume' of air was judged as that at which the mucosal outline was easily seen, and in most cases was between 500 and 800 ml. There was excellent agreement between radiological assessment of depth of mucosal ulceration and that demonstrable histologically in the resected colon – overall accuracy 86%. It is not clear whether the technique was useful in those who did not need surgery, and the paper does not entirely exclude a relationship between the procedure and a subsequent adverse prognosis (such as perforation). It is likely, but unproven, that the technique is as safe as instant barium enema which has a very impressive safety record [14]. It is almost certainly safer than colonoscopy in this setting, with a major complication incurred in one of only 46 patients with severe disease in a report from the latter technique's principal protagonists [15]. It is nevertheless surprising that air enema was necessary in such a high proportion of patients, since the required information would be expected from the unenhanced plain film much more often than in the 22% of cases (11 of 49) reported.

A suggested framework of clinical and investigatory monitoring is given in Table 4.3. Most of the elements are standard observations, but it is surprisingly informative to collect the various items on to a single 'colitis observations proforma'. Although there is implicit benefit in a daily assessment of the fulminant colitic by a senior clinician, who will often be able to provide a reliable overall assessment from clinical review alone, the global assessments made by the well-supported junior using the proforma are rarely different. Measurement of abdominal girth is notoriously irreproducible and is not recommended.

Early surgery should be considered for fulminant colitis if any complication develops, or if there is an overall deterioration despite appropriate medical therapy. Surgery should also be planned if there has been no improvement by around 5 days from the initiation of aggressive steroid therapy. Surgery is probably indicated in all patients in whom any monitoring criterion worsens, even if the overall status appears quite reasonable, and particularly so when the CRP fails to fall, or if one of the key radiological signs emerges. An aphorism, learnt early and no less valid today, runs as follows: 'When the patient feels well but the signs are bad, the colon is usually a mess, and should be removed', or more simply: 'If in doubt – operate'.

There is probably only one operation to be considered in this context – the subtotal colectomy with ileostomy formation (and probably a mucous fistula to vent the recto-sigmoid). This aborts the emergency, avoids the dangers of extensive pelvic dissection in the acute situation, and permits elective pouch surgery to be considered at leisure. Even with this approach, colectomy for fulminant colitis has a mortality in the region of 5% (compared to less than 1% even for taxing, pouch creating, elective surgery) (see below).

Table 4.3   Fulminant colitis: suggested framework for clinical and investigatory monitoring

Pulse	6 hourly
Temperature	6 hourly
Stool frequency	Recorded on daily basis
Stool consistency	Recorded on daily basis
Presence of blood?	Recorded on daily basis
Abdominal tenderness?	Recorded on daily basis
Nature of bowel sounds	Recorded on daily basis
Serum electrolytes	Daily
Full blood count	Daily
Plain abdominal radiograph	Daily
Serum CRP (or ESR)	Thrice weekly
Serum albumin	Thrice weekly
'Global assessment'	Daily – recorded as better, same or worse

The place of cyclosporin in management of the fulminant colitic is dealt with in detail in Chapter 3, but neither its use nor that of other medical therapies should be permitted to delay laparotomy in the unresponsive patient if we are to retain the improved prognosis that has come from the earlier and safer surgery practised through the past quarter of a century.

It should be recognized that a single episode of fulminant colitis – however catastrophic – once survived without surgery, ceases to have any direct bearing on surgical planning for that patient. Although such patients do not escape future severe exacerbations, their risk thereof and of needing surgery is no greater than for other individuals with similar disease extent (and may be less) [16] (Chapter 2).

PROBLEMATIC DISTAL ULCERATIVE COLITIS

In most cases distal ulcerative colitis will respond well to the simple measures outlined in Chapter 3, the northern European emphasis on topical steroids for acute disease gradually being eroded by increasing use of topical 5-ASA, with probable greater efficacy if also greater cost. Unfortunately there are patients in whom the disease is manifestly limited to a short segment of distal bowel, but in whom symptom control is not achieved. In many cases this is because the problem is a functional one akin to irritable bowel syndrome rather than predominantly the result of uncontrolled inflammation. In this event endoscopic examination reveals unremarkable macroscopic features, although care should be taken to ensure that active disease does not exist proximal to the lowermost zone within range of the rigid sigmoidoscope where disease has been controlled by topical therapy. If symptoms do appear out of proportion to objective criteria, it is reasonable to consider symptomatic measures in addition to continuing topical 5-ASA (or steroid) therapy. Loperamide or another opioid may be sufficient, but many patients obtain greater benefit from increased fibre (for example as ispaghula) or lactulose, as proximal constipation is just as often the cause of distress (Chapter 2). There is also some evidence that lactulose may have a therapeutic effect on colitis in its own right (unpublished observations). Other strategies used for irritable bowel syndrome can also be valuable.

When the distal disease is macroscopically active, the combination of topical steroid and 5-ASA is worth trying (Chapter 3), and patience can also be rewarded, many patients coming into remission over 6–8 weeks simply by continuing a regime that was not initially helpful. Alternative topical regimes based on the various agents outlined in Chapter 3 have their advocates, and it will often be appropriate to conduct therapeutic trials. Reliable data are lacking, especially in this context of resistant disease. When a selection of such measures have failed, and especially if there are indicators of systemic disease such as an elevated platelet count or CRP, I am increasingly inclined to manage the patient as if the colitis was more extensive and am accordingly happy to consider systemic steroids and azathioprine. Azathioprine has not been subjected to controlled trial in this context but appears to yield a response rate comparable to that in patients with more extensive disease.

Surgery is obviously a less attractive proposition when much of the colon is felt to be normal, but will be appropriate in some resistant patients. The correct operation is total colectomy, since more limited resection is almost always followed by aggressive relapse in the previously normal bowel (see below). Between 10 and 15% of the colectomies performed for ulcerative colitis at St Mark's are currently in patients with intractable limited disease, and at least 5% might be expected for this indication in a more general colorectal surgical practice.

SURGERY

Surgery is rarely the first therapy considered in inflammatory bowel disease but often proves an important component of overall management in affected patients. The indications for early and occasionally emergency surgery for fulminant colitis have been enumerated above, but in other circumstances the decision will be more of an elective one, with contributions to the decision-making process from the three key parties: physician, surgeon and patient.

Ulcerative colitis

Surgery is required in ulcerative colitis for one of three main indications:

1.　uncontrolled severe acute disease and especially so if there are complications;
2.　uncontrolled chronic disease, with either a lack of adequate response to medical therapy, or steroid dependence;
3.　the development of long-term complications such as dysplasia or frank malignancy (see Chapter 8).

At least 70% of procedures are performed for the second indication in all the major centres. This is also the most patient-dependent indication, and careful analysis of the severity of symptoms and realistic expectations of surgery are essential in management planning.

Surgery for ulcerative colitis should be almost synonymous with total colectomy because partial colectomy is usually followed by problematic relapse in the retained colon, and because the patient is otherwise left at risk of colorectal carcinoma. In a typical series of seven elderly patients in whom deliberately conservative surgery with segmental resection was performed, even limited follow-up revealed troublesome recurrence in all [17]. This recurrence of colitis is a problem even when documented distal disease has been fully resected, leaving apparently healthy proximal colon. A report from Varma and colleagues lends support to the numerous anecdotes to this effect [18]. All four patients treated by segmental resection had a major relapse in the neoterminal colon within 11 months (median 6 months), and no fewer than three required early completion colectomy and proctectomy. Initial pouch surgery after pancolectomy would have been predicted to be successful in these patients, further emphasizing the poor final outcome.

Total proctocolectomy with formation of an end-ileostomy remains a viable option with relatively low (but significant) immediate complication rates, and a short period of perioperative morbidity; the cancer risk is eliminated and colitic symptoms are abolished. However, the presence of a permanent ileostomy is unacceptable to many, and the lifetime complication rate is well in excess of 50%. In a detailed actuarial analysis of 150 patients with an end-ileostomy, the 20 year frequency of stomal complications reached 75% in ulcerative colitis (and 56% in Crohn's disease) [19]. There were a variety of skin problems, with retraction and/or herniation of the stoma, with overt intestinal obstruction in 23%. Revisional surgery had been necessary in 28% of those where the stoma had been performed for ulcerative colitis (and 16% in Crohn's disease).

Good though the results of proctocolectomy and ileostomy generally are, it has been understandable that patients seek more normal continence. Kock devised a continent ileostomy by fashioning a pouch from the terminal ileum secured to the abdominal wall. Parks took this idea a step further in the 1970s by anastomosing a similar pouch to the anal canal, thus creating the pelvic ileo-anal pouch and a more truly restorative procedure which has changed surgical practice. This has become the most frequently performed surgical procedure for ulcerative colitis in specialist centres (75 of 145 operations at St Mark's through 1986–1990 and still increasing) [20]. This is not the place for a detailed analysis of the surgical techniques, but an awareness of the principal options is worthwhile. The first decision is whether the surgery should be performed in a single operation or spread over two or more sessions. The patient with fulminant colitis should almost certainly have a simple (and safe) colectomy and ileostomy, with the later option of pouch creation when in remission. A consensus is otherwise forming that a single-stage procedure in which the colectomy, proctectomy and pouch creation are done together (with no defunctioning ileostomy) is appropriate for the majority of patients undergoing elective surgery. All defunctioning ileostomies need to be closed at some stage and are not themselves without complications; the experienced pouch surgeon increasingly tends to reserve ileostomy creation for the patient in whom there is technical difficulty with the pouch formation or greater than average anxieties about pelvic sepsis – the principal early hazard of the pelvic pouch. The pouch may be made from a single loop or from multiple loops of ileum (the so-called 'J', 'S' or 'W' pouch, Figure 4.3), may be stapled or hand-sewn, and may be secured to the anal canal with a varying degree of stripping of the distal rectal and transitional mucosa. Stapling devices lend some degree of technical simplicity and speed in pouch creation, and aid the creation of a very distal anastomosis without damage to the anal sphincters.

There is a tendency for the healthy pouch to take on a number of characteristics of normal colon (Plate 8). The normal villous pattern of the terminal ileum becomes somewhat blunted with shortening and broadening of the villi. It is unclear to what extent this represents an appropriate accommodation to the new reservoir function and the altered bacterial flora, and to what degree it may be considered pathological. However, the magnitude of this colonic metaplasia does not appear to predict short- or long-term complications.

The most common reasons for pouch failure are perianal and/or pelvic sepsis and unknowing pouch creation in Crohn's disease (but see below), with some patients falling prey to intractable inflammation within the pouch – pouchitis (Chapter 1 and below). Pelvic sepsis affects around 15% of patients to some extent, and although it rarely leads to loss of the pouch, it is responsible for considerable distress and protracted hospital stays. Early postoperative intestinal obstruction is seen in around 10% and may also delay discharge substantially, up to half of affected patients needing further laparotomy [21]; however, the longer-term outcome of this complication is good. Even including early cases at St Mark's (when the institution was still on the 'learning curve') the cumulative rate of pouch failure was only 12% at 5 years [22]. However, the magnitude of the

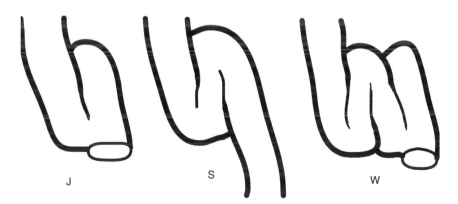

Figure 4.3 Three formats used in creation of the ileo-anal pouch The more 'folds' made in the terminal ileum, the greater the volume of the pouch and the less the need for frequent evacuation. The efferent limb of the 'S' pouch has been associated with a higher incidence of outlet obstruction and is now less favoured.

undertaking from the patient's perspective should not be underestimated, as 68% of patients had required re-admission during those 5 years for reasons other than for ileostomy closure, and roughly half of those had required further laparotomy. Typically, 3 months' morbidity can be expected even when things go well. It should be recognized that defaecatory function is not normal in patients with a satisfactory pouch, as the frequency of evacuation is usually 3–6 times daily. However, this is not associated with urgency nor with much night-time waking, and patients can usually adapt well to this constraint, which is so much more predictable than their prior experiences with colitis. Comparisons with patients' own assessments of outcomes from proctocolectomy and ileostomy are heavily in favour of the reconstructive operation [23]. Even those patients unlucky enough to be troubled by some degree of incontinence report a preference for their new state compared to the prior colitis (and tend to wish that their surgery had been performed sooner) [24]. A nice contrast is posed by patients having a restorative proctocolectomy for polyposis coli (for cancer prevention) in whom there were no previous colonic symptoms and in whom these restrictions are perceived less favourably.

Very few units now recommend colectomy with ileorectal anastomosis because rectal symptoms may still be a problem (to the extent of compromising continence) and because of the continuing concern about neoplasia. This may, however, be an option in the young patient who is very keen to avoid an ileostomy but who is not ready to invest the time required for pouch creation. In this circumstance a relatively generous portion of distal bowel should be left in continuity to avoid the need for two pelvic procedures. These patients need careful follow-up with attention to neoplastic risk, as if total colitis still persisted, until the rectum is finally removed (Chapter 8).

Pouchitis

Inflammation within the newly created ileo-anal pouch may be the result of gastrointestinal infection, surrounding sepsis in the pelvis, or of mechanical deficiencies such as outlet obstruction, but also occurs when these factors are absent. This 'pouchitis' must be defined carefully and requires histological as well as clinical and endoscopic evidence for its confirmation. Publications and clinical decisions on pouchitis in the absence of these criteria should be treated with great reserve. Pouchitis is recognized in the Kock pouch as well as in the pelvic pouch at a comparable frequency [25], and is presumed to have little or nothing to do with the location of the pouch, but more to do with the underlying disease, as it hardly ever occurs in patients having pouch surgery for familial polyposis coli. It remains poorly understood, but several strands of evidence favour the idea that to some extent it represents ulcerative colitis of the ileal cells

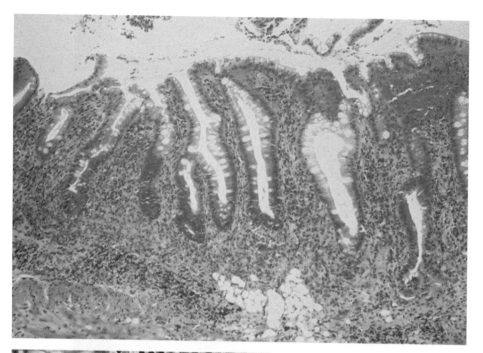

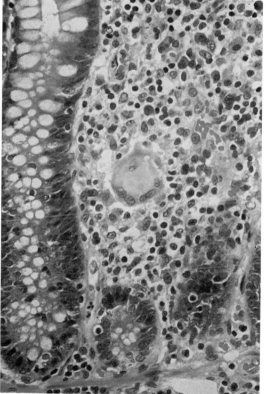

Plate 1 Histology of a rectal biopsy in ulcerative colitis. Note the loss of the normal architectural organization, the relative depletion of goblet cells and the beginnings of crypt abscess formation.

Plate 2 Colonic histology in Crohn's disease. The presence of giant cell granulomata, together with better preserved goblet cell content and overall mucosal architecture, are almost pathognomonic of Crohn's.

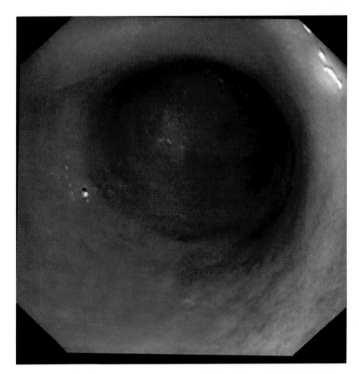

Plate 3 Colonoscopic view of the descending colon in relatively inactive ulcerative colitis – the disease is confluent with a generalized granular appearance.

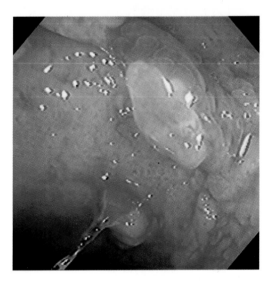

Plate 4 Post-inflammatory polyposis in a patient with inactive ulcerative colitis – biopsies from the raised areas showed non-specific inflammation.

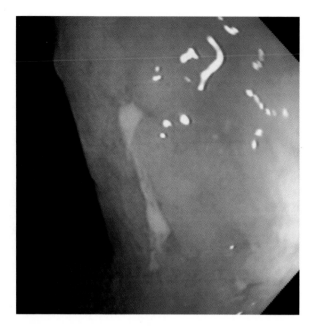

Plate 5 Relatively deep linear ulcer typical of Crohn's disease as seen at colonoscopy.

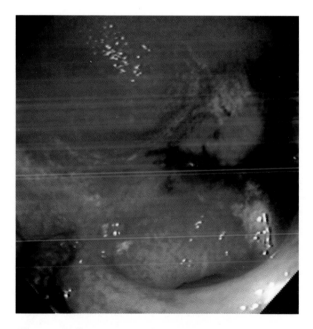

Plate 6 Inflammation of the caecum in Crohn's disease – the relative fixity of the anatomy enables a partial view through the ileocaecal valve across which runs a shallow linear ulcer.

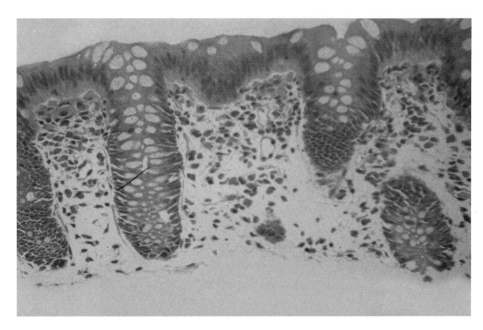

Plate 7 Histological appearance of collagenous colitis. The overall mucosal architecture and the mild inflammatory infiltrate are typical but the diagnosis is clinched by the thick band of collagen immediately beneath the epithelium.

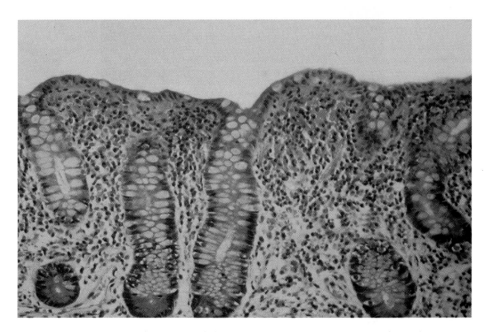

Plate 8 Histology of the normal ileo-anal pouch. The ileal mucosa has taken on many colonic features, most obvious of which is the loss of villi; there is a minimal inflammatory infiltrate. (Courtesy of Professor I.C. Talbot.)

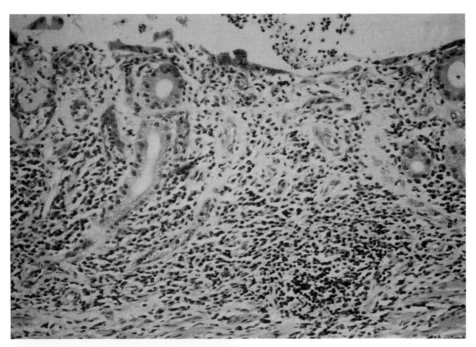

Plate 9 Histology of the ileo-anal pouch with pouchitis. The colonified mucosa now exhibits destruction of the normal glandular structure and a marked inflammatory infiltrate. (Courtesy of Professor I.C. Talbot.)

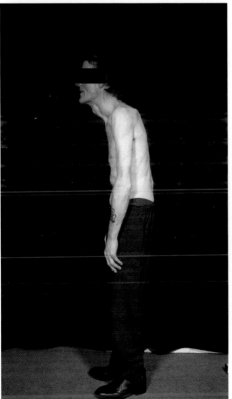

Plate 10 The characteristic stooped posture of ankylosing spondylitis, here in a patient with troublesome ulcerative colitis.

Plate 11 Characteristic appearance of erythema nodosum, which in this case was on the shin of a patient with ulcerative colitis and measured 3 cm in diameter.

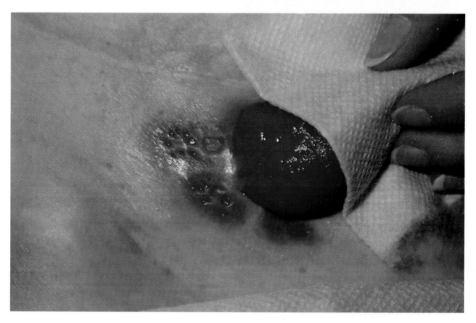

Plate 12 Pyoderma gangrenosum may occur at any site but is over-represented at sites of previous trauma (pathergy). In this case it developed shortly after the creation of an ileostomy in a patient with extensive Crohn's disease.

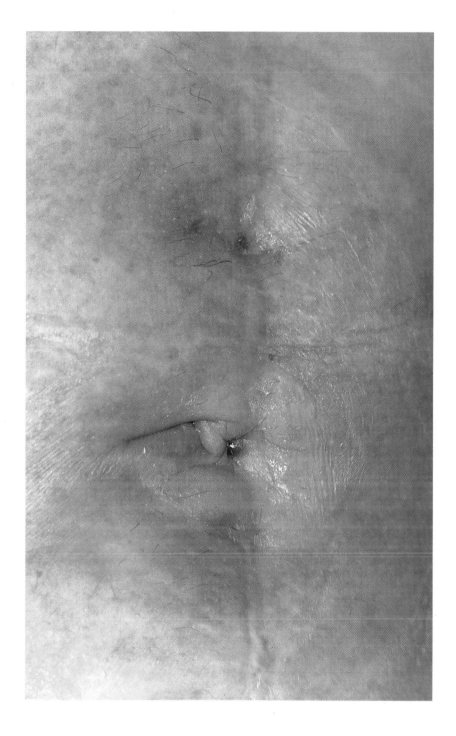

Plate 13 Small postoperative fistula in the scar of a patient with Crohn's disease. Resolution with conservative therapy might reasonably be expected.

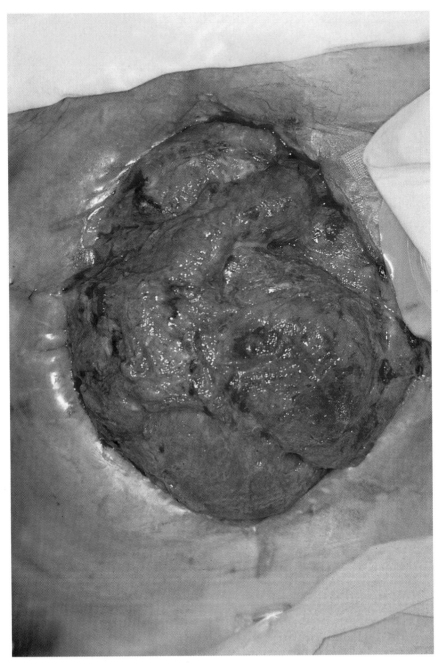

Plate 14 Catastrophic fistulation in a patient with Crohn's disease in whom surgical resection was complicated by dehiscence of the abdominal wound and by numerous enteric fistulae. At the time of this photograph, meticulous wound care and exclusive parenteral nutrition have led to the covering of the initial virtual laparostomy by clean, healthy granulation tissue, despite the continuing presence of at least four fistulous openings. Further surgery was required later.

transformed by colonic metaplasia (Chapter 1). It is possible that an imbalance in the intestinal flora is aetiologically important in the pathogenesis of pouchitis and the microflora of the ileal reservoir have accordingly been analysed [26]. Patients with pouchitis proved to have an increased number of aerobes and *Clostridia*, with fungal species that were not found in controls, and relatively fewer anaerobes and lactobacilli. The prevailing pH was also more alkaline in those with pouchitis (6.5 v. 5.4). Unfortunately, these authors do not make the crucial distinction between the effects of pouchitis and the situation prior to its onset; these findings may all be secondary to pouchitis that has arisen for an unconnected reason. Serial estimations and challenge with the patients' own faecal stream prior to ileostomy closure (studies in progress at St Mark's) will hopefully clarify this. Pouchitis may or may not be more common in those with pANCA (Chapter 1). This has been debated by Estève *et al.*, who themselves find no difference in pouchitis risk between those positive for pANCA preoperatively and those who lacked the antibody [27]. Better serial data are needed.

A frequency of pouchitis (at some time) in the region of 20% is to be expected, but problematic disease is much less common, and leads to pouch excision in well under 5% of patients in most series. There do not appear to be any reliable clinical pointers to a higher risk of pouchitis in ulcerative colitis patients apart from a higher risk in males [28] and in those with initially the most extensive colitis [29].

Pouchitis most commonly presents acutely with proctitis-like symptoms which settle rapidly with or without intervention, but in about half of those affected there are recurrent relapsing or continual symptoms. It leads to a loss of the normal vascular pattern at endoscopy, with a variable degree of inflammation, contact bleeding and occasionally frank ulceration. None of these features is sufficiently specific for the diagnosis to be made without supportive histology. The microscopic changes include a prominent polymorphonuclear cell infiltrate in the acute phase, with a greater involvement of lymphocytes and other mononuclear inflammatory cells with developing chronicity (Plate 9). The histological features may be patchy and tend to affect the most distal part of the pouch preferentially [30]. Infective causes should be excluded by appropriate microbiological investigation.

Pouchitis therapy is still at a relatively primitive stage. Metronidazole (400 mg thrice daily) has been shown in a small, blinded, cross-over study of relatively intractable pouchitis, to offer a significant advantage in terms of a reduced frequency of evacuation but without histological or other objective improvements [31]. This remains, nevertheless, the first intervention of most clinicians and often appears valuable; it is unclear whether its apparent effect is primarily an antimicrobial one or whether it is acting in some other fashion. Various alternatives have been utilized,

including topical and systemic steroids, topical and oral 5-ASA preparations, and a range of other topical agents otherwise thought valuable in
the management of proctitis. Careful trials with controlled data are seriously needed. Fortunately, despite this therapeutic quagmire, most
patients finally do well and excision of a pouch for intractable pouchitis is
a rare event.

Functional disorders of the pouch also exist and deserve brief comment, not least because the affected patient is perhaps the most likely to
be referred on from the specialist in pouch surgery. The most common
functional disorder is the early postoperative intestinal obstruction in
which no mechanical cause can be demonstrated. Although laparotomy
may occasionally be necessary to prove this, the prognosis is generally
good and continuing action unnecessary. Frequency of pouch action is
greatest in the first weeks after surgery and usually settles to the 3–6 times
daily alluded to above. Higher frequency in the absence of pouchitis is
usually relatively readily overcome by incremental therapy with loperamide or other opioids. Occasionally patients behave as if the small
bowel were a great deal shorter than it is known to be, exhibiting 'short
bowel syndrome'. Although this tends to be a transient phenomenon, it
may last for some weeks and require intensive fluid and nutritional support during this time (Chapter 7).

Difficulty in pouch evacuation was a much more common problem in
the early days of pouch surgery, and particularly in the case of the 'S'
pouch with its efferent limb (Figure 4.3), an operation now avoided by
most surgeons for this reason. There remain a few patients (<5%) who
need to intubate with a soft catheter to achieve defaecation, and others
who continue to have a major problem with unpredictable evacuation.
Postoperative problems are not predicted by preoperative physiological or
other assessments, with the proviso only that preoperative sphincter function must be reasonably normal: however successful the pouch, the reservoir contents will never have the solidity of a normal stool. Investigation
of the problematic pouch by contrast pouchography (analogous to the
defaecating proctogram) will usually permit the exclusion of pouch outlet
obstruction, and may demonstrate oddities of pouch configuration (such
as a floppy pouch that twists on itself), that help to determine the place, if
any, for revisional surgery. When no structural abnormality can be identified, the patient can at least be reassured that the pouch is viable, itself a
cause of great relief to many who fear pouch excision and ileostomy more
even than substantial difficulties with the pouch. Continuing management is then symptom orientated, and may include the careful use of enemas or behavioural techniques such as biofeedback. More authoritative
advice will no doubt become available with time.

One of the main justifications for pouch surgery in ulcerative colitis, as
opposed to ileorectal anastomosis, is to avoid the risk of rectal carcinoma.

Theoretically, the pouch eliminates this risk, but there are two notes of caution. Since the mucosa of the pouch usually takes on a number of colonic characteristics, it is possible that it may also become at risk of colonic-type neoplasia with the passing of time (or indeed independently of colonic metaplasia, given the stasis and altered flora which are alien to the normal distal small bowel). Secondly, there remains the possibility of rectal mucosal cells being retained (accidentally from inadequate mucosal stripping, or unavoidably in the transitional zone above the anal canal). Although the literature contains a small collection of case reports of so-called pouch cancers, careful reading indicates that these generally (and perhaps exclusively) reflect incomplete rectal excision. It is too soon to be sure, however, that the first risk is only hypothetical, especially in the light of a recent report from Huddinge [32]. Dysplasia was found in a subgroup of pouch patients in whom the postoperative course was complicated by continuing severe pouchitis associated with permanent subtotal or total villous atrophy, which constituted 9% of the series. Dysplasia was low grade and affected three patients (3.4% of all pouch patients) at a mean follow-up of 6.3 years. It affected mucosa of apparently small bowel origin, and was present at numerous sites (on eight occasions, in 63 biopsies in the three patients). The prognostic significance of this observation is not yet known, but continued clinical surveillance and regular pouch biopsy is evidently warranted.

Crohn's disease

There are important differences in approach when surgery for Crohn's disease is considered. Key amongst these are the high lifetime frequency of surgery in this disease (>50%), involvement of the small bowel, the potential for permanent nutritional dependency if a major proportion of the intestine is removed, the absence of any confident expectation of 'cure' of the underlying condition, and the possibilities pre- and postoperatively of other complications. Emergency surgery is less often required for colonic Crohn's than for ulcerative colitis, as fulminant colitis and its complications are much less common (see above). However, urgent surgical intervention may be required for intestinal obstruction from stenotic disease, or for the effects of sepsis and abscess formation (see below). Fistula surgery is rarely best embarked upon on an emergency footing (Chapter 7).

The high postoperative relapse rates in all forms of Crohn's disease (see also Chapter 3) should not be allowed to denigrate the excellent surgical results that can be obtained, and especially in the first-time patient with localized ileocaecal disease failing to respond to standard medical measures. At least 40% of such patients will have uncomplicated surgery and prolonged remission, which will be lifelong in a sizeable minority.

Representative data include those of the Cleveland Clinic, where resection led to prolonged surgery-free survival in 47–56%, depending on the site of the original disease [33]; of the Leuven group, who record 66% of patients symptom-free at 3 years postoperatively [34]; and the Leiden group, where 44% remained free of further surgery at 20 years [35]. Patients who have already had surgery, those with fistulae and those with other complications cannot be given such a good prognosis. Although good results are certainly still achieved, the proportion decreases with each additional procedure and complication. There is a curious phenomenon influencing the nature of postoperative recurrence which has been documented clearly by the Chicago group [36]. For reasons yet to be explained, when Crohn's disease recurs after resection, it affects a similar length of intestine, with a remarkable degree of consistency (26 cm v. 24 cm; correlation coefficient: 0.70), but is not then progressive with time. The risk of relapse has much to do with the continuity of small and large bowel. When a terminal ileostomy is created, the frequency of relapse is low, reverting to the general risk of relapse if the ileostomy is subsequently closed. Some possible mechanisms for this phenomenon are discussed in Chapter 1. In practice, patient management is not greatly influenced by this knowledge, as there is a natural tendency of patients and surgeons alike to avoid stoma formation if at all possible, reserving it for the patient with pancolitis, especially when there is intractable perianal disease implicating the sphincter zone, and when continence has been prejudiced or entirely lost. A stoma may be created with the intention that it will be temporary (to be closed when the perineum or distal colorectum has recovered), but it is my experience that in almost 50% of such cases, closure never becomes feasible. Patients undergoing surgery for difficult Crohn's disease should always be aware that a stoma may be a necessary intervention, and that even an intentionally temporary stoma may become permanent.

Conservative surgery in small bowel Crohn's disease has an important place nevertheless, and is generally to be preferred precisely because of the high risk of recurrence (despite improving postoperative maintenance with pharmacological agents (Chapter 3)) and the concern that future surgery will lead to borderline or actual short bowel syndrome. Most surgeons will therefore choose to perform reparative stricturoplasty unless there is a very well-defined (and relatively short) section of diseased small bowel. This procedure entails a longitudinal division of the stricture with a transverse anastomosis of the enterotomy created (Figures 4.4 and 4.5). Sites for surgical attention can be identified by the peroperative passage of a 2.5 cm balloon along the small bowel with stricturoplasty (or resection) performed at each site that the balloon will not pass. There is a low immediate morbidity from stricturoplasty, with a postoperative dehiscence rate of around 5%, which is more impressive when one considers that a single patient may have upwards of 10 stricturoplasties at one operative session, but depressing when this so often means an enterocutaneous fistula [37, 38]. The postoperative recurrence rate is unsurprisingly substantial; at 12 months, over 96% of Tjandra's patients were without obstructive symptoms, but in continuing follow-up, 13% required further stricture surgery [37]. Although one might expect the best results for stricturoplasty to be confined to patients in whom the predominant problem is fibrous stricturing with little current inflammation, this does not seem universally to be the case. Not only do some stenoses with an active inflammatory component do well, but the inflammation may also settle with apparent recovery of the bowel at the site of the surgical incision, with future relapses just as, or more, likely to affect previously unaffected parts of the small bowel [37]. It is perhaps for similar reasons that endoscopically detected but surgically inapparent lesions do not appear to impart a worse prognosis if left undisturbed [39].

The situation in respect of the lower bowel is a little different. The colon has a role in preserving fluid and electrolyte balance (especially in short bowel syndrome; Chapter 7), but in most circumstances it is nutritionally less essential. However, there is a continuing controversy as to the place of segmental colonic resection, because there is a concern that disease will not only recur in the residual colon but that (as in ulcerative colitis) it will prove more aggressive, more difficult to control and will probably lead to completion colectomy soon afterwards. There are no controlled data to help us, although a trial between segmental resection and ileorectal anastomosis would be entirely legitimate. A controlled trial comparing segmental resection to colectomy and ileostomy would also be of interest, but this would be most unlikely to be acceptable to patients or ethical committees. Personal experience indicates that some patients do well with segmental resection and some do badly, but it is rarely at all clear preoperatively which outcome is to be expected. The Tübingen group has tried to help with a long-term analysis of 142 patients with segmental resections performed at a single centre [40], comparing this with 28 patients who had an initial colectomy (often with retention of the rectum). Based on a mean of nearly 12 years' follow-up from the time of first surgery, they constructed actuarial statistics for the first 10 years. Only 37% of the patients with pancolitis and an initial segmental resection needed further resection

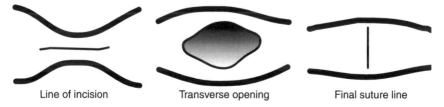

| Line of incision | Transverse opening | Final suture line |

Figure 4.4 The Heineke–Mikulicz stricturoplasty for conservational ileal stricture surgery.

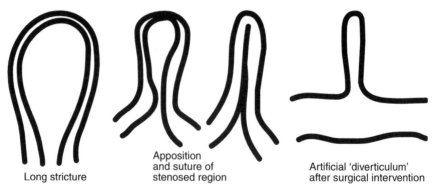

Figure 4.5   The Finney stricturoplasty for the more lengthy ileal stricture.

by the 10-year mark, of whom 12% would by then have an end-ileostomy. Of the entire cohort treated initially by segmental resection, only 11% had an ileostomy at 10 years. These figures compare with a need for further surgery in 40%, and an overall ileostomy rate of 50% in the group undergoing initial colectomy. The authors advocate a more liberal policy towards segmental colectomy, but it must be accepted that there has been a high degree of selection leading to the initial surgical decision. Contemporary French data on the place of ileorectal anastomosis in Crohn's surgery reach a less encouraging conclusion, with a high failure rate, leading on to proctectomy in 50% of their patients during as little as 2 years' follow-up [41]. Patients with anorectal disease were least likely to do well, and poorer outcomes were recorded in those with extra-intestinal manifestations of their disease. The state of the rectum and the perianal region clearly should have a major influence on surgical planning but, as in all inflammatory bowel disease surgery, the informed patient will often be the final arbiter.

Diversion colitis

When the rectum has been defunctioned but not resected there is a frequency of relapse divided uncertainly between defunction/diversion proctitis and reactivated Crohn's, which together affect around half of the patients so treated. It may be difficult to distinguish accurately between the two forms of proctitis clinically or histologically (Chapter 2). The recognition and diagnosis of diversion colitis is plagued by inconsistencies, but histological abnormalities are almost always to be found on biopsy. In a well-documented series in which the final conclusions were drawn from resection specimens, 14 of the 15 cases had many features in common [42]. There was diffuse, mild, chronic inflammation, with a variable extent of mild architectural abnormality of the crypts, minor crypt abscesses, and follicular lymphoid hyperplasia. In other words, the changes are those of mild ulcerative colitis rather than ones suggestive of Crohn's disease. A French series of 48 patients indicates that, over 8 years' follow-up, one-third of these patients can be expected to come to proctectomy – most of whom will have had preoperative proctitis – and that prolonged rectal remission is the fortunate outcome in only about 30% [43].

Pouches in Crohn's disease

Ileo-anal pouch construction in Crohn's has been vetoed by most inflammatory bowel disease practitioners because of the anxieties in respect of pelvic sepsis, pouch breakdown and the potentially catastrophic effects of disease recurrence. However, for reasons alluded to elsewhere (Chapter 2), it is not always possible to exclude Crohn's disease as a cause of colitis, and sometimes a confident diagnosis of ulcerative colitis proves incorrect (or changes, or the patient has both diseases?). Some of these patients have had 'accidental' pouch surgery and the results are not as bad as might be expected. The Paris group has been heavily criticized for a recent paper which records respectable results in 13 such patients, the criticism being levelled not for their inclusion of these patients, but for the use of pouch surgery in a further 18 patients in whom the diagnosis was known to be Crohn's disease and in whom the operation was a deliberate 'high risk' strategy [44]. There has also been some surprise that so many patients could be found to fulfil the stated criteria of colonic Crohn's without either ileal or anorectal disease. Follow-up is still relatively short (mean 59 months) and caution is certainly required, but the 6% relapse rate (Crohn's disease affecting the pouch in two patients) and the 19% complication rate are remarkably good. As the authors note, the complication rate is neither statistically nor numerically different from their own results in ulcerative colitis, and is comparable to that for ulcerative colitis series at other centres. When it is remembered that the appropriate comparitor is not pouch surgery in ulcerative colitis but alternative surgery in Crohn's disease with generally higher overall relapse and complication rates even for terminal ileostomy – the surgical 'best option' – the possibility of pouch construction for the Crohn's patient with severe but isolated colonic disease should no longer be dismissed out of hand.

Laparoscopy in inflammatory bowel disease surgery

A section on surgery in inflammatory bowel disease can no longer stand without comment on the role of laparoscopy. Colorectal surgeons were late to enter the laparoscopic arena, but are now doing so with a highly variable degree of enthusiasm. Fazio's group have been publishing on laparoscopically assisted resections for Crohn's disease for several years [45], and techniques for ileostomy creation have also been developed [46].

At present it would be reasonable to conclude that laparoscopic methodology is technically possible in some patients, and may permit an easier
convalescence [47] but with the proviso that it will rarely be suitable for
those with extensive previous surgery, adhesions and complex fistulae,
and has yet to prove itself in anything approaching a formal comparison
with the more established methods employed at open surgery.

Endoscopic stricture dilatation

Anorectal strictures have been dilated by surgeons and patients since
mythological times with good results. There is always concern that strictures of the large bowel complicating inflammatory bowel disease have
neoplastic potential (Chapter 8), but with initial and periodic histological
assessment their dilatation can also be undertaken routinely with the
expectation of good results [48]. More proximal strictures can now be
reached endoscopically, and with reliable, modern, through-the-scope
balloons, endoscopic therapy became a technical possibility. The problem
with earlier balloons was not so much their small calibre but their short
length, which led to them slipping proximally or distally as they were
inflated. Now that balloons of 5 cm or more in length and up to 25 mm in
diameter are routinely available, this is much less of a problem. Virtually
all colonic and anastomotic strictures are theoretically accessible. There is
still a technical failure rate (stricture too tight or its distal opening too
angled for access) and a perforation rate, both in the region of 5–10%,
depending on selection criteria. There are no clear comparative data for
long-term results from dilatation. My clinical impression has been that
patients with inactive disease and entirely or mainly fibrous stricturing
can achieve good and long-lasting results, but those with any degree of
inflammatory activity get little benefit, apart perhaps from a placebo
response which is lost after 2 or 3 weeks. Accordingly, I reserve this
approach for patients with negative inflammatory markers and negative
white cell scans. The literature is a little more positive, but inclusion criteria are not uniform and there has been no controlled trial. Papers
inevitably come from endoscopy enthusiasts, and there may be a publication bias towards better results. The Leuven group probably has most
experience and reported on their technical success in dilating 16 of 18
strictures in 1992 [49]. Their more recent review includes 55 patients with
59 strictures (average length 40 mm) treated on 78 occasions [50]. All of
these patients were considered resistant to medical therapy and would
otherwise have been treated surgically. Dilatation, with a water-filled balloon, was to 18 mm, and to 25 mm in the more recent patients. It was possible to pass a colonoscope through 73% of the strictures after dilatation,
and a further 17% of procedures were considered technical successes.
There were six perforations, only two of which necessitated laparotomy

and resection; there was no mortality. Kaplan–Meier estimation of recurrence-free survival time indicated that around 40% of patients remained well to 3 years, and that surgery had been avoided in more than 60% at 3 years. The results compare favourably with those to be expected from surgical stricturoplasty [37] but there are important identifiable differences between the patients included in surgical and endoscopic series, not least the higher frequency of multiple strictures in the former. There is a continuing case for both forms of intervention in appropriately selected patients.

REFERENCES

1. Chapman RW, Selby WS, Jewell DP. Controlled trial of intravenous metronidazole as an adjunct to corticosteroids in severe ulcerative colitis. *Gut* 1986; **27**: 1210–1212.
2. Truelove SC, Willoughby CP, Lee EG, Kettlewell MGW. Further experience in the treatment of severe attacks of ulcerative colitis. *Lancet* 1978; **ii**: 1086–1088.
3. McIntyre PB, Powell-Tuck J, Wood SR *et al.* Controlled trial of bowel rest in the treatment of severe acute colitis. *Gut* 1986; **27**: 481–485.
4. Panos MZ, Wood MJ, Asquith P. Toxic megacolon: the knee–elbow position relieves bowel distension. *Gut* 1993; **34**: 1726–1727.
5. Present DH, Wolfson D, Gelernt IM *et al.* Medical decompression of toxic megacolon by rolling. A new technique of decompression with favorable long-term follow-up. *J Clin Gastroenterol* 1988; **10**: 485–490.
6. Travis SPL, Farrant JM, Ricketts C *et al.* Predicting outcome in severe ulcerative colitis. *Gut* 1996; **38**: 905–910.
7. Meyers S, Lerer PK, Feuer EJ *et al.* Predicting the outcome of corticoid therapy for acute ulcerative colitis. Results of a prospective, randomized, double-blind clinical trial. *J Clin Gastroenterol* 1987; **9**: 50–54.
8. Lennard-Jones JE, Ritchie JK, Hilder W, Spicer CC. Assessment of severity in colitis: a preliminary study. *Gut* 1975; **16**: 579–584.
9. Chew CN, Nolan DJ, Jewell DP. Small bowel gas in severe ulcerative colitis. *Gut* 1991; **32**: 1535–1537.
10. Oshitani N, Kitano A, Fukushima R *et al.* Predictive factors for the response of ulcerative colitis patients during the acute phase treatment. *Digestion* 1990; **46**: 107–113.
11. Caprilli R, Frieri G, Latella G *et al.* Faecal excretion of bicarbonate in ulcerative colitis. *Digestion* 1986; **35**: 136–142.
12. Caprilli R, Vernia P, Latella G, Torsoli A. Early recognition of toxic megacolon. *J Clin Gastroenterol* 1987; **9**: 160–164.
13. Almer S, Bodemar G, Franzen L *et al.* Use of air enema radiography to assess depth of ulceration during acute attacks of ulcerative colitis. *Lancet* 1996; **347**: 1731–1735.

14. Bartram CI. Barium radiology. *Scand J Gastroenterol* 1994; **203**(suppl): 20–23.
15. Carbonnel F, Laver GNEA, Lémann M *et al.* Colonoscopy of acute colitis: a safe and reliable tool for assessment of severity. *Dig Dis Sci* 1994; **39**: 1550–1557.
16. Järnerot G, Rolny P, Sandberg-Gertzen H. Intensive intravenous treatment of ulcerative colitis. *Gastroenterology* 1985; **89**: 1005–1013.
17. Condie JD Jr, Leslie KO, Smiley DF. Surgical treatment for inflammatory bowel disease in the older patient. *Surg Gynecol Obstet* 1987; **165**: 135–142.
18. Varma JS, Browning GGP, Smith AN *et al.* Mucosal proctectomy and coloanal anastomosis for distal ulcerative proctocolitis. *Br J Surg* 1987; **74**: 381–383.
19. Leong AP, Londono-Schimmer EE, Phillips RK. Life-table analysis of stomal complications following ileostomy. *Br J Surg* 1994; **81**: 727–729.
20. Melville DM, Ritchie JK, Nicholls RJ, Hawley PR. Surgery for ulcerative colitis in the era of the pouch: the St Mark's Hospital experience. *Gut* 1994; **35**: 1076–1080.
21. Wexner SD, Jagerman D, Lavery D, Fazio V. Ileoanal reservoir. *Am J Surg* 1990; **159**: 178–185.
22. Setti-Carraro P, Ritchie JK, Wilkinson KH *et al.* The first 10 years' experience of restorative proctocolectomy for ulcerative colitis. *Gut* 1994; **35**: 1070–1075.
23. Kohler L, Pemberton JH, Zinsmeister AR, Kelly KA. Quality of life after proctocolectomy: a comparison of Brooke ileostomy, Kock pouch and ileal pouch-anal anastomosis. *Gastroenterology* 1991; **101**: 679–684.
24. Keighley MRB. Review article: the management of pouchitis. *Aliment Pharmacol Ther* 1996; **10**: 449–457.
25. Svaninger G, Nordgren S, Oresland T, Hulten L. Incidence and characteristics of pouchitis in the Kock continent ileostomy and the pelvic pouch. *Scand J Gastroenterol* 1993; **28**: 695–700.
26. Ruseler-Van Embdem JG, Schouten WR, Van Lieshout LM. Pouchitis: result of microbial imbalance? *Gut* 1994; **35**: 658–664.
27. Estève M, Mallolas J, Klaasen J *et al.* Antineutrophil cytoplasmic antibodies in sera from colectomised ulcerative colitis patients and its relation to the presence of pouchitis. *Gut* 1996; **38**: 894–898.
28. Setti-Carraro P, Talbot IC, Nicholls RJ. Long-term appraisal of the histological appearances of the ileal reservoir mucosa after restorative proctocolectomy for ulcerative colitis. *Gut* 1994; **35**: 1721–1727.
29. Luukkonen P, Jarvinen H, Tanskanen M, Kahri A. Pouchitis – recurrence of the inflammatory bowel disease? *Gut* 1994; **35**: 243–246.
30. Moskowitz RL, Shepherd NA, Nicholls RJ. An assessment of inflam-

mation in the reservoir after restorative proctocolectomy with ileoanal ileal reservoir. *Int J Colorect Dis* 1986; **1**: 167–174.

31. Madden MV, McIntyre AS, Nicholls RJ. Double-blind crossover trial of metronidazole versus placebo in chronic unremitting pouchitis. *Dig Dis Sci* 1994; **39**: 1193–1196.

32. Veress B, Reinholt FP, Lindquist K *et al.* Long-term histomorphological surveillance of the pelvic pouch: dysplasia develops in a subgroup of patients. *Gastroenterology* 1995; **109**: 1090–1097.

33. Whelan G, Farmer RG, Fazio VW, Goormastic M. Recurrence after surgery in Crohn's disease. Relationship to location of disease (clinical pattern) and surgical indication. *Gastroenterology* 1985; **88**: 1826–1833.

34. Rutgeerts P, Geboes K, Vantrappen G *et al.* Predictability of the postoperative course of Crohn's disease. *Gastroenterology* 1990; **99**: 956–963.

35. Shivananda S, Hordijk ML, Pena AS, Mayberry JF. Crohn's disease: risk of recurrence and reoperation in a defined population. *Gut* 1989; **30**: 990–995.

36. D'Haens GR, Gasparaitis AE, Hanauer SB. Duration of recurrent ileitis after ileocolonic resection correlates with presurgical extent of Crohn's disease. *Gut* 1995; **36**: 715–717.

37. Tjandra JJ, Fazio VW. Stricturoplasty without concomitant resection for small bowel obstruction in Crohn's disease. *Br J Surg* 1994; **81**: 561–563.

38. Spencer MP, Nelson H, Wolff BG, Dozois RR. Stricturoplasty for obstructive Crohn's disease: the Mayo experience. *Mayo Clin Proc* 1994; **69**: 33–36.

39. Klein O, Colombel JF, Lescut D *et al.* Remaining small bowel endoscopic lesions at surgery have no influence on early anastomotic recurrences in Crohn's disease. *Am J Gastroenterol* 1995; **90**: 1949–1952.

40. Makowiec F, Paczulla D, Schmidtke C *et al.* Crohn's colitis: segmental resection or colectomy? *Gastroenterology* 1996; **110**: A1402.

41. Cattan P, Lémann M, Fritsch S *et al.* Criteria predicting rectal conservation failure after subtotal colectomy in Crohn's disease. *Gastroenterology* 1996; **110**: A880.

42. Geraghty JM, Talbot IC. Diversion colitis: histological feature in the colon and rectum after defunctioning colostomy. *Gut* 1991; **32**: 1020–1023.

43. Quandalle P, Tryohen F, Gambiez L *et al.* Long term follow up of patients with excluded rectum in Crohn's disease. *Gastroenterology* 1996; **110**: A996.

44. Panis Y, Poupard B, Nemeth J *et al.* Ileal pouch/anal anastomosis for Crohn's disease. *Lancet* 1996; **347**: 854–857.

45. Milsom JW, Lavery IC, Böhm M, Fazio VW. Laparoscopically assisted ileocolectomy in Crohn's disease. *Surg Laparosc Endosc* 1993; **3**: 77–80.
46. Roe AM, Barlow AP, Durdey P *et al*. Indications for laparoscopic formation of intestinal stomas. *Surg Laparosc Endosc* 1994; **4**: 345–347.
47. Bauer JJ, Harris MT, Grumbach NM, Gortine SR. Laparoscopic-assisted intestinal resection for Crohn's disease. *Dis Colon Rectum* 1995; **38**: 712–715.
48. Linares L, Moreira LF, Andrews H *et al*. Natural history and treatment of anorectal strictures complicating Crohn's disease. *Br J Surg* 1988; **75**: 653–656.
49. Breysem Y, Janssens JF, Coremans G *et al*. Endoscopic balloon dilation of colonic and ileo-colonic Crohn's strictures: long-term results. *Gastrointest Endosc* 1992; **38**: 142–147.
50. Couckuyt H, Gevers AM, Coremans G *et al*. Efficacy and safety of hydrostatic balloon dilatation of ileocolonic Crohn's strictures: a prospective longterm analysis. *Gut* 1995; **36**: 577–580.

5

Obstetrics and paediatrics

FERTILITY AND PREGNANCY IN INFLAMMATORY BOWEL DISEASE

Fertility and pregnancy are perennial concerns of patients of both sexes with inflammatory bowel disease. Fortunately it is possible to be quite reassuring in both regards.

Males

In males there appear to be few problems aside from the temporarily reduced fertility in the obviously sick individual requiring in-patient care. Overall male fertility in inflammatory bowel disease has not been shown to be different from that of the general population [1]. However, sulphasalazine is responsible for reversible oligospermia. The remaining spermatozoa are probably normal, and many normal pregnancies have occurred in the partners of men taking the drug. It is no longer acceptable to continue this drug in a man planning a family, given that the available alternative aminosalicylate (5-ASA) drugs are without this side-effect.

There are hypothetical dangers to the fetus from preconception exposure of the father to immunosuppressive drugs such as azathioprine. These dangers have not been demonstrated in any reported series and it is likely that any adverse effect is negligible or extremely rare (see also Francella's data below). It is a reasonable practice to inform prospective parents of the potential hazard and, whenever possible, to withdraw these drugs in the preconception period.

Female fertility

The fertility of women with inflammatory bowel disease is probably nearly normal, but fewer children are born to such women than to their peers without disease, and it is difficult to be sure whether this reflects social choices (obviously influenced by having to cope with a chronic disease) and medical advice, or a failure of desired conception. The mean of 0.4 further infants born after a diagnosis of Crohn's disease was made (despite less use of contraception) compared to 0.7 born to controls in the same time-interval in one survey suggests a true inhibiting effect of the disease [2]. Good data for ulcerative colitis are lacking. Infertility occurs for all the reasons that may affect other women, with a small additional group of those with Crohn's disease in whom pelvic sepsis-related infertility is the direct result of the disease. Accurate numerical data do not exist to determine the frequency of this.

The menarche usually occurs at a normal age in girls with well-controlled inflammatory bowel disease, but is delayed in those with problematic Crohn's disease and growth retardation. Occasionally, delayed onset of periods is the presenting feature that prompts the investigations leading to its diagnosis. For reasons that are not clear, the menopause occurs about 4 years early in Crohn's disease and 2 years sooner than in the general population in ulcerative colitis.

Pregnancy

Inflammatory bowel disease typically runs a relatively benign course in pregnancy, with around half of women finding that quantity and quality of remission are at their best. Equally, there is a small proportion (10–15%) in whom the bowel is obviously more troublesome during pregnancy, and in a very few women the inflammatory bowel disease presents for the first time during pregnancy. For reasons that presumably have something to do with the very rapid hormonal shifts that occur after delivery, it is common for the post-puerperal period to represent a peak time for relapse in both Crohn's disease and ulcerative colitis. I routinely book a follow-up appointment for my patients 2–4 weeks after the expected date of delivery in anticipation of this.

Fortunately, the drugs most often used in inflammatory bowel disease are relatively innocuous in pregnancy. Mesalazine does not cross the placenta to any great extent, and there are no data indicating a risk to the fetus at any stage in gestation [3], even should larger amounts be transferred for whatever reason. All of the newer 5-ASA drugs, including olsalazine, can, in my view, safely be used throughout pregnancy, with the usual proviso that the regulatory authorities will continue to advise caution (e.g. British Committee on Safety of Medicines). Equally, the risk/benefit equation will be shifted away from drug use, for situations (such as prophylaxis of Crohn's disease relapse) where the indications are less clear-cut; the prospective parent should clearly be involved in this decision process. Sulphasalazine has the longest track-record for safe use in pregnancy, but poses an additional risk of neonatal haemolysis and methaemoglobinaemia because of the sulphonamide component. It is my practice to switch expectant mothers from sulphasalazine to one of the newer agents (or to stop therapy) prior to term in order to avoid this slight risk.

Steroid use in pregnancy is especially emotive. Hydrocortisone obviously crosses the placenta freely, and prednisolone hardly less so. There have been suggestions that cleft palate and hare lip are more common in infants born to mothers on steroids, but the evidence for this is not compelling. With daily systemic doses of less than 10 mg prednisolone (or 50 mg hydrocortisone) the risk of adrenal suppression in the infant is negligible, but adrenal problems can certainly affect the fetus and the neonate if larger doses are required for the mother's health. Alternatives to steroids should therefore be employed in inflammatory bowel disease care whenever possible, defined liquid diet being an especially attractive option in Crohn's disease [4], but as in other potentially maternal-life-threatening conditions the infant's health is best served by full attention to its mother's needs. Paediatric advice and a reducing steroid regime for the neonate with actual or potential adrenal suppression should be sought.

None of the immunosuppressives should be used in pregnancy unless essential for maternal health. However, there are reassuring data on the use of azathioprine. To Alstead's work summarizing 16 successful pregnancies in 14 women on the drug [5] can now be added data (in abstract form) from Francella and colleagues [6] in respect of no fewer than 155 patients (male and female) with inflammatory bowel disease who had had 6-mercaptopurine (6MP) and had also conceived (on a total of 347 occasions). This constituted about one-third of all their patients on the drug, who in turn represented 17% of all their inflammatory bowel disease patients. There were four groups – those who became pregnant having already stopped 6MP (95 pregnancies), those who discontinued the drug after pregnancy was established (64 pregnancies), those who continued the drug throughout pregnancy (eight pregnancies), and a control group who commenced the drug only after completing one or more pregnancies (180 pregnancies). There were no significant differences between any of the groups in terms of premature delivery, spontaneous abortion, congenital anomaly, neonatal infection or childhood neoplasia. There was, however, a trend towards higher rates for spontaneous abortion (19.2% v. 16.7%), congenital anomaly (4.2% v. 2.8%) and infection (4.2% v. 1.1%) in pregnancies of patients exposed to the drug. Whether the treated parent was the father or the mother seemed to have no influence on outcome, although the one childhood malignancy in the series (a Wilm's tumour) was in the son of a man on 6MP. The numbers of each complication were low and complete confidence is not appropriate, especially given the very small number of women who continued the drug throughout pregnancy, but it is encouraging that all the figures reported are very similar to those for the general healthy population. Immunosuppression and pregnancy remain very uneasy bed-fellows. If it is possible to withdraw immunosuppression successfully prior to conception, then this should be done. If attempts at withdrawal lead to rapid and uncontrolled relapse, then it is reasonable for the patient and his or her partner to make an informed choice to remain on the drug, recognizing that there is a risk, but for their particular case that the chance of a successful pregnancy is greater with the patient in remission on the drug than potentially or actually in relapse off it. I am unaware of pregnancy-related data for other immunosuppressives used in inflammatory bowel disease, but transplant recipients on cyclosporin appear to achieve normal outcomes for their pregnancies.

Surgery for inflammatory bowel disease may be needed during pregnancy. The desire to avoid potentially toxic drugs paradoxically increases the likelihood that surgery will be considered. There are, unsurprisingly, no controlled data on the safety and success of such surgery in comparison to comparable surgery performed outwith pregnancy, but expectations can be similar. Any abdominal procedure poses risks to the fetus but the decision to operate for inflammatory bowel disease will only be taken as a lesser of evils and it is most unlikely that a major pelvic procedure such as pouch creation will be considered.

The delivery of the infant will usually be a matter for the woman and her obstetric advisers. However, Caesarean section is strongly advised in the patient who has active perianal Crohn's, or who has needed previous surgery for anorectal fistula. Questionnaire data suggest that vaginal delivery (especially with episiotomy) poses a substantial risk of provoking perianal Crohn's disease even in those previously unaffected, with a 17.9% frequency of new occurrences of disease occurring within 2 months of pregnancy ($n = 179$), but these were unvalidated data and probably overestimate the association [7]. Few would argue that elective Caesarean section should be carefully considered in the woman with an ileo-anal pouch (Chapter 4), but good obstetric outcome and subsequent pouch function after vaginal delivery are recorded by at least one prominent centre [8].

Breast feeding

All drugs are sources of anxiety for the nursing mother, and with good reason, because most find their way into breast milk and thus to the infant to some extent. Amongst those most likely to be used in inflammatory bowel disease there need be no greater anxiety than while the mother is pregnant. Moderate doses of systemic steroids given to the mother put the infant at risk of cosmetic changes and adrenal suppression (and possibly subject to other steroid toxicity) but this is rarely a major medical issue.

Breast feeding is highly desirable but is not essential. If it is not possible for the mother to be satisfactorily maintained on a regime that is obviously safe for the infant, then bottle feeding is probably to be preferred.

PAEDIATRIC INFLAMMATORY BOWEL DISEASE PRACTICE

It is inappropriate for this volume to pretend a major role in guiding the paediatrician with a specialist interest in inflammatory bowel disease, but since the adult gastroenterologist will occasionally be asked to advise on the management of inflammatory bowel disease affecting children, and since a comprehensive service in paediatric gastroenterology is rarely available, a brief section is included. Referral to a tertiary centre is always wise if any doubt exists. However, much of paediatric inflammatory bowel disease practice is remarkably similar to that in adults. The main point of management difference is in respect of growth and growth retardation – an issue in many children with Crohn's disease but rarely a problem in ulcerative colitis.

The combined incidence of inflammatory bowel disease in those under 16 was around 5 per 100 000 in the mid 1980s in Sweden, with a rough equivalence of ulcerative colitis and Crohn's disease, given the number with unconfirmed Crohn's disease and the 23% with indeterminate colitis at the time of reporting [9]. There is a trend to earlier recognition and diagnosis of inflammatory bowel disease, which probably coincides with a true change in incidence. Numerous centres have confirmed that the continuing increase in incidence of Crohn's disease is most obvious in the paediatric age range, and perhaps most of all in children of immigrants to Western countries from the Indian subcontinent (Chapters 1 and 2). It is unlikely, however, that the aetiology of inflammatory bowel disease is different in children.

The clinical features of childhood disease are similar to those of adults, with the obvious difference that the very small child is unable to provide the history that is often so important in making a prompt diagnosis. In a series of 31 patients aged 10 or younger [10] there was no striking difference from what might be expected in terms of distribution of disease, the proportion of ulcerative colitis and Crohn's, or the clinical severity in an adult cohort: most were managed as out-patients. In the under-fives Crohn's disease is more likely to present late with growth retardation alone, while features of ulcerative colitis remain more typical [11]. In the latter series, eight under-fives with Crohn's disease had predominantly colonic involvement, with perianal disease in four, and with terminal ileal disease in only one; three had extra-intestinal manifestations. Of 11 patients with ulcerative colitis, nine had pancolitis and five needed surgery at a mean of 12 months from presentation. However, the Leiden group [12] found more anorexia, more general malaise and, predictably, more growth disturbance in the under-16s. Most of the differences they identify are less striking than the similarities, and the greater delay before diagnosis probably accounts for those that do exist. There is a general perception that Crohn's disease proves to be the final diagnosis more often than anticipated at first investigation; even when colectomy has been performed for (presumed) ulcerative colitis, the final diagnosis was Crohn's in no less than 53% of a Canadian series [13]. This difficulty is most pronounced for emergency colectomy, which reflects this difficulty in adult practice (Chapters 2 and 4).

The differential diagnosis is a little different in paediatric practice. Adult gastroenterologists are, for example, unlikely to see cow's milk protein colitis and will incorrectly assume that this sometimes florid haemorrhagic condition is ulcerative colitis, only to be surprised when a better-informed paediatric colleague achieves complete resolution simply by switching the infant to an amended milk formula. Reference to a paediatric gastroenterologist is recommended whenever diagnostic doubt exists.

Disease distribution in children with ulcerative colitis is comparable to that in adults, but children with Crohn's disease are more likely to have extensive and proximal small bowel disease. This is borne out by endoscopic assessment of the upper gastrointestinal tract; abnormalities are typically found in more than two-thirds of children with inflammatory bowel disease if both gastroscopy and colonoscopy are performed, regardless of the localization of symptoms and signs. In one such study the upper gastrointestinal signs were instrumental in making the diagnosis of Crohn's disease in no less than 41% of patients [14]; this study showed involvement of the upper gastrointestinal tract in 71%, of the terminal ileum in 53% and colon in 86%. The severity of disease probably encompasses the same spectrum as in adult practice. Complications of inflammatory bowel disease such as toxic megacolon, sclerosing cholangitis and the various extra-intestinal manifestations (Chapter 6) occur in children at similar frequency. Malignancy complicating inflammatory bowel disease is almost never seen in children, but this probably simply reflects the major influence of disease duration, and that most children have become adult before becoming at significant risk. Nevertheless, it is precisely those that present in childhood that are ultimately most likely to develop malignancy.

Growth retardation is a substantial problem in children with Crohn's disease. The following points are drawn from a fairly consistent literature. More than a third of juvenile patients with inflammatory bowel disease can be expected to fall below the fifth centile for height at some time [15], and two-thirds of those with Crohn's will have a growth velocity more than two standard deviations below normal [16]. Final adult height is notably deficient in 7%, and falls at least one standard deviation below normal in 29% [16]. Impaired growth velocity is the more sensitive measure of growth impairment, and should be sought even if growth centiles are maintained [17]. Concomitant reduction in childhood bone mass and bone density is also demonstrable in Crohn's disease [18].

Whether growth retardation in inflammatory bowel disease is steroid related is much less clear. The Motil and Griffiths studies [15, 17] failed to demonstrate a link with past or present steroids, Hildebrand *et al.* [16] attributed a weak link to current steroid usage, but felt that almost all of the growth deficit was after the onset of the disease but prior to its diagnosis (and treatment). The Issenman study [18] considered that steroid therapy had no effect on growth, which improved with time whether or not steroids were used. There is an increasing consensus that the main reason for growth failure is caloric insufficiency [19].

Nevertheless, therapy in children with inflammatory bowel disease is devised to minimize steroid usage, with a relative favouring of primary nutritional therapy in Crohn's disease (Chapter 3), and with a somewhat lower threshold for surgical intervention. Azathioprine and 6-mercaptopurine come under consideration relatively frequently, but there is understandable reserve about their actual use. In fact, safety appears good, and if surgery is not strongly indicated then they should be utilized more or less as in adults. It is probable that (as for steroids) a higher dose per kilogram body weight is required in the prepubertal child; a ratio of 1.5 to 1 is suggested [20]. Most specialist paediatricians now consider surgery early, especially when there is growth retardation, as this can be the crucial intervention to re-establish the patient on the appropriate centile of the growth chart. Very convincing clinical data have been presented by the Bart's group in London [21]. In other respects surgical series indicate strong similarities with adult practice (Chapter 4), most units now feeling confident to consider pouch creation for the older child with ulcerative colitis, although generally preferring an ileorectal anastomosis in the smallest, with the option to convert to a pouch in adolescence or early adulthood. A word of warning is sounded by the paediatricians in Montréal [13] who are concerned that ulcerative colitis is still erroneously diagnosed in some children with Crohn's disease. Although some of their data go back to 1961 and can hardly be considered contemporary, that no less than 15 of 28 children treated by colectomy for ulcerative colitis subsequently proved to have Crohn's disease should not be neglected. The reasonable comment is made that error is less likely if preoperative colonoscopy has been performed, and especially if the terminal ileum has been visualized and biopsied; this is already preferred practice in most paediatric gastrointestinal units.

Surgery in children with inflammatory bowel disease

The majority of decisions about surgery in children with inflammatory bowel disease will be similar to those in adults, although the patient's voice will be supported or substituted for by that of the parent. However, there is a greater urgency for surgical intervention in the child with Crohn's who is not growing. The St Bartholomew's group has made a compelling case for major improvement in growth velocity if the bulk of the diseased intestine can be removed, quite apart from the more obvious advantages to be expected from appropriate surgical intervention [21]. However, a degree of controversy remains, with the Toronto group considering that surgery made little difference (albeit with the caution that these patients would reasonably have been expected to do worse) [17]. Perhaps here one should follow the watchwords in fulminant colitis, and advise whenever there is doubt about surgery in a child with Crohn's disease and impaired growth that the choice should be surgery.

ADOLESCENTS

Adolescents pose problems distinct from both adults and children, and are unfortunately rather neglected by most health-care systems. Between 15 and 20% of all patients with inflammatory bowel disease present at this age, so there is even less excuse for the continued ignoring of this group. In most cases physicians more used to dealing with adults will be called upon to provide care. The adolescent with inflammatory bowel disease, like the child, remains prey to impaired growth and development, but practice here becomes influenced by the adolescent's desire (and need) for personal autonomy. Very easily this can lead to rejection of parental advice and encouragement (for example with nutrition) and a degree of bloody-mindedness that spills over into the patients' dealings with their medical advisers. In a partially controlled study of growth-retarded peripubertal individuals, 8 of 14 agreed to and were compliant with an overnight nasogastric tube feed. Linear growth and weight increased significantly over the next 12 months in those eight (by 7 cm and 11.7 kg, respectively), but remained unchanged in the six who declined nasogastric therapy [22]. It is not suggested that this was the only reason for the differences in outcome, as those choosing to reject care may well have a different prognosis for other reasons also, but it highlights some of the problems that must be tackled in adolescent management. In this context, the results of the Scottish follow-up of growth and development are reassuring for doctors, and should permit useful transmission of that information to adolescents when their anxieties about failed growth are at their peak. The study identified 105 individuals admitted for inflammatory bowel disease during 1968–83 and contacted all 87 of those that by the time of the study were at least 18 years of age and 5 years or more from the time of admission [23]. All of the patients were by then sexually mature, and all those with ulcerative colitis were of normal height and body mass index. Patients with Crohn's disease were about 8 kg lighter than their normal contemporaries (mean 67 kg in men, 51 kg in women), but only three were pathologically short. The strong implication is that although the pubertal growth spurt tends to be delayed in Crohn's disease it is usually, ultimately, effective in achieving normal height.

Concern that immunosuppressive therapy might be unduly hazardous in adolescence has not been borne out by experience [24], efficacy and safety appearing similar to that recorded in adults. The greater difficulties that I find in persuading this age group to have regular blood counts when on azathioprine and in remission do not seem to translate into problematic myelosuppression, but there must be some concern about this. Steroids are better avoided for all the reasons applicable in paediatric and adult practice, and with the additional pressing need to preserve normal appearance as the patient becomes sexually aware.

REFERENCES

1. Narendranathan M, Sandler RS, Suchindran CM, Savitz DA. Male infertility in inflammatory bowel disease. *J Clin Gastroenterol* 1989; **11**: 403–406.
2. Mayberry JF, Weterman IT. European survey of fertility and pregnancy in women with Crohn's disease: a case control study by European collaborative group. *Gut* 1986; **27**: 821–825.
3. Trallori G, D'Albasio G, Bardazzi G *et al*. 5-Aminosalicylic acid in pregnancy: clinical report. *Ital J Gastroenterol* 1994; **26**: 75–78.
4. Teahon K, Pearson M, Levi AJ, Bjarnason I. Elemental diet in the management of Crohn's disease during pregnancy. *Gut* 1991; **32**: 1079–1081.
5. Alstead EM, Ritchie JK, Lennard-Jones JE *et al*. Safely of azathioprine in pregnancy in inflammatory bowel disease. *Gastroenterology* 1990; **99**: 443–446.
6. Francella A, Dayan A, Rubin P *et al*. 6-Mercaptopurine is safe therapy for child bearing patients with inflammatory bowel disease: a case controlled study. *Gastroenterology* 1996; **110**: A909.
7. Brandt LJ, Estabrook SG, Reinus JF. Results of a survey to evaluate whether vaginal delivery and episiotomy lead to perineal involvement in women with Crohn's disease. *Am J Gastroenterol* 1995; **90**: 1918–1922.
8. Juhasz ES, Fozard B, Dozois RR *et al*. Ileal pouch-anal anastomosis function following childbirth. An extended evaluation. *Dis Colon Rectum* 1995; **38**: 159–165.
9. Hildebrand H, Fredrikzon B, Holmquist L *et al*. Chronic inflammatory bowel disease in children and adolescents in Sweden. *J Ped Gastroenterol Nutr* 1991; **13**: 293–297.

10. Chang CH, Heyman MB, Snyder JD. Inflammatory bowel disease in children less than 10 years old: is severe disease common? *Gastroenterology* 1996; **110**: A795.
11. Integlia M, Weiselberg B, Polk B *et al.* Features of inflammatory bowel disease in children less than 5 years old. *Gastroenterology* 1996; **110**: A807.
12. Wagtmans MJ, Van Hogezand RA, Mearin ML *et al.* The clinical course of Crohn's disease differs between children and adults. *Gastroenterology* 1996; **110**: A1041.
13. D'Agata ID, Deslandres C. Outcome of pediatric patients after subtotal colectomy for presumed ulcerative colitis. *Gastroenterology* 1996; **110**: A797.
14. Cameron DJ. Upper and lower gastrointestinal endoscopy in children and adolescents with Crohn's disease: a prospective study. *J Gastroenterol Hepatol* 1991; **6**: 355–358.
15. Motil KJ, Grand RJ, Davis-Kraft L *et al.* Growth failure in children with inflammatory bowel disease: a prospective study. *Gastroenterology* 1993; **105**: 681–691.
16. Hildebrand H, Karlberg J, Kristiansson B. Longitudinal growth in children and adolescents with inflammatory bowel disease. *J Ped Gastroenterol Nutr* 1994; **18**: 165–173.
17. Griffiths A, Nguyen P, Smith C *et al.* Growth and clinical course of children with Crohn's disease. *Gut* 1993; **34**: 939–943.
18. Issenman RM, Atkinson SA, Radoja C, Fraher L. Longitudinal assessment of growth, mineral metabolism, and bone mass in pediatric Crohn's disease. *J Ped Gastroenterol Nutr* 1993; **17**: 401–406.
19. Polk DB, Hattner JA, Kerner JA Jr. Improved growth and disease activity after intermittent administration of a defined formula diet in children with Crohn's disease. *J Parent Ent Nutr* 1992; **16**: 499–504.
20. Cuffari C, Théôret Y, Lahaie R, Seidman E. 6-Mercaptopurine metabolite levels in adult and pediatric IBD: correlation with drug efficacy. *Gastroenterology* 1996; **110**: A890.
21. Shand WS. Surgical therapy of chronic inflammatory bowel disease in childhood. *Baillières Clin Gastroenterol* 1994; **8**: 149–180.
22. Aiges H, Markowitz J, Rosa J, Daum F. Home nocturnal supplemental nasogastric feedings in growth-retarded adolescents with Crohn's disease. *Gastroenterology* 1989; **97**: 905–910.
23. Ferguson A, Sedgwick DM. Juvenile onset inflammatory bowel disease: height and body mass index in adult life. *Br Med J* 1994; **308**: 1259–1263.
24. Markowitz J, Rosa J, Grancher K *et al.* Long-term 6-mercaptopurine treatment in adolescents with Crohn's disease. *Gastroenterology* 1990; **99**: 1347–1351.

6

Extra-intestinal manifestations

EXTRA-INTESTINAL MANIFESTATIONS OF INFLAMMATORY BOWEL DISEASE

The extra-intestinal manifestations of inflammatory bowel disease fall into two broad groups. On the whole, those which follow an acute course are also those that run in parallel with the associated inflammatory bowel disease. The more chronic and potentially progressive extra-intestinal manifestations generally behave more independently, and are relatively uninfluenced by the activity of the gastrointestinal disorder. Although it is more convenient to consider individual problems according to the particular organ site involved, it will be noted that many of the extra-intestinal manifestations occur together, and that each may be associated with other non-gastrointestinal problems.

All of the extra-intestinal manifestations tend to occur in patients with disease of the colon, and rarely complicate Crohn's disease confined to the small bowel. There are a number of hypotheses for this observation, but no confirmed factual data. The 40 kDa colonic epithelial antigen discussed in Chapter 1 is expressed also in the epithelial tissues of the common extra-intestinal sites, suggesting that it may be of some general relevance, but is absent in Crohn's disease whether or not there is colonic involvement. A relevance of the faecal stream, with or without intestinal permeability disruption (see Chapter 1 and below), is suggested by the close link with colonic disease, and it is possible that a similar mechanism accounts for the finding that those with perforating Crohn's are the most likely to develop extra-intestinal manifestations [1].

JOINTS IN INFLAMMATORY BOWEL DISEASE

Patients with inflammatory bowel disease are at increased risk of a number of specific joint conditions and remain subject to (for example) degenerative arthritides and rheumatoid arthritis at frequencies typical of the general population. Ankylosing spondylitis and other spondarthritides are over-represented, and there is an important, though poorly understood, condition peculiar to those with inflammatory bowel disease, to be described here as inflammatory bowel disease-related arthropathy, a term preferred to alternatives such as enteropathic arthritis because it is not necessarily the case that the intestinal disorder is the cause of the joint problems, and because many overtly disabled patients lack objective evidence of an arthritis despite obvious symptoms focused on the joints.

Ankylosing spondylitis (AS) affecting patients with inflammatory bowel disease runs a relatively independent course typical of spondylitis in patients without gastrointestinal problems [2] (but see below). Modest morning stiffness and low back pain may progress to a stooped posture (Plate 10) and an increasingly immobile spine which can eventually impair ventilation. The sacro-iliac joint margins become blurred radiologically, with associated patchy sclerosis, and are later lost; the vertebrae pass through a parallel course from being 'squared', to exhibiting entheses, syndesmophytes and finally the bamboo spine. Patients with ulcerative colitis carry a 30-fold increased risk of spondylitis, but it remains an uncommon association as AS itself has a prevalence of only 150 per 100 000 in Western populations. Interestingly, although almost all patients with spondylitis have the HLA B27 genotype, only between 60 and 80% of those with both ulcerative colitis and spondylitis are positive. Treatment of progressive spondylitis is never easy, the emphasis resting with physiotherapy and non-steroidal anti-inflammatories. Unfortunately the latter are less well tolerated in inflammatory bowel disease.

Inflammatory bowel disease patients much more frequently develop sacroiliitis without generalized spondylitis. A prevalence in the region of 10% is recorded [3] and this is therefore a relatively frequent incidental finding on radiography (as, for example, in barium series). If asymptomatic, no action is necessary as it is often not progressive. Other forms of spondarthritis (psoriatic, etc.) are over-represented in inflammatory bowel disease, but require no special measures. All of these tend to behave independently of the intestinal disorder.

IBD-related arthropathy is more common still. It was described as long ago as 1929, and there is a quoted prevalence ranging between 10% [1] and 22% [4]. It usually presents as a polyarthropathy, symmetrically affecting medium-sized joints; deforming arthritis is rare. It is said to be more common in Crohn's affecting the colon than in entirely small bowel disease, and in Crohn's colitis than in ulcerative colitis. If there is no concurrent sacroiliitis, radiological features are few, and may even then be confined to the demonstration of soft tissue swelling. IBD-related arthropathy follows a close but not identical activity profile to the associated intestinal disease, tends to respond along with the bowel to gastrointestinal therapy (perhaps especially to steroids), but may also have its onset or relapse as steroids are withdrawn. Occasionally patients are seen with a condition clinically more similar to rheumatoid arthritis, but without the characteristic antibodies; they probably constitute an IBD-related arthropathy subgroup [5]. The condition may predate the onset of inflammatory bowel disease symptoms, and can occur at a very early age indeed [6]. We have recently completed a prospective survey of IBD-related arthropathy at St Mark's [7] and, given the incompleteness of the literature, a brief summary is in order.

Consecutive attenders at the inflammatory bowel disease clinic (55 with Crohn's disease and 46 with ulcerative colitis) were studied. Arthropathy was sought clinically and by questionnaire. As there are no agreed diagnostic standards for IBD-related arthropathy, and because radiology is often normal in symptomatic patients, the following definitions were employed. Spinal (or axial) arthropathy was recorded if continuing, disabling back pain began before age 30, or if radiological signs were present; peripheral arthropathy was diagnosed if joints were involved on more than five occasions for more than 12 weeks, or from radiographic abnormalities. Arthropathy affected 31% of Crohn's patients and 30% of those with ulcerative colitis. It was peripheral in 22% and 24%, respectively, and spinal in 22% and 6% (40% and 0% of whom, respectively, had radiological evidence of sacroiliitis). There were no positive radiographs in those without symptoms. Compared to Crohn's patients without arthropathy, those with joint symptoms exhibited a higher prevalence of smoking (59% v. 29%), of perianal disease (70% v. 45%) and more frequent colonic involvement (100% v. 74%). In both Crohn's and ulcerative colitis there were significantly higher frequencies of other extra-intestinal manifestations in those with arthropathy (e.g. erythema nodosum 28% v. 3%; oral ulcers 82% v. 47%; conjunctivitis 46% v. 26%; symptomatic gallstones 14% v. 5%). This observation has also been made by others with (for example) erythema nodosum affecting 35% of Crohn's patients with arthritis compared to 6% of those without [4]. Only 12 of our 31 patients with arthropathy had received specific therapy (including only 7 of the 12 who had had rheumatological consultations). Non-steroidals were effective in about two-thirds of those in whom they were tried, but had to be withdrawn because of intestinal side-effects in half. Steroid injections were effective on the six occasions on which they had been employed. There was no apparent advantage from the use of sulphasalazine compared to other 5-ASA drugs in treatment of the inflammatory bowel disease, despite the value of the former in other rheumatological conditions. It was concluded (with acknowledgement of the potential biases of reporting from a tertiary referral centre) that disabling joint symptoms are more common in inflammatory bowel disease than the literature suggests, and might be considered to warrant closer involvement of rheumatologists. The substantially higher prevalence in our series than in a comparable study (limited to Crohn's disease) which found only 22% of patients to have joint disease [4] most probably reflects our deliberately less stringent criteria for diagnosis, rather than a bias from the nature of referral practice. The higher proportion of the Münch patients with overt sacroiliitis (14%) supports this view. Our position is defended on the basis that it reflects patients' symptoms rather than our ability to attach a firm, objectively verifiable diagnosis, but this is clearly only a point of view.

Taken from the perspective of the rheumatologist, the issue of inflammatory bowel disease in relation to the seronegative arthropathies is quite as compelling, with a frequency of gastrointestinal involvement in at least 50% of these patients. De Vos and her colleagues have now reported on 123 patients with well-defined spondyloarthropathy, but who failed to meet criteria for ankylosing spondylitis; all were investigated gastroenterologically [8]. Patients with previously known inflammatory bowel disease were excluded. All patients had a rectal examination and biopsy, and only 40 were found to lack histological evidence of proctitis. Nearly 50 of the patients were then subjected to 'routine' serial colonoscopy. In keeping with the literature, there appeared to be virtual independence of activity of gut and joints in those in whom gastrointestinal disease became overt. However, initial macroscopic and histological inflammation of the intestine predicted a higher risk of progression to formal established ankylosing spondylitis; of the 19% who progressed, all but one had initial colitis. In 7.3% of the study group, frank inflammatory bowel disease developed during follow-up (seven of the nine subjects having histological changes at presentation). Sulphasalazine was successfully used for the joint symptoms but had no apparent influence on the likelihood of development of intestinal symptoms.

Parallel data come from a scintigraphic study of patients with seronegative spondyloarthropathy compared with those with inflammatory bowel disease [9]. HMPAO scans (Chapter 2) were positive (as expected) in a high proportion of those with intestinal disease (67% in Crohn's disease and 66% in ulcerative colitis) but were also abnormal, showing increased intestinal uptake, in 53% of those with spondyloarthropathy who were previously considered to be free of intestinal involvement.

The potential importance of pouchitis as a human model of inflammatory bowel disease has been discussed in general terms (Chapter 1); it has relevance also to IBD-related arthropathy. Although most patients with ulcerative colitis and arthropathy improve after colectomy, a small percentage of those having an ileo-anal pouch then develop an arthropathy similar to IBD-related arthropathy, despite having had no joint symptoms prior to colectomy [10, 11]. This is not explained, and the finding itself is disputed by another group [12] .

Several lines of evidence suggest that altered intestinal permeability may contribute to the onset of IBD-related arthropathy. These include the clinical observations in pouch patients, the obvious parallels with septic arthritis (characteristically with gastrointestinal pathogens such as *Salmonella*) and the reactive arthritides (again linked to organisms such as *Campylobacter jejuni* or *Giardia lamblia* that are also harmful to the gastrointestinal tract) [2]. A role of abnormal permeability is also suggested for the reactive arthritides that occur in conjunction with infection of the genitourinary tract, in which bacterial antigens are often detectable in the synovium of affected joints. In a study of patients with seronegative arthritis and subclinical gastrointestinal involvement, the histological and immunological features of the gastrointestinal inflammation appeared to follow one of two patterns [13]. Patients had either an acute inflammatory response, and increases predominantly in ileal IgA and IgG, or more chronic inflammation, with elevation of mucosal IgM as well as IgA and IgG. The former group had the clinical features of a reactive, peripheral arthritis, while the latter had a more spondylitic arthritis. While these patients had no evidence of intra-articular bacterial antigens, it is certainly possible to show that such translocation of bacteria (and presumably other potential pathogens) from the gut to systemic sites can occur (A. Keat, personal communication; [14]). In the HLA B27 transgenic rat model, Rath *et al.* have shown that not only were extra-intestinal manifestations (including arthritis) produced by exposure to organisms such as *Bacteroides* and a variety of streptococci, but that treatment with metronidazole was protective against these effects [15]. The strong correlation in all published series of IBD-related arthropathy with the presence of other extra-intestinal manifestations, and now with smoking in Crohn's, points to further areas of potentially fruitful research and may indicate new therapeutic strategies.

OSTEOPOROSIS AND OTHER BONE DISEASE IN INFLAMMATORY BOWEL DISEASE

Bone density is undoubtedly reduced in patients with inflammatory bowel disease. This appears to reflect chronicity of disease activity at least as much as any particular therapeutic intervention or other complications. Typical studies find negative Z scores for the majority of patients with both ulcerative colitis and Crohn's disease [16, 17]. Although Bischoff *et al.* found a 65% prevalence of diminished bone mineral density in the forearm bones, which was more than two standard deviations below the normal range in 19% [17], the larger Finnish study found deficiency of this degree in only 5.3% [16]. Serum calcium is usually normal, but evidence of parathyroid overactivity and markers of excess osteoclastic activity are common. Bischoff's study was able to link evidence of bone breakdown with activity of the inflammatory bowel disease. The relevance of steroids is not certain, but the Finnish study showed very weak but statistically significant associations between lower bone density and cumulative exposure to prednisolone ($r = 0.16$–0.24, depending on bone site). It was felt that steroids were relevant to this, especially since the effect was most obvious in those who had received more than 10 g prednisolone, but this does not help us to distinguish the effect of the disease and its chronic inflammation from that of the drugs used to treat it. Data of particular relevance here come from a Scottish study of 30 newly diagnosed inflammatory bowel disease patients (who had obviously not received steroids) [18]. Spine and forearm bone mineral density was normal in all of 15 patients with ulcerative colitis, while significant defects were apparent in 15 patients with Crohn's disease (mean Z scores of below –1 at both bone sites). Significantly, in 23 patients reinvestigated after 12 months, there was no marked individual change nor significant overall change in Z score regardless of whether or not patients had received steroids during this time.

In children (see also Chapter 5), there is the additional concern of failed growth and that subnormal bone mass will be associated with osteoporosis and a lifelong increased risk of fractures. This is an appropriate concern given that the risk of osteoporotic fractures in the elderly appears to be strongly influenced by the peak bone mass of early adulthood. Clearly, there are other factors, but this is one that can potentially be manipulated by exercise programmes, and arguably no less so in inflammatory bowel disease patients. Herzog *et al.* have been concerned at the profound osteopenia uncovered on investigation of children with Crohn's disease and growth retardation [19] but identify a need to correct the extent of bone mineralization for the bone age, or in other words to use a score for osteoporosis where instead of chronological age adjustment (as for a Z score), the bone age is utilized. When such corrections are made, the degree of osteoporosis is considerably less alarming but still constitutes an important reason for remedying growth retardation as soon as possible.

It is possible to reverse osteopenia associated with coeliac disease by dietary intervention [20], from which should be taken the concept that intervention has the potential to do more than merely prevent further deterioration.

RENAL AND URINARY TRACT PROBLEMS ASSOCIATED WITH INFLAMMATORY BOWEL DISEASE

Urinary tract stones, particularly calcium oxalate stones, are over-represented in patients with inflammatory bowel disease. Most at risk are those with extensive small bowel Crohn's yet with a retained colon, in whom the proportion affected by stone formation may exceed 25% [21]. Intestinal luminal oxalate is normally calcium-bound and poorly available.

In fat malabsorption calcium becomes preferentially bound to free fatty acids, and oxalate accordingly becomes sodium-bound. Sodium oxalate is soluble and is absorbed in the colon. This increased absorption predisposes to hyperoxaluria, and thus to an increased risk of renal stones [22]. This is particularly a problem in patients with short bowel syndrome (Chapter 7); avoidance of foodstuffs rich in oxalate, such as spinach, parsley, rhubarb, strawberries, beetroot, cocoa and tea, should be advised.

Urate stones are less common, and usually reflect continual dehydration associated with high volume intestinal losses. Again, they are seen most often in those with short bowel syndrome, but here the association is with the high jejunostomy and problematic fluid and electrolyte loss [23]. Prevention, from adequate hydration and good urine flow, forms part of standard good management. Nephrological advisers will often need advice on the management of short bowel syndrome if inappropriate advice simply to drink more is to be avoided (Chapter 7).

Hydronephrosis and retroperitoneal fibrosis are described in Crohn's disease. Simple hydronephrosis is evidently not a rare complication, affecting perhaps 2% of all Crohn's patients ([24] and unpublished observations.) It usually affects the right side, and is related (weakly) to contiguous inflammatory disease. It seems to be a benign complication and rarely requires intervention in its own right, but intra-ureteric stenting and surgical reconstruction are then effective.

The continuing question of nephropathy as an important potential complication of aminosalicylate (5-ASA) therapy has been discussed in Chapter 3, and although most data are reasonably reassuring, this will no doubt remain a discussion point. Comparisons of patients with human volunteers and animal models are not necessarily relevant, however, as inflammatory bowel disease itself predisposes to intrinsic renal disease affecting both glomeruli and tubules independently of therapy.

Morphological changes in the glomeruli of patients with inflammatory bowel disease have long been recognized [25, 26]. The prevalence is uncertain but low; reporting authors generally seem to believe that the associations are of a causal nature, and unrelated to pharmacological intervention. Minor elevations of serum creatinine are also often demonstrable in inflammatory bowel disease, but are not progressive and should probably not be considered sufficient to be of major clinical concern.

Kreisel *et al.* [27] have examined renal status in inflammatory bowel disease patients using a selection of urinary enzymes as markers for tubular function. Pathological enzymuria (corrected for renal excretory function) was almost exclusively linked with active disease in ulcerative colitis and not with current or past exposure to 5-ASA. In Crohn's disease there was no strong relationship between disease activity and enzymuria, but nor was there any link between enzymuria and 5-ASA exposure. The authors conclude that subtle tubular damage is a common feature of inflammatory bowel disease (found in 20–25% of cases) that appears independent of therapy, and is not obviously associated with other extra-intestinal manifestations of disease (although the number of cases with other non-gastrointestinal features was probably too small for the latter to be a confident conclusion). Urinary β-N-acetyl-D-glucosaminidase was the most sensitive marker of those studied. The authors speculate that the problem is related to high circulatory levels of inflammatory cytokines, and that differences from previous studies are probably explicable on the basis of their smaller numbers and the previous inclusion predominantly of patients with ulcerative colitis in remission. It does not appear that the tubular damage now being identified has major prognostic significance, and two major studies of all-causes mortality have failed to demonstrate excess deaths from renal failure (Chapter 2).

Amyloidosis of the reactive AA type is seen in some patients with long-standing Crohn's disease, but there is probably no increased incidence in ulcerative colitis. The kidney is the most common site for clinically significant amyloid deposition, affecting around 1% of patients with Crohn's disease on a lifetime basis [28]. It is probable that it is more frequent when control of Crohn's-related inflammation has not been good, and it is suggested that anti-inflammatory therapy might be justified on this basis even in the asymptomatic patient who continues to exhibit a high level of acute-phase reactants (L.B. Lovat and M.B. Pepys, personal communication). Once renal amyloidosis is established it is most often responsible for nephrotic syndrome, although the magnitude of this is very variable. It runs a course independent of the Crohn's disease once it has arisen, and occasionally leads to a need for renal replacement therapy.

SKIN PROBLEMS IN INFLAMMATORY BOWEL DISEASE

Erythema nodosum presents as painful, raised, red lesions, typically on the shins, in the relatively young patient with active inflammatory bowel disease (Plate 11). It is the most common dermatological manifestation of inflammatory bowel disease and is more often seen in Crohn's disease than in ulcerative colitis, affecting around 15% of Crohn's patients [29] compared to only about 2% of those with ulcerative colitis [30]. It is the result of a subcutaneous septal panniculitis and is associated with a neutrophil infiltrate that evolves through a more chronic inflammatory process before complete resolution. Biopsy, though of reasonably characteristic nature, is very rarely appropriate given the clear clinical pointers to the diagnosis in inflammatory bowel disease patients. It usually appears during active inflammatory bowel disease (only 10% of Mir-Madjlessi's patients having inactive colitis, for example), and runs a broadly parallel course which does not normally require specific therapy. Although it may recur with further exacerbations of the intestinal disease, it very rarely, if ever, recurs after proctocolectomy.

Pyoderma gangrenosum is less common, affecting no more than about 2% of inflammatory bowel disease patients [30, 31], but it is more common in long-standing disease, and is usually associated with active colitis in patients with Crohn's disease. About 55% of all patients with pyoderma have underlying inflammatory bowel disease, but it is also seen in a variety of other inflammatory conditions and in isolation. When it is the presenting feature of inflammatory bowel disease it may be misinterpreted, not least since the histological findings are non-specific. The lesions are typically single, affecting the lower limb. They develop into deep ulcers with a necrotic base, undermined purple edges, with a purulent sterile discharge. Pyoderma gangrenosum may respond to therapy for inflammatory bowel disease, but may require this at an intensity out of proportion to that needed for the bowel. Especially when there are many large lesions, prolonged high-dose steroids, other forms of immunosuppression, or colectomy may be indicated, but controlled data are lacking. There is good anecdotal response, also, for the use of intralesional steroids, and the application of potent steroid preparations beneath an impermeable dressing seems particularly helpful. Long-term scarring may remain. The pathogenesis is not clear, but the strong association of pyoderma lesions with sites of surgical and other trauma, especially the peristomal area [32], suggests that pathergy is an important factor (Plate 12).

The rare condition known as Sweet's syndrome, or acute pyrexial neutrophilic dermatosis, is also described in both ulcerative colitis and Crohn's disease [33]. It presents with purple/red plaque-like lesions of the skin with pyrexia and a high neutrophil count, as the name suggests. It is more commonly associated with malignant disorders (especially haematological ones) and most of the data on its therapy come from that context. It is probable that simple short courses of prednisolone by mouth suffice in most cases but metronidazole and a variety of other agents have also been suggested.

OPHTHALMIC COMPLICATIONS IN INFLAMMATORY BOWEL DISEASE

In common with many of the other extra-intestinal manifestations, involvement of the eye is more often seen in patients with colitis, and on the whole is associated with active intestinal disease [34, 35]. It appears to be more common in Crohn's colitis than in ulcerative colitis, and a disturbing paediatric report suggests that the frequency of asymptomatic anterior uveitis may be as high as 6.2% in Crohn's disease [36]. Iritis and uveitis present clinically, as when unassociated with inflammatory bowel disease, with impaired visual acuity and a painful red eye. The diagnosis can be confirmed by slit-lamp examination if it is not otherwise obvious clinically; topical steroids are usually sufficient therapy (with a mydriatic), but there is a risk of permanent damage if prompt treatment is not initiated. Pain will usually respond to simple analgesics or to non-steroidal anti-inflammatories [37].

Episcleritis is the most common ophthalmic association of inflammatory bowel disease. It is usually responsible for redness and discomfort with a conjuctivitis-like syndrome, but there are occasionally disturbances of vision and, more rarely still, superficial ulcers may develop. Treatment is not normally required, other than that for the concurrent exacerbation of the intestinal inflammation, but for the more severe cases topical steroids almost always suffice [37].

HEPATOBILIARY DISEASE IN INFLAMMATORY BOWEL DISEASE

Cholelithiasis

Gallstones are more common in patients with ileal Crohn's disease and particularly so when there has been terminal ileal resection. The prevalence in Birmingham was 28% in relatively unselected patients with Crohn's disease screened by ultrasonography [38] if those who had already had a cholecystectomy were included, and reaches 45% in those with established short bowel syndrome [39]. A population-controlled study suggests, at first sight, that these figures may overemphasize the attributable risk, as 9.7% of the normal population also had stones [40]. However, after age and sex matching, the odds ratio for cholelithiasis proved significant for both ulcerative colitis (OR, 2.5; CI, 1.2–5.2) and for Crohn's disease (OR, 3.6; CI, 1.2–10.4), with, as expected, the highest rate in those with ileal involvement (OR, 4.5). The duration of the intestinal disorder also correlates with the risk of stone formation. The Birmingham group was unable to demonstrate a direct link with ileal involvement [38], but curiously found an association with the number of laparotomies rather than with the cumulative magnitude of intestinal resection, and suggested that biliary stasis and/or dysmotility are therefore more important than the bile salt malabsorption and reduced bile salt pool that have previously been implicated. In general, patients with previous intestinal resection for Crohn's disease have low biliary cholesterol saturation, and a higher than normal ratio of ursodeoxycholic to deoxycholic acid [41]. Cholesterol stones are not therefore to be expected in Crohn's disease, and gallstones in inflammatory bowel disease are indeed usually predominantly of pigment type. However, predominantly cholesterol stones are described in patients with ileo-anal anastomoses [42]. Crohn's-induced stones may also result from a competition for binding between excess (malabsorbed) colonic bile salts and bilirubin, promoting an enterohepatic circulation of bilirubin, a higher concentration of bilirubin in gallbladder bile and a predisposition to pigment stones [43]. The management of cholelithiasis in patients with inflammatory bowel disease is that of cholelithiasis in general, but it may prove difficult or impossible safely to perform laparoscopic cholecystectomy in the patient who has already had extensive surgical intervention for Crohn's disease.

Intrinsic liver disease

Parenchymal liver disease occurs to some extent in primary sclerosing cholangitis (see below) but is also over-represented in other respects, with upwards of 10% of patients with inflammatory bowel disease having abnormal liver function tests at some time [44]. In most cases these reflect active intestinal disease and have no other significance. Patients with inflammatory bowel disease appear similarly susceptible to viral hepatitis, and the effects of alcohol abuse, but those with ulcerative colitis in particular are more prone to certain hepatic disorders. Liver disease tends to affect those with more severe inflammatory bowel disease, so the 50% with abnormal liver histology at prospective liver biopsy in a series of patients having colectomy for ulcerative colitis might be thought to be unrepresentative [45] were it not for a 50% rate of abnormal histology in biopsies from 74 colitics with normal liver function [46]. There were, however, higher proportions of specific diagnoses in Mattila's study [45], with steatosis affecting 28%, sclerosing cholangitis 41%, hepatitis 21%, and only 10% with the ill-defined abnormalities more typical of the Swedish study [46].

Steatosis is accordingly a common intrinsic condition of the liver in inflammatory bowel disease, and is found in Crohn's as well as in ulcerative colitis. It probably reflects chronic inflammation and possibly a degree of malnutrition, and does not appear to be progressive. Hepatic fibrosis and cirrhosis may be seen as complications of long-term parenteral nutrition, and will, as such, occasionally be seen in patients with Crohn's disease who have had massive resections, but they also occur in unresected inflammatory bowel disease. The incidence of cirrhosis attributable to the intestinal disorder is not known, given confounding factors such as transfusion-related hepatitis, sclerosing cholangitis, and alcohol abuse, but is probably in the region of 1% on a lifetime basis. Appropriate management and prognosis are most probably those of cirrhosis in general.

Chronic active hepatitis affects patients with ulcerative colitis more than those with Crohn's disease – at a frequency in the region of 2%. There has been some confusion in the literature over the distinction between chronic active hepatitis and pericholangitis, not least since the two may occur together. It is increasingly recognized that the latter is predominantly a feature of primary sclerosing cholangitis, and is of little consequence in its own right. From a large series of patients with severe autoimmune chronic hepatitis, Perdigoto *et al.* identified no less than 16%

with associated ulcerative colitis, half of whom also had sclerosing cholangitis [47]. The colitics appeared to have more severe disease and worse prognosis than those with isolated liver disease, but this adverse influence was lost when the patients with sclerosing cholangitis were excluded. Such patients usually respond to steroids and azathioprine similarly to those without intestinal disease.

The only hepatic lesion that appears to be more common in Crohn's disease than in ulcerative colitis is granulomatous hepatitis. The prevalence is not certain, there having been no biopsy study of unselected patients comparable to the Swedish studies in ulcerative colitis. Clinically significant disease affects about 1% of those with Crohn's, with a cholestatic enzyme profile, sometimes associated with hepatic discomfort and pyrexia [48].

Primary sclerosing cholangitis

Primary sclerosing cholangitis (PSC) is a chronic cholestatic condition, variable both in its severity and its tendency to progress. There is a characteristic pattern of inflammation and fibrosis which can affect any part of the biliary tree, where it can be responsible for a combination of stricturing and duct dilatation. A considerable majority of patients with PSC also have ulcerative colitis – most series reporting the association in about 80% or more (the diagnosis of PSC occasionally preceding the diagnosis of colitis). In a recent Swedish study of 76 patients with PSC, 65 were previously known to have inflammatory bowel disease. Nine of the remaining 11 agreed to be investigated by a protocol colonoscopy. This revealed ulcerative colitis in six, Crohn's disease in one, and non-specific changes in two [49].

In inflammatory bowel disease clinics PSC can be expected in about 2.5% of colitics. It is described in Crohn's disease, but most patients with PSC have ulcerative colitis. It is usual that the colitis is extensive, and often the case that it is relatively inactive. Given the relative rarity of PSC with Crohn's disease it is odd that the Mayo Clinic should find a much higher than expected association of PSC with another granulomatous disorder – namely sarcoidosis – which was present in 0.7% of their PSC cases [50].

Potential aetiological associations
A strong association between primary sclerosing cholangitis and the HLA haplotype A1-B8-DR3-DQ2 has been known to exist for some time, and has been refined to the subtyped haplotype DRB1*1301, DQA1*0103, DQB1*0603 [51], genetic probing indicating that the determinant for this lies close to the DRB locus [52].

An association has also been established between PSC and the presence of antineutrophil cytoplasmic antibodies. This exceeds the expected degree of association for their prevalence in ulcerative colitis (Chapter 1) and has been reported at frequencies up to 82% [53]. It is probable that (as in the colon) the antibody has no clinical, pathogenic or prognostic significance [54]. However, detectable pANCA has also been described in 25% of healthy relatives of those with primary sclerosing cholangitis [53].

The association of non-smoking with ulcerative colitis (Chapter 1) holds good for patients with PSC, whether or not they also have ulcerative colitis, although it should be conceded that the data for PSC without colitis are based on rather small numbers [55, 56].

Clinical features

PSC should be considered in all colitic patients who develop abnormal liver biochemistry. In the absence of firmly established useful therapy it is probably not yet justifiable to seek it in the asymptomatic patient with normal liver function, despite the probability that by doing this it might prove possible to diagnose the condition at an earlier stage. Early PSC is almost always asymptomatic. With progression it becomes more common for the patient to describe periodic cholestasis (pruritus, dark urine, pale stools), with or without evidence of cholangitis and right upper quadrant abdominal pain. There are no characteristic physical signs until liver failure and the non-specific signs of portal hypertension and decompensated cirrhosis supervene. Diagnosis of PSC requires moderately invasive procedures (usually endoscopic retrograde cholangiography (ERCP) and often liver biopsy), and it is therefore appropriate to check first for other causes of liver dysfunction that are identifiable by serology or biochemical tests. If such testing is unhelpful or negative, then ERCP is probably indicated (Figure 6.1).

Imaging

There are data indicating that PSC can be inferred from biliary abnormalities identified on ultrasonographic scanning [57], but the reliability is as yet insufficient to be confident of either positive or negative outcomes. Magnetic resonance imaging of the biliary tree is at an exciting phase of its evolution, and may soon reduce the need for diagnostic ERCP, but its undoubted ability to identify intraductal stones may not be associated with sufficient resolution to confirm or refute the changes of PSC. The radiological diagnosis of PSC requires evidence of biliary changes at at least two sites, with evidence of mucosal damage and a combination of stenosis and dilatation of the biliary tree. It is conventional to confine the diagnosis to individuals in whom there has been no history of cholelithiasis, as the changes of sclerosing cholangitis secondary to chronic duct stone retention are not possible to distinguish from those of PSC. The sclerosing cholangitis peculiar to HIV infection and AIDS [58] deserves brief comment as this variant almost certainly has an infective aetiology

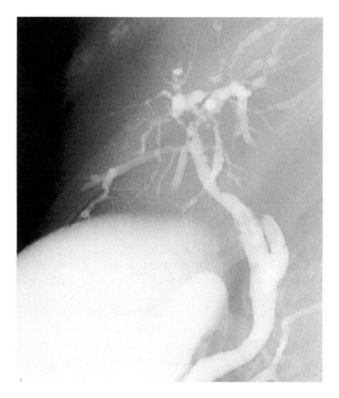

Figure 6.1 ERCP in primary sclerosing cholangitis. The distended gallbladder is characteristic and helps to confirm that the scrawny stenotic intrahepatic ducts are diseased and that the appearances are not simply those of an underfilled system. In this case the slight irregularities of the common bile duct should anyway lead to the correct diagnosis.

(*Cryptosporidium* or cytomegalovirus are most implicated). The radiological features of AIDS-related sclerosing cholangitis are virtually identical to those of PSC, apart from the AIDS-related condition being associated at times with intraluminal polypoidal lesions which are not seen in PSC. Although the radiographic similarity might suggest comparable aetiopathogenesis in PSC, it may simply reflect the fact that the biliary tree (like the liver) has only a limited repertoire of responses to chronic inflammation of whatever cause.

Pathology
When only small biliary radicals are involved, liver biopsy is necessary to make the diagnosis of PSC. Some authorities would always seek histological support for a radiographic diagnosis, but this is not necessarily a productive course as large-duct disease may be associated with virtually normal histology, or that which simply confirms a more distal cholestasis

without providing further evidence as to its cause. However, when present, the specific histological findings are characteristic. The so-called onion-skin or lamellar periportal fibrosis is unmistakable, and is associated with a variable degree of chronic inflammatory response, progressing to hepatic fibrosis and cirrhosis in its later stages.

Therapy

Treatment of PSC was not hitherto possible other than by liver transplantation for endstage liver failure. Two routes to improving this situation are now under active exploration and exploitation. If a single dominant stricture is identified at ERCP, it is technically possible to dilate it with transendoscopic balloons (with or without infusion of steroids or other substances, or of subsequent stenting) [59]. The endoscopic route is also applicable for patients with a small number of major strictures, especially when a single, long stent can be expected to span them all. The use of the expandable metal stent has been taken up with enthusiasm, as the smaller calibre of the unexpanded stent allows negotiation of tighter strictures, while its larger final lumen leads to less blocking with biliary debris during follow-up. Numerous case reports describing these advances have appeared but, as is so often the case with new 'surgical' interventions, there are still no controlled data with which to compare the encouraging outcomes described. This is of more than average concern, as PSC usually follows a remitting and relapsing course, and will tend to provoke intervention at times of maximal expression, when spontaneous improvement is concurrently also at its most likely.

A number of pharmacological agents have been employed in PSC but, with one exception, have had very limited success. Formal controlled data are few, but of the studies yet reported none shows results of sufficient promise to justify large-scale trials other than those using ursodeoxycholic acid. Recently reported data from the Dutch multicentre study are typical of those in the literature [60], demonstrating reductions in enzyme levels, with no change in bilirubin or synthetic markers of liver function over 2 years, but at least one author and reviewer has been convinced that the drug reduces the need for transplantation [61].

Prognosis

Some patients have little trouble from their PSC, while others follow a rapidly deteriorating course culminating in cirrhosis, hepatic failure and death if successful liver transplantation is not possible. Several prognostic models have accordingly been devised based on standard clinical criteria, with or without inclusion of liver biopsy data. Details of the different models may reflect case selection in the originating centres, but although each model is fallible [62], there is some measure of agreement that female gender, increasing age, decreasing albumin and increasing bilirubin level are poor prognostic markers. A still simpler strategy has been adopted at the Cleveland Clinic where the Childs–Pugh score has been compared with and found to be superior to other models [63]. A multicentre Italian study suggests that high cholesterol, low albumin and anaemia may also be of adverse prognostic value, but the data come from a predominantly symptomatic population (70%) and may not be generalized [64]. Activity of associated colitis has little, if any, bearing on the progress of primary sclerosing cholangitis, and even colectomy affects the biliary status very little. Clearly, patients with established parenchymal liver disease run a greater operative risk if they come to later colectomy, with three of eight such patients perishing in one series [65]. Overall transplant-free survival has improved since early studies and is now typically in excess of 75% at 10 years [66], which probably reflects earlier diagnosis and better case ascertainment rather than any influence of therapeutic strategies.

Neoplasia in primary sclerosing cholangitis

Patients with primary sclerosing cholangitis are at substantially increased risk of cholangiocarcinoma, and perhaps also at an increased risk of colorectal malignancy over and above the increased risk determined by their extent and duration of colitis. This is discussed in more detail in Chapter 8.

REFERENCES

1. Maeda K, Okada M, Yao T *et al*. Intestinal and extra-intestinal complications of Crohn's disease: predictors and cumulative probability of complications. *J Gastroenterol* 1994; **29**: 577–582.
2. Keat A. Spondyloarthropathies. *Br Med J* 1995; **310**: 1321–1324.
3. Gravellese EM, Kantrowitz FG. Arthritic manifestations of inflammatory bowel disease. *Am J Gastroenterol* 1988; **83**: 703–709.
4. Münch H, Purrmann J, Reis HE *et al*. Clinical features of inflammatory joint and spine manifestations in Crohn's disease. *Hepatogastroenterology* 1986; **33**: 123–127.
5. Norton KI, Eichenfield AH, Rosh JR *et al*. Atypical arthropathy associated with Crohn's disease. *Am J Gastroenterol* 1993; **88**: 948–952.
6. Israel DM, Olson AD, Ilowite NT, Davidson M. Arthritis as the initial manifestation of inflammatory bowel disease in early infancy. *J Ped Gastroenterol Nutr* 1989; **9**: 123–125.
7. Yahia B, Dave U, Keat A, Forbes A. Arthropathy in inflammatory bowel disease; an under-estimated problem? *Gastroenterology* 1996; **110**: A1048.
8. De Vos M, Mielants H, Cuvelier C *et al*. Long-term evolution of gut inflammation in patients with spondyloarthropathy. *Gastroenterology* 1996; **110**: 1696–1703.

9. Alonso JC, Lopez-Longo FJ, Lampreave JL *et al.* Different abdominal scintigraphy pattern in patients with ulcerative colitis, Crohn's disease and seronegative spondylarthropathies. *Br J Rheumatol* 1995; **34**: 946–950.
10. Axon JM, Hawley PR, Huskisson EC. Ileal pouch arthritis. *Br J Rheumatol* 1993; **32**: 586–588.
11. Andreyev HJN, Nicholls RJ, Forbes A, Kamm MA. Joint symptoms after restorative proctocolestomy in ulcerative colitis and familial polyposis coli. *J Clin Gastroenterol* 1996; **23**: 35–39.
12. Naughton M, Young H, Hughes L, Williams BD. Is the construction of an ileoanal pouch associated with the development of arthritis? *Br J Rheumatol* 1994; **33**: 64–66.
13. Cuvelier C, Mielants H, De Vos M *et al.* Immunoglobulin containing cells in terminal ileum and colorectum of patients with arthritis related gut inflammation. *Gut* 1988; **29**: 916–925.
14. Lichtman SN. Translocation of bacteria from gut lumen to mesenteric lymph nodes – and beyond? *J Ped Gastroenterol Nutr* 1991; **13**: 433–434.
15. Rath HC, Ikeda JS, Herafarth HH *et al.* Anaerobic bacteria, especially *Bacteroides* species stimulate colitis and gastritis in HLA-B27 transgenic rats. *Gastroenterology* 1996; **110**: A998.
16. Silvennoinen JA, Karttunen TJ, Niemelä SE *et al.* A controlled study of bone mineral density in patients with inflammatory bowel disease. *Gut* 1995; **37**: 71–76.
17. Bischoff SC, Herrmann A, Evers J *et al.* Bone density and bone metabolism in inflammatory bowel diseases. A clinical study in 90 patients. *Gastroenterology* 1996; **110**: A865.
18. Ghosh S, Cowen S, Hannan WJ, Ferguson A. Low bone mineral density in Crohn's disease but not in ulcerative colitis at diagnosis. *Gastroenterology* 1994; **107**: 1031–1039.
19. Herzog D, Bishop N, Glorieux F, Seidman EG. Normal bone mineral density values corrected for bone age in pediatric patients with Crohn's disease and growth failure. *Gastroenterology* 1996; **110**: A805.
20. Valdimarsson T, Löfman O, Toss G, Ström M. Reversal of osteopenia with diet in adult coeliac disease. *Gut* 1996; **38**: 322–327.
21. Andersson H, Bosaeus I, Fasth S *et al.* Cholelithiasis and urolithiasis in Crohn's disease. *Scand J Gastroenterol* 1987; **22**: 253–256.
22. Chadwick VS, Modka K, Dowling RH. Mechanism for hyperoxaluria in patients with ileal dysfunction. *N Engl J Med* 1973; **289**: 172–176.
23. Grossman MS, Nugent FW. Urolithiasis as a complication of chronic diarrheal disease. *Am J Dig Dis* 1967; **12**: 491–493.
24. Present D, Rabinowitz JG, Banks PA, Janowitz HD. Obstructive hydronephrosis – a frequent but seldom recognized complication of granulomatous disease of the bowel. *N Engl J Med* 1969; **280**: 523–528.

25. Glassman M, Kaplan M, Spivak W. Immune-complex glomeru-lonephritis in Crohn's disease. *J Ped Gastroenterol Nutr* 1986; **5**: 966–969.

26. Wilcox GM, Aretz HT, Roy MA, Roche JK. Glomerulonephritis asso-ciated with inflammatory bowel disease. *Gastroenterology* 1990; **98**: 786–791.

27. Kreisel W, Wolf LM, Grotz W, Grieshaber M. Renal tubular damage: an extra-intestinal manifestation of chronic inflammatory bowel dis-ease. *Eur J Gastroenterol Hepatol* 1996; **8**: 461–468.

28. Greenstein AJ, Sachar D *et al.* Amyloidosis and inflammatory bowel disease: a 50-year experience with 25 patients. *Medicine* 1992; **71**: 261–270.

29. Jorizzo JL. Blood vessel-based inflammatory disorders. In: Moschella SL, Hurley HJ, eds. *Dermatology,* 3rd edn. Philadelphia: Saunders, 1992: 584–586.

30. Mir-Madjlessi SH, Taylor JS, Farmer RG. Clinical course and evolu-tion of erythema nodosum and pyoderma gangrenosum in chronic ulcerative colitis: a study of 42 patients. *Am J Gastroenterol* 1985; **80**: 615–620.

31. Schoetz DJ Jr, Coller JA, Veidenheimer MG. Pyoderma gangrenosum and Crohn's disease. Eight cases and a review of the literature. *Dis Colon Rectum* 1983; **26**: 155–159.

32. Tjandra JJ, Hughes LE. Parastomal pyoderma gangrenosum in inflammatory bowel disease. *Dis Colon Rectum* 1994; **37**: 938–942.

33. Fett DL, Gibson LE, Su WPD. Sweet's syndrome: systemic signs and symptoms and associated disorders. *Mayo Clin Proc* 1995; **70**: 234–240.

34. Salmon JF, Wright JP, Murray AD. Ocular inflammation in Crohn's disease. *Ophthalmology* 1991; **98**: 480–484.

35. Billson FA, De Dombal FT, Watkinson G, Goligher JG. Ocular com-plications of ulcerative colitis. *Gut* 1967; **8**: 102–106.

36. Hofley P, Roarty J, McGinnity G *et al.* Asymptomatic uveitis in chil-dren with chronic inflammatory bowel disease. *J Ped Gastroenterol Nutr* 1993; **17**: 397–400.

37. Soukiasian SH, Foster CS, Raizman MB. Treatment strategies for scleritis and uveitis associated with inflammatory bowel disease. *Am J Ophthalmol* 1994; **118**: 601–611.

38. Hutchinson R, Tyrrell PN, Kumar D *et al.* Pathogenesis of gall stones in Crohn's disease: an alternative explanation. *Gut* 1994; **35**: 94–97.

39. Nightingale JM. The short-bowel syndrome. *Eur J Gastroenterol Hepatol* 1995; **7**: 514–520.

40. Lorusso D, Leo S, Mossa A *et al.* Cholelithiasis in inflammatory bowel disease. A case-control study. *Dis Colon Rectum* 1990; **33**: 791–794.

41. Lapidus A, Einarsson K. Effects of ileal resection on biliary lipids and bile acid composition in patients with Crohn's disease. *Gut* 1991; **32**: 1488–1491.

42. Mibu R, Makino I, Chijiiwa K. Gallstones and their composition in patients with ileoanal anastomosis. *J Gastroenterol* 1995; **30**: 413–415.

43. Brink MA, Slors JFM, Carey MC *et al.* Enterohepatic cycling of bilirubin in patients with ileal Crohn's disease: a pathophysiological mechanism for pigment gallstone disease. *Gastroenterology* 1996; **110**: A1159.

44. Broomé U, Glaumann H, Hellers G *et al.* Liver disease in ulcerative colitis: an epidemiological and follow up study in the county of Stockholm. *Gut* 1994; **35**: 84–89.

45. Mattila J, Aitola P, Matikainen M. Liver lesions found at colectomy in ulcerative colitis: correlation between histological findings and biochemical parameters. *J Clin Pathol* 1994; **47**: 1019–1021.

46. Broomé U, Glaumann H, Hultcrantz R. Liver histology and follow up of 68 patients with ulcerative colitis and normal liver function tests. *Gut* 1990; **31**: 468–472.

47. Perdigoto R, Carpenter HA, Czaja AJ. Frequency and significance of chronic ulcerative colitis in severe corticosteroid-treated autoimmune hepatitis. *J Hepatol* 1992; **14**: 325–331.

48. Maurer LH, Hughes RW Jr, Folley JH, Mosenthal WT. Granulomatous hepatitis associated with regional enteritis. *Gastroenterology* 1967; **53**: 301–305.

49. Broomé U, Löfberg R, Lundqvist K, Veress B. Subclinical time span of inflammatory bowel disease in patients with primary sclerosing cholangitis. *Dis Colon Rectum* 1995; **38**: 1301–1305.

50. Joseph JK, Porayko MK, Steers JL *et al.* The association of primary sclerosing cholangitis and sarcoidosis. *Gastroenterology* 1996; **110**: A1224.

51. Olerup O, Olsson R, Hultcrantz R, Broomé U. HLA-DR and HLA-DQ are not markers for rapid disease progression in primary sclerosing cholangitis. *Gastroenterology* 1995; **108**: 870–878.

52. Underhill JA, Donaldson PT, Doherty DG *et al.* HLA DPB polymorphism in primary sclerosing cholangitis and primary biliary cirrhosis. *Hepatology* 1995; **21**: 959–962.

53. Seibold F, Slametschka D, Gregor M, Weber P. Neutrophil autoantibodies: a genetic marker in primary sclerosing cholangitis and ulcerative colitis. *Gastroenterology* 1994; **104**: 532–536.

54. Lo SK, Fleming KA, Chapman RW. A 2-year follow-up study of antineutrophil antibody in primary sclerosing cholangitis: relationship to clinical activity, liver biochemistry and ursodeoxycholic acid treatment. *J Hepatol* 1994; **21**: 974–978.

55. Loftus EV Jr, Sandborn WJ, Tremaine WJ *et al.* Primary sclerosing cholangitis is associated with non-smoking: a case-control study. *Gastroenterology* 1996; **110**: 1496–1502.

56. Van Erpecum KJ, Smits SJHM, Van de Meeberg PC *et al.* Risk of primary sclerosing cholangitis is associated with nonsmoking behaviour. *Gastroenterology* 1996; **110**: 1503–1506.

57. Majoie CB, Smits NJ, Phoa SS *et al.* Primary sclerosing cholangitis: sonographic findings. *Abdom Imaging* 1995; **20**: 109–112.

58. Forbes A, Blanshard C, Gazzard B. Natural history of AIDS related sclerosing cholangitis: a study of 20 cases. *Gut* 1993; **34**: 116–121.

59. Gaing AA, Geders JM, Cohen SA, Siegel JH. Endoscopic management of primary sclerosing cholangitis: review and report of an open series. *Am J Gastroenterol* 1993; **88**: 2000–2008.

60. Van Hoogstraten HJF, Wolfhagen FJH, Van de Meeberg PC *et al.* Single versus three times daily ursodeoxycholic acid for primary sclerosing cholangitis: results of a randomized controlled trial. *Gastroenterology* 1996; **110**: A1352.

61. Stiehl A. Ursodeoxycholic acid therapy in treatment of primary sclerosing cholangitis. *Scand J Gastroenterol Suppl* 1994; **204**: 59–61.

62. Broomé U, Eriksson LS. Assessment for liver transplantation in patients with primary sclerosing cholangitis. *J Hepatol* 1994; **20**: 654–659.

63. Shetty K, Carey WD, Rybicki L. Childs–Pugh score as a prognostic indicator for survival in primary sclerosing cholangitis. *Gastroenterology* 1996; **110**: A1322.

64. Okolicsanyi L, Fabris L, Viaggi S *et al.* Primary sclerosing cholangitis: clinical presentation, natural history and prognostic variables: an Italian multicentre study. *Eur J Gastroenterol Hepatol* 1996; **8**: 685–691.

65. Post AB, Bozdech JM, Lavery I, Barnes DS. Colectomy in patients with inflammatory bowel disease and primary sclerosing cholangitis. *Dis Colon Rectum* 1994; **37**: 175–178.

66. Loftus EV, Sandborn WJ, Tremaine WJ *et al.* Risk of colorectal neoplasia in patients with primary sclerosing cholangitis. *Gastroenterology* 1996; **110**: 432–440.

7

Complications of inflammatory bowel disease

INTRA-ABDOMINAL SEPSIS AND ABSCESS FORMATION IN CROHN'S DISEASE

The perianal and perineal abscesses, fissures and superficial fistulae of Crohn's disease can usually be treated adequately by local measures. More complex perineal disease and the multiple fistulous openings of the 'watering can perineum' pose more difficulty and will often only respond to defunctioning by a more proximal stoma (Chapter 4). Chronic intra-abdominal and pelvic abscesses may represent still greater problems.

Drainage of septic foci is as necessary in Crohn's disease as in other situations, but whether drainage alone can be sufficient therapy is controversial. Several major centres consider that drainage should be considered only as an immediate measure to overcome septicaemia, restore cardio-vascular stability and general well-being, before proceeding to later more definitive surgery to resect the implicated segment of bowel. There is a related debate as to the place of open surgery as opposed to non-surgical methodologies to achieve drainage. The argument in favour of drainage alone is supported by the general desire to minimize surgery and quantity of bowel resection, and the fact that many of these patients appear to do extremely well in the short term, and are then keen to avoid further intervention when they seem to have recovered.

The relatively limited numerical scale of the problem is clear from the literature, but the difficulty of management should not be underestimated. The Birmingham group published a surgical series on sepsis in Crohn's disease [1], referring to 124 resections in 111 patients, 13 of whom had abscesses preoperatively (unsuspected in eight). These were mostly localized and all 13 affected patients 'requiring urgent surgery'. A further 17 abscesses (six multiple) occurred postoperatively, five in patients with preoperative lesions. In New York, Ribeiro et al. [2] recorded 129 abscesses (21%) in 610 patients with small bowel Crohn's disease, which were intraperitoneal in 109 cases and retroperitoneal in the remainder; all were considered to have required operative intervention. Fifteen required further surgery for abscess and 26 developed postoperative enterocutaneous fistulae; there were three deaths from sepsis.

The particular case of psoas abscess has attracted attention because of its potential to mislead clinically (presenting, for example, with pain in the knee or hip rather than with an obviously abdominal problem), and also because it may be the presenting feature of Crohn's disease – 11 of 46 cases in one series [3]. Although Crohn's disease is probably the single most common predisposing factor for psoas abscess, it still accounts for less than half of those that occur; the 14 of 43 in another series being typical [4].

At St Mark's, having excluded perineal abscesses and those occurring within 3 months of surgery (because it was otherwise difficult to make the distinction from postoperative wound infection) we identified 35 patients with Crohn's-related abscesses from a prospective database of 531 Crohn's patients admitted on a total of 1156 times in a 4-year period [5]. The age and sex distribution (median age 35 years, 14 male) was typical of our patient group and the affected patients had had Crohn's disease for a median of 12 years. The abscesses were abdominal in 61%, retroperitoneal in 22%, and pelvic in 17%, and were associated with abdominal masses in 64% of cases and with enterocutaneous fistulae in 26% (see below). Three-quarters of the patients had chronically active Crohn's disease and 18% had subacute obstruction at the time of presentation with abscess. Nearly half had been on steroids for more than 6 months and most had had previous surgery (in 36% of cases for previous abscess or fistula). A communication between the bowel and the abscess was demonstrable in 61%, in 35% originating from a previous anastomosis. Similar observations were made recently in Montreal [6]. Microbiological investigation is not particularly helpful in these patients as mixed growths are usual. In almost all cases, aerobic intestinal organisms will be demonstrated, with anaerobes as well in about a third.

There is no ideal method to investigate and localize abscesses in Crohn's disease, nor are there controlled trials to guide the clinician. There is an obvious case for ultrasonographic scanning, given its availability and non-invasiveness, but this may yield poor views in the patient with intestinal distension and when there has been a recent abdominal incision. Protagonists for the CT scan [7] will probably soon concede that the ability of MR scanning to detect inflammation relatively specifically (on spin-echo sequences) is preferable (see also Chapter 2), when adequate information is unavailable from ultrasound. It is unclear that endoscopic ultrasound will be useful to the general radiologist but Tio provides encouraging data from one specialist centre which compare well with all other forms of imaging and with surgical assessment [8].

Percutaneous and surgical drainage of Crohn's-related abscesses

Percutaneous drainage of a Crohn's-related abscess was first described by Bluth and co-workers in 1985 [9] and by Millward *et al.* in 1986 [10], with success in three of these four patients. Doemeny *et al.* reviewed its use in nine cases and reported technical and short-term success in eight, with long-term resolution in five, only three patients needing elective surgery at some stage [11]. Percutaneous drainage was also technically possible in the London and Montreal series (see above) when attempted, and led to resolution of the acute problem in around half of the treated patients, the others coming to later surgery.

The results for percutaneous drainage were, of course, in selected patients, and conclusions should be guarded, but it is instructive to examine the results in the contemporaneous patients at St Mark's treated initially by open surgery. Of 23 such patients, 10 had a drainage procedure, and 13 a more definitive resection (with stoma creation in four). There were nine postoperative recurrences, recurrent fistulae in two, new enterocutaneous fistulae in two and new presentation of short bowel syndrome in six, two of whom are now on long-term home parenteral nutrition. There were no deaths, but at 3 months only two-thirds were well and free from sepsis and fistulae. Surgical data from other centres, with a substantial rate of new enterocutaneous fistulae [2], and relapse in 19 of 26 surgically drained patients compared to only 4 of 18 resected [3], taken together with the St Mark's data, begin to suggest that surgical drainage should be avoided. Given that none of the data sets is controlled, and that in each case a considered clinical decision was taken to follow one option or another, it is pertinent to examine other possible prognostic factors and alternative therapeutic strategies.

Pre-intervention steroids have not appeared to influence outcome. Even when an abdominal mass was identified and high-dose steroids were used in therapy (albeit in the absence of overt sepsis) Felder *et al.* were able to reassure us that of 24 patients so treated, none required urgent surgery or developed life-threatening sepsis, even though 13 of the 24 masses were finally shown to include an abscess component [12]. No other generalizable factors have emerged.

Drainage by radiologically guided percutaneous methods is technically possible in the great majority of Crohn's-related abscesses, and although a clinically useful result is usual, nearly 50% of patients will still need surgical intervention. Similar success, but a higher complication rate, is associated with surgical drainage procedures. Controlled trial of the two forms of drainage is probably feasible, but will not be easy given the relative rarity of the condition and the great difficulty in ensuring matching between groups (these are not especially homogeneous groups of patients) and may never be done. A pragmatist might reasonably take the view that within the limitations indicated, percutaneous drainage is no more or less successful than open surgical drainage. As percutaneous drainage is less invasive and possibly has a lower complication rate than open drainage, it should be the first choice if the surgical option would (at that time) be drainage alone. A percutaneous approach would seem especially appropriate for the patient who is unfit for surgery, or who is still recovering from previous intervention. Percutaneous drainage is less likely to be helpful in patients with obviously multilocular abscesses and those in whom fistulation has already occurred. In each case, there should be a plan for more definitive surgery once the acute septic event has resolved, with the intention of minimizing the chance of recurrence. When there is a reasonable prospect of definitive surgery at the first intervention, then immediate excisional surgery offers the best chance of long-term remission and may be a sensible course to follow. However, reconstructive surgery with primary closure in the presence of current sepsis is less likely to be wise, and defunctioning stoma creation will often be necessary, reducing the apparent benefit of combining drainage with resection.

ENTEROCUTANEOUS FISTULA

The management of an enterocutaneous fistula is heavily influenced by the underlying aetiology and its anatomical nature, which together mainly determine the likelihood of resolution without surgical intervention. A simple single fistula with no obstruction which follows colectomy for ulcerative colitis, for example, stands a hugely greater chance of closing with good medical care, than multiple complex fistulae occurring spontaneously in Crohn's disease. Closure is impeded by continuing sepsis, malnutrition and, particularly, by distal obstruction or bowel discontinuity.

Enterocutaneous fistulae always have their origins in adherent abscess-related disorders and sepsis. There is always an associated penetrating bowel disorder, and the most common single association is with recent surgery. Fistulae may be classified conveniently according to their anatomical nature, taking into account both the site of the intestine involved and the nature of the openings on the skin. Simple, single openings clearly have less significance than the more complex fistula where the two ends of bowel have become disrupted or where communication with the skin is via a continuing abscess cavity (Figure 7.1). The presence of distal obstruction is also most important, as such a fistula will not heal without surgical intervention.

We do not know the true incidence of postoperative fistulae in inflammatory bowel disease as they are considered by many surgeons to be indicative of a technical failing and are therefore not widely reported. The data available come from referral centres which are thereby unable to give truly representative data. Interestingly, in one such series [13] in which

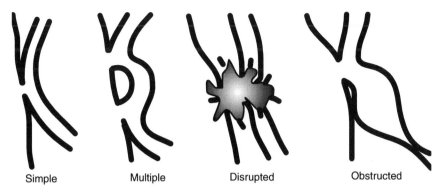

| Simple | Multiple | Disrupted | Obstructed |

Figure 7.1 A classification of enterocutaneous fistulae. In the disrupted (or complex) fistula the two ends of intestine are no longer in direct contact or communicate only via an abscess cavity.

6.3% of enterocutaneous fistulae were in patients with Crohn's disease, 4.2% occurred in ulcerative colitis, a condition not normally associated with this complication. Enterocutaneous fistulae are associated with significant mortality (around 4%) but this is rarely a direct result of the fistula itself, more a reflection of the patient's overall poor state. In Crohn's disease fistulae can be expected in up to 15% of patients at some stage in their disease [14]. At least 80% of these episodes occur shortly after surgery and up to one-quarter of laparotomies may be expected to be complicated in this way. The fistula is usually at the site of the surgical incision [15]. It is valuable to distinguish the relatively straightforward fistula occurring after satisfactorily comprehensive surgery (Plate 13), from those occurring in patients with extensive Crohn's and involving actively diseased bowel (Plate 14). The former stand a reasonable chance of closing with medical therapy, whereas the latter will very rarely heal without surgical intervention. Failure to make this distinction has led to conflicting statements in the literature claiming spontaneous closures in anything from 0 to 60% of cases. There is also the frequent occurrence of an fistula closing over, but without true resolution, which can lead to overestimations of therapeutic success if follow-up is inadequate [16].

The imaging of enterocutaneous fistulae is far from ideal, but ultrasound scanning, barium studies, CT and MR scanning all have a place. Endoscopic evaluation is not normally very contributory. However, the 'fistulogram', in which water-soluble contrast is instilled into the cutaneous opening, is helpful in most cases (Chapter 2).

The immediate management of the patient with an acute enterocutaneous fistula follows resuscitation, which may require fluid replacement and the drainage of abscesses (see above). Care of the skin around the fistulous opening should be an early priority, especially when the fistula is from the jejunum and the effluent accordingly rich in enzymes and acid.

The patient will then usually also need nutritional support. Total parenteral nutrition may be necessary, but when the fistula is low ileal or colonic, enteral feeding will often allow sufficient bowel rest without the hazards of the parenteral approach or the loss of the protective/trophic effects that luminal nutrients have on the small bowel mucosa. The high-output fistula may lead to grave problems in assessment of fluid and sodium balance, but the principles outlined for management of short bowel syndrome can then usefully be applied (see below). Patients with less than 1 m of reasonably normal intestine above the fistula will generally require parenteral support. If the fistula patient is not nil by mouth, the 'antisecretory' regime proposed for short bowel syndrome patients will usually be indicated (see below).

Consideration of parenteral nutrition in patients with short bowel syndrome and enterocutaneous fistula will follow early resuscitation and immediate fluid replacement. In most circumstances, the patient can be evaluated over several days, and it will often be appropriate to perform a trial of enteral therapy. In a survey of similar patients treated with parenteral nutrition and enteral tube-based regimes, there was no difference in mortality, nor an obvious difference in fistula outcome [17]. There were, however, almost 50% more septic episodes in the patients treated with parenteral nutrition compared to those with the enterally based regimes. We know that enteral feeding has significant advantages in intestinal protection and in encouraging its growth and recovery. Enteral regimes also have the great advantage of avoiding central catheter related problems and (as above) in reducing the overall rate of infection. Enteral regimes are most likely to be successful when given slowly, and in most cases continuously, by nasogastric or gastrostomy tube. The volume should be kept low and additional sodium will often need to be added. High-energy feeds (those with more than 1 kcal/ml) are less appropriate as they may provoke an osmotic diarrhoea and increase the fistula (or stomal) output.

The place of parenteral nutrition in enterocutaneous fistula may be summarized as being mandatory in patients in whom true intestinal failure is present, and in whom it is impossible to achieve positive nutritional balance without enteral regimes. It is usually indicated in those with a high site of fistula and/or those with a high output (for example, >2000 ml daily). Parenteral nutrition will probably be indicated if spontaneous closure of the fistula is a reasonable expectation, since then the time needed to that closure can be expected to be shorter. It may be indicated if the patient is malnourished, since the duration of malnutrition may then be shortened, but it is unlikely to be appropriate in the patient with a fistula which is low in the bowel (especially in the colon), when the output is low and the fistula well tolerated. If parenteral nutrition is required, standard regimes may be used, although they will require modification to allow for the greater fluid requirements (up to 6 litres daily) with additional sodium (often around 300 mmol/day) and additional magnesium. Even when parenteral nutrition is being employed, the patient should continue oral antisecretory therapy using opioids, proton pump inhibitors and probably octreotide also (see below).

Immunosuppressive agents such as azathioprine may be valuable in selected patients with enterocutaneous fistulae complicating active Crohn's disease [18]. The place of cyclosporin [19] is less clear as the small number of patients apparently helpfully treated is insufficient to provide confidence that the potential for impaired healing has truly been overcome; there are no controlled data.

Somatostatin and its more stable analogue, octreotide, show promise. Their actions include the reduction of intestinal and pancreatic secretion, and of the speed of intestinal transit. As they also increase water and electrolyte absorption, it is understandable that therapeutic trials have been conducted in patients with high fistulae. Both agents will reduce fistula output reliably and reproducibly by about 500 ml/day [20]. If the combination of fluid restriction, electrolyte solution supplementation and opioids is insufficient, then the addition of octreotide may be considered. When compared against placebo in three studies of patients with postoperative fistulae, there was no improvement in the percentage of fistulae which healed without surgery, but the speed at which this healing took place was much faster (by about 10 days) [21]. There were also fewer infective complications in the patients treated with octreotide.

A somewhat more controversial approach is taken by one group who report the beneficial use of reinfusion of intestinal secretions lost from the fistula site to reduce hepatic dysfunction, perhaps via a reduction in endotoxaemia [22]. This is not a technique with which most units have felt comfortable, and it is probably significant that there have been no more recent publications on its use.

Surgery is often required in patients with enterocutaneous fistulae. It is particularly strongly indicated if the fistula is unrelated to recent surgery, if the bladder is involved and when the fistula is high in the bowel or of particularly high output. The results of surgery can be expected to be good when there is localized disease and when it is possible to excise the involved bowel and the fistula track completely. Drainage procedures are probably not sufficient alone, although they may form a part of initial resuscitation (see above). The best results from surgery are achieved when it is unhurried and follows meticulous preoperative attention to fluid and sodium balance, adequate nutrition and good skin care. At St Mark's it is strongly advised that no patient with a fistula should have elective surgery within 6 weeks of a previous laparotomy [23]. It must be emphasized that the management of the patient with an enterocutaneous fistula is a team effort. No one discipline, however skilled, can hope to manage these patients to their best advantage. The skills of the physician, surgeon and ward nurse need the supplementary skills of the stoma care therapist, the nutrition nurse and often members of the psychological support team, given the chronic and emotionally damaging nature of these unpleasant conditions.

SHORT BOWEL SYNDROME

Intestinal failure or short bowel syndrome (SBS) results from a deficiency in the ability of the intestine to handle nutrients and its own secretions. Excessive water and electrolyte losses and malnutrition result. SBS usually follows major resection, typically leaving less than 200 cm of small bowel, but also when the relatively intact intestine is unable to function because of severe inflammation (or disorders of motility). In many Crohn's patients with SBS both causes coexist.

Short bowel syndrome is unusual, with a prevalence of less than one case per 100 000 population in the UK and North America, and with an incidence around one-tenth of that. Crohn's disease accounts for around half of all benign causes of long-term intestinal failure. Short-term intestinal failure is, of course, seen in many postoperative inflammatory bowel disease patients with prolonged 'ileus', and in a few patients after the apparently straightforward creation of an end-ileostomy for ulcerative colitis. It is also a relatively frequent cause for medical referral in the patient after one-stage pouch surgery (Chapter 4) who seems to be at above-average risk of this complication – presumably from the combination of a lengthy procedure (with more than average handling of the small intestine) with a modest loss of effective small bowel length from the creation of the pouch.

The management of SBS is influenced to a considerable extent by the expected duration of the problem. In the short term, parenteral nutrition will be required for any patient unable to achieve nutritional adequacy with enteral feeding, but many such patients will later achieve sufficient intestinal function to become partially or totally independent of parenteral nutrition. The ileum is more adaptable than the jejunum and, as will be demonstrated, the continued presence of the colon will help in attainment of fluid/electrolyte balance and to some extent in nutrition also. The process of intestinal adaptation begins soon after injury, and continues for at least 6 months and probably up to 2 years [24].

Short bowel syndrome is best managed when anticipated. The length of the remaining small bowel should be measured at the time of surgery, and both its anatomical identity and integrity recorded. The variable length of the normal small intestine and the frequent history of previous resections in patients with Crohn's disease make measurements of the resected segment much less helpful. When there is no record of the length of remaining bowel, an approximate measurement can be made on barium follow-through.

Patients with a high jejunostomy can be expected to lose upwards of 3 litres of fluid each day, with a sodium loss of at least 90 mmol/l. This follows from the physiological, secretory response of the upper gastrointestinal tract and jejunum, as only when the luminal sodium concentration reaches 90 mmol/l or more does net absorption commence. Since almost all spontaneously consumed drinks have very little sodium content, salt and water deficiency becomes almost inevitable. Unfortunately, the consequent onset of thirst will exacerbate the problem, as the patient drinks more, yet more intestinal secretion is provoked, amplifying the already high stomal losses. Daily parenteral fluid and electrolyte supplements are likely to be required in all those with less than 100 cm of small bowel above a stoma [25]. If all or part of the colon remains in continuity with the small intestine, then there is more opportunity for restitutive distal reabsorption of sodium and water, and regular intravenous fluids are less likely to be necessary.

Absorption of nutrients also correlates inversely with jejunal length. In Nightingale's study [26], every patient with less than 85 cm of small bowel terminating in a stoma required parenteral nutrients as well as intravenous fluids. Those with a normal small bowel of length greater than 100 cm can often be maintained in a reasonable state of nutrition with oral food and supplements. Of course, if a short small bowel remains in continuity with a functional large intestine, malabsorption of nutrients still occurs, and these patients are also placed at potential risk by the passage of larger than normal amounts of bile salts and non-absorbed constituents of food into the colon, but the colon is able to utilize short-chain fatty acids derived from unabsorbed carbohydrate as a source of energy [27]. There is accordingly some advantage in ensuring a higher proportion of total oral energy from carbohydrate in these patients. For the same total energy provision, the SBS patient with a colon will absorb more when the diet contains more carbohydrate and less fat, in contrast to the SBS patient who lacks a colon, in whom the distribution of fat and carbohydrate calories in the diet makes no difference to retention of energy [28]. Although there may also be a theoretical advantage in avoiding fats in SBS patients to reduce steatorrhoea, this is rarely a clinical issue and most patients should be encouraged to eat as they wish [29, 30].

Retention of all or most of the colon may be considered roughly equivalent to an additional 50 cm of small bowel in respect of the absorption of nutrients (as well the more dramatic advantage in respect of easier fluid and electrolyte management alluded to above) [26]. All of 71 patients studied with greater than 50 m of small bowel and retained colons were supported with enteral supplements alone at 5-year follow-up. It is probable that part of this benefit is vested in the functional ileocaecal valve, and unfortunate that this is the part of the bowel most often resected in Crohn's disease. The greater potential of the terminal ileum for adaptation, the preservation of the 'ileal brake', normal absorption of bile salts and vitamin B_{12}, are also usually denied the postoperative patient with Crohn's.

Symptoms and signs

Weight loss despite good appetite and food consumption, especially in the presence of profuse diarrhoea (or high stomal losses), will be obvious pointers to intestinal failure, but the early symptoms of sodium deficiency are often missed, as patients find them difficult to describe and may not volunteer them. In addition to features suggestive of postural hypotension, thirst and relative oliguria, patients may experience curious echo-like sensations. Examination will include weight and height, enabling computation of the body mass index, but taking into account the presence of dehydration or oedema, the latter in particular being a source of potential confusion. A search for signs of specific nutrient deficiencies is appropriate but will usually be unproductive, as intestinal failure presents with obvious macronutrient deficiency before the more subtle features from lack of micronutrients become apparent. Salt and water deficiency is more reliably indicated by postural hypotension than assessment of skin turgor or venous filling. Tetany provoked by the sphygmomanometer cuff provides confirmation of calcium or (much more often) magnesium deficiency.

Arguably the most important investigation in SBS (and one of the most underutilized) is the urine sodium concentration. This need not be a timed collection, as random samples will usually give the necessary information. If the sodium content is less than 20 mmol/l, salt deficiency is likely. Only in the presence of established renal failure does the urine sodium content become unreliable. Other laboratory data are almost superfluous. It is difficult to monitor fluid and sodium balance in short bowel syndrome, especially if there are stomal or fistula leakages, but daily weighing (on the same scales), lying and standing blood pressure, and daily urine sodiums, are reproducible, practical and sufficiently informative in most cases.

Therapy

The aim of SBS management is to provide a good quality of life with effective but minimally invasive medical interventions which prevent thirst and dehydration and permit maintenance of an acceptable body weight. It is often difficult for Crohn's disease patients to achieve pre-morbid body weight, but it should always be possible to attain a weight that is acceptable to patient and physician, and it is practical to aim for a body mass index of around 20 kg/m². Additional quantifiable objectives include an average stomal output of no more than 2 litres a day, or the absence of disabling diarrhoea in the patient without a stoma. The daily urine output should ideally exceed 1 litre, although in practice as little as 700 ml is acceptable so long as the patient is healthy in other respects and has a urine sodium of at least 20 mmol/l. The serum magnesium should be in the normal range. Normal levels of other nutritional markers are usually achieved surprisingly easily.

Many SBS patients will come to attention while still in serious trouble from their inflammatory bowel disease, with uncontrolled stoma or enterocutaneous fistula output and problematic skin care (see above). The immediate involvement of the stoma therapist is an essential part of good intestinal failure management, and may be the team's first opportunity to gain the patient's trust and confidence. This is especially true when referral follows a long sequence of unsuccessful or partially successful operative interventions. The peri-stoma/fistula skin needs careful handling, with preventive methods to protect it from necrosis or infection. Correction of zinc deficiency may be particularly helpful in this context whether or not the characteristic rash is seen.

Most patients with a short bowel will take food orally despite their substantially incomplete absorption. Only if eating causes severe symptoms, or if in management of a high fistula there has been a decision to continue a deliberate nil-by-mouth policy to maximize chances of closure, should it not be positively encouraged. Patients should be advised to concentrate on normal foods high in energy and protein [31], and most will need to avoid large fluid volumes (see above). They need not avoid fatty food, since the high energy content is valuable, tolerance is rarely a problem and excess losses of divalent cations (calcium, zinc and magnesium) do not occur, as was once thought [30]. Elemental feeds should not be used as their high osmolarity will increase the stomal output. Certain foods such as tomatoes or onions will also have this effect in some individuals. Patients with a high jejunostomy should add salt to their food within the limits of palatability to minimize sodium secretion into the gut and thereby to minimize stomal losses of both sodium and water. This may be the only nutritional measure required in patients in whom the stomal losses average less than 1200 ml/day. High oxalate consumption is, nevertheless, best avoided to minimize the risk of urinary tract oxalate stones (Chapter 6).

Patients who are unable to maintain their normal weight on a high calorie diet with frequent meals and between-meal snacks may achieve this goal by use of one of the specially prepared liquid or semi-solid food supplements, perhaps given overnight via a nasogastric or gastrostomy tube, as the slower but more continuous administration maximally utilizes the absorptive potential of the remaining bowel. There has been concern about the use of percutaneous gastrostomy tube insertion in Crohn's disease given the high frequency of upper gastrointestinal disease and a perceived risk of gastrocutaneous fistula. However, our experience at St

Mark's has been uniformly positive, and although numbers and duration of follow-up are still small, we are increasingly optimistic that gastrostomy feeding can be utilized safely when it seems indicated in inflammatory bowel disease.

When absorption falls below about one-third of all energy taken enterally, it becomes impossible to achieve positive nutritional balance, or to maintain a satisfactory weight [25]. Parenteral supplements then become necessary. For practical purposes, any patient with a stomal output of greater than 2500 ml/day is likely to be dependent on fluids, electrolytes and nutrients, all given by the parenteral route [32]. The nutrient regimens to be considered differ very little from those used for other conditions. The differences reflect the frequent need for large volumes and generous amounts of magnesium and sodium rather than specific nutritional issues. Parenteral nutrition is almost inevitably a long-term concern in these patients and should always be administered via a dedicated tunnelled catheter inserted into a central vein, or via one of the implantable devices. It is usual to commence with a continuous 24-hour infusion regimen, but quickly increasing the rate to permit a steadily lengthening nutrition-free period each day. This cyclical regimen has many advantages, enables mobility and is surprisingly important in psychological rehabilitation [33].

The concept of non-total parenteral nutrition is important and not always fully appreciated even by those engaged in the regular care of patients such as these. Most patients with intestinal failure from Crohn's disease are able to eat, and most are able to absorb a useful proportion of the nutrients that are taken orally, even if this is inadequate to sustain life without intravenous support. These patients accordingly do not require *total* parenteral nutrition, as they can and do absorb some of their daily requirements from the gut. In general nutritional practice, enteral feeding is encouraged (to maintain normal gastrointestinal flora, to increase gastrointestinal adaptation, to prevent gallbladder sludge accumulation, etc.). This principle holds good in the patient requiring parenteral nutrition for SBS. Once malnutrition is corrected, and if there is not a compelling daily need for fluids and electrolytes, it will often prove possible to reduce the parenteral feeding to three or four nights a week to maintain body weight.

Fluid balance in SBS patients is frequently poorly managed. This results from basic misapprehensions and inappropriate extrapolation from other conditions in which thirst and dehydration coexist. The remedy in the patient with intestinal failure is almost always to restrict fluid intake, and to prescribe a glucose–electrolyte solution to drink whenever thirsty, or on a regular basis to prevent thirst in the more severely affected individual [34]. The more crucial element of the strategy is the restriction of sodium-poor fluids, but the prescription of a rehydration solution is often easier to explain and compliance easier to ensure. Experimental work indicates that the solution should contain at least 90 mmol of sodium per litre, but it must also be palatable, easy to prepare and (preferably) cheap, to promote its long-term use by the patient. Studies at St Mark's Hospital have suggested that the use of the World Health Organization formula (without potassium chloride) is a good compromise on theoretical and experimental grounds [35].

The St Mark's oral rehydration solution consists of: glucose powder, 20 g (110 mmol); sodium chloride, 3.5 g (60 mmol); sodium bicarbonate, 2.5 g (30 mmol), measured using standard scoops, and made up to 1 litre in tap water. The inclusion of sodium bicarbonate is to increase palatability (and perhaps absorption) [35] rather than for an effect on pH, and may be replaced by sodium citrate (2.9 g = 30 mmol) if the patient prefers. Most find it easiest to drink if chilled, but palatability can also be improved by flavouring with fruit drink concentrates. Restriction of all other fluids to 500–750 ml each day, but with emphasis on drinking at least as much of the electrolyte solution, is recommended.

Intravenous fluids will often be required in the initial resuscitation of short bowel patients. These should be given mainly as sodium chloride 0.9% (150 mmol/l of sodium) as sodium deficiency is as much a problem as lack of water. For practical purposes, the patient with overt clinical dehydration, postural hypotension or biochemical evidence of pre-renal uraemia can be considered to need intravenous fluids. If these features are absent, an oral regime as above should at least be attempted. Sodium should be replaced to provide around 90 mmol for each litre of measured urine and gastrointestinal losses from the previous 24 hours. Potassium will often not be needed if the patient continues to receive enteral nutrition, but magnesium is frequently necessary. If it proves impossible to wean from parental fluids, training in the self-administration of intravenous supplements becomes necessary, unless adequate control can be reliably achieved with the addition of less than 1 litre daily. In this case the simpler and safer option of self-administration of subcutaneous saline can be employed.

Magnesium deficiency is common in SBS patients with a terminal jejunostomy, and may be confounded by hypocalcaemia (which it renders untreatable until the low magnesium is corrected). Once recognized, its deficiency can be remedied rapidly by the administration of intravenous magnesium, 10–12 mmol, repeated as necessary until the serum magnesium has returned to within the normal range. Oral magnesium supplements at a dose of 12–24 mmol daily will usually be tolerated without worsening diarrhoea or increasing stomal output. If the patient requires more magnesium, then the dose can be increased until side-effects become intolerable or the therapeutic dose is reached. Heavy magnesium oxide capsules (160 mg) are found easier and no less effective than magnesium glycerophosphate, nevertheless tolerance is variable, and therapeutic trials are worthwhile if the first salt tried is not acceptable. In some patients tolerance is so poor that compliance is negligible; intravenous magnesium becomes necessary, and in some cases is the main justification for long-term parenteral access.

Some control can be exercised over the absence of the ileal brake and consequently rapid gastric emptying and intestinal transit with opioids [36]. They act on receptors in the gastrointestinal tract, reduce loss of water and electrolytes [37, 38] and may contribute to increased nutrient absorption [39]. Loperamide is preferred as it is thought to act only on the opioid receptors in the gut, and therefore has negligible addictive potential. Codeine phosphate is frequently used either alone or in combination with loperamide, and may be preferred by some patients. Diphenoxylate is prescribed occasionally as, although double-blind trial has shown it to be less effective [40], some patients find it helpful. Very large doses of opioids may be required. A prescription for 64 mg loperamide *and* 480 mg codeine phosphate each day is neither unusual nor inappropriate in SBS patients without a colon. The resultant reduction in stool or stomal losses can make a crucial difference to quality of life (as, for example, by permitting an undisturbed night's sleep), without risk of physical or psychological dependence. The drugs should be taken 30–60 min before meals for maximal effect.

Proton pump inhibitors such as omeprazole and lansoprazole, and to a lesser extent the H_2 blockers, reduce gastric acid secretion, but there is also a parallel reduction in the volume of gastric secretion, rendering these agents of considerable value in SBS. Reduced jejunostomy output and increased absorption of nutrients can be achieved [41]. Although neither effect is itself dramatic (typically a jejunostomy output will be reduced by no more than 15% or 500 ml per day) it can be sufficient to have meaningful impact on quality of life. For reasons that are not entirely clear, doses much larger than in standard therapeutic regimes are frequently needed to obtain maximal benefit.

Somatostatin and its analogues reduce gastric, biliary and pancreatic secretions [42] and slow gastro-jejunal transit time [43]. Although there is also evidence that they have an adverse effect on the uptake of nutrients, possibly on wound healing and may interfere with the physiological process of adaptation to resection [44], it is natural that their effects on stomal and fistula output have been studied (see above). Sodium and water losses are not significantly affected in patients who are net absorbers (or in positive gastrointestinal balance), but a reproducible reduction in stomal output can be achieved in net secretors, averaging around 500 ml/day. There does not seem to be any difference in efficacy between somatostatin and the more convenient octreotide. Twice or thrice daily subcutaneous injections of octreotide 50–100 μg have usually been used, with little evidence for greater effect from daily doses in excess of

300 μg. Major side-effects are not recorded, although the high risk of gall-stone formation is important, given the already increased frequency of gallstones in SBS patients.

A series of other agents thought to be of potential use in SBS have been tried and found to be of very limited effect. The bulking agents such as ispaghula decrease the fluidity of gut effluent, but increase the loss of water and electrolytes and aggravate their depletion [37]. Cholestyramine is of value in patients with a retained colon with either bile salt-related diarrhoea without steatorrhoea, or with hyperoxaluria. Its negative influence on absorption of fat-soluble vitamins and its lack of palatability militate further against its use.

Professionals more peripherally involved in the care of SBS patients are often ill-informed and intimidated by the problems posed, leading to suboptimal care. The most damaging effects arise when the dehydrated patient is incorrectly advised to drink more fluid. Each patient should be educated about the condition and its management, and should have written details which can be shown to new health-care personnel. The anger and general distress of patients and relatives should not be underestimated; formal psychological support and counselling may be appropriate in some cases.

ANAEMIA IN INFLAMMATORY BOWEL DISEASE

It may seem odd to include a separate section on anaemia as a complication of inflammatory bowel disease, this being a common presenting feature of the new patient, and usually rapidly responsive to therapy which controls inflammation and curtails intestinal blood loss. Short- to medium-term supplementation with the appropriate haematinics will provide the necessary supportive role, with indefinite vitamin B_{12} for those with no terminal ileum. However, there are patients in whom chronic low-grade blood loss, or the anaemia of chronic disease, is not easily overcome. This will sometimes be sufficient to justify colectomy in the chronic colitic, but more rarely to warrant resection in the patient with extensive Crohn's who is usually the very patient who is anaemic partly because of an existing degree of intestinal failure. It is obviously important to define the nature of the anaemia. Vitamin B_{12} deficiency is easily diagnosed and overcome, but will normally have been anticipated and pre-empted in patients with terminal ileal resection. Folate and iron deficiency often coexist in patients with extensive small bowel Crohn's, and an apparently normocytic anaemia should not be attributed to chronic disease until their status has been established (the patient with folate and iron deficiency will normally have an elevated red cell distribution width even if there is not overt anaemia). Adequate folate restitution, also, is usually straightforward with oral administration (or intravenous in those with overt short bowel syndrome, as above). Iron replacement is more often problematic. Many inflammatory bowel disease patients find iron salts intolerable, and many have specific gastrointestinal side-effects that limit use. It is always worth a trial of liquid oral iron (as Sytron® in the UK) which some patients seem to tolerate better and which may lead to useful absorption even in those with short bowel syndrome. Transfusion is of limited application, tends to be of short-lived value, and has its own hazards. Similar strictures apply to the use of total dose iron therapy by infusion, and to prolonged courses of intramuscular injections. Although intravenous iron is effective in around 75% of otherwise intractable iron-deficient patients, it is not without risk. In a small audit at St Mark's (unpublished data) 25% of Crohn's patients treated with intravenous iron developed a clinically significant anaphylactoid reaction. As, in the view of the supervising physician, half of these required adrenaline therapy, alternative regimes are clearly needed!

Study of anaemic patients with Crohn's disease demonstrates a defect in erythropoietin production which is inadequate for the magnitude of anaemia, regardless of iron status or the current degree of disease activity [45]. In other medical contexts, both intractable iron deficiency and the anaemia of chronic disease have been significantly helped by exogenous erythropoietin. Early data in inflammatory bowel disease suggest that there may be a place for this expensive parenteral therapy in difficult cases, both in adults and children [46, 47]. In Schreiber's study, 15 patients with ulcerative colitis and 19 with Crohn's disease were randomized to oral iron with or without subcutaneous erythropoietin (150 units/kg twice weekly) [46]. Over 12 weeks there was a mean 1.7 g/dl gain in haemoglobin in those receiving both drugs, compared to a loss of 0.85 g/dl in those on iron alone. Significance was achieved both for patients with Crohn's disease and with ulcerative colitis.

THROMBOSIS AND THROMBOEMBOLIC PHENOMENA IN INFLAMMATORY BOWEL DISEASE

Thrombosis and thromboembolic phenomena are important causes of morbidity and mortality in active inflammatory bowel disease [48]. Although strict comparative data are lacking, deep vein thrombosis in the legs and pelvis, pulmonary embolism, mesenteric and intracranial thromboses all appear to be more common than in other groups of in-patients with benign disease. Mesenteric microvascular thrombosis, postulated as a pathogenic factor for inflammatory bowel disease (Chapter 1), and possible abnormalities in heparan status (Chapter 3), may be contributory factors, as may the thrombocytosis typical of the patient with active disease. Spontaneous platelet aggregation, and high levels of thromboxane B_2, platelet factor 4, fibrinopeptide A and β-thromboglobulin are demonstrable in Crohn's disease [48, 49]. There are substantially reduced, and therefore prothrombotic, levels of antithrombin III in some but not all patients with active inflammatory bowel disease [50, 51]. Acquired deficiency of protein C and S may also occur. There is evidence for abnormality also of the tissue plasminogen system [49, 52]. In a recent study from the Royal Free in London patients with Crohn's disease were found to have pathological levels of plasma factor VII:C, lipoprotein (a) and fibrinogen. In ulcerative colitis levels of lipoprotein (a) and fibrinogen were normal, but factor VII:C again exceeded the normal range [53]. The probable increased risk of arterial thrombosis in inflammatory bowel disease may be linked to a strikingly increased prevalence of IgG anticardiolipin antibodies in Crohn's disease (43% of patients positive compared to 2.5% of matched controls), and hardly less so in ulcerative colitis (at 20%) [54].

The issue of thrombosis in inflammatory bowel disease is beginning to take on medicolegal significance, and it will be difficult to refute future claims arising from thrombotic events if prophylactic measures were not taken, since it will be argued that such an event was sufficiently predictable that these measures should have been taken, or that the reason for not so doing should have been recorded. All patients admitted for inflammatory bowel disease should be on a prophylactic regime (quite apart from any potential therapeutic benefit from heparin in ulcerative colitis (Chapter 3)); those with septic or other complications of their disease appear to be at especial risk [3]. However, if thrombosis occurs, there does not appear to be any particular need for inflammatory bowel disease patients to be managed differently from those with thrombosis complicating other medical conditions. Apart from during the immediate postoperative period, standard anticoagulation with heparin and then a coumarin such as warfarin is safe and will not normally lead to excessive gastrointestinal bleeding (indeed, the opposite is suggested for heparin in ulcerative colitis (Chapter 3)). Patients with short bowel syndrome are sometimes difficult to anticoagulate satisfactorily, but cautious use of warfarin with haematological monitoring at a fixed interval from exposure to nutrient solutions (particularly lipid) will usually suffice. Difficulty in achieving anticoagulation with heparin in inflammatory bowel disease probably reflects concurrent antithrombin III deficiency – it is possible that leeches may be able to help here as their anticoagulant, hirudin, unlike heparin, is independent of antithrombin III [55].

REFERENCES

1. Keighley MRB, Eastwood D, Ambrose NS *et al.* Incidence and microbiology of abdominal and pelvic abscess in Crohn's disease. *Gastroenterology* 1982; **83**: 1271–1275.

2. Ribeiro MB, Greenstein AJ, Yamazaki Y, Aufses AH Jr. Intra-abdominal abscess in regional enteritis. *Ann Surg* 1991; **213**: 32–36.
3. Ricci MA, Meyer KK. Psoas abscess complicating Crohn's disease. *Am J Gastroenterol* 1985; **80**: 970–977.
4. Leu SY, Leonard MB, Beart RW Jr, Dozois RR. Psoas abscess: changing patterns of diagnosis and etiology. *Dis Colon Rectum* 1986; **29**: 694–698.
5. Jawhari A, Ong C, Kamm MA, Forbes A. Abdominal and pelvic abscesses in Crohn's disease: a review of non-invasive and surgical management. *Gastroenterology* 1995; **108**: A843.
6. Sahai A, Gianfelice D, Bélair M *et al.* Percutaneous drainage of abscesses in Crohn's disease: success or failure? *Gastroenterology* 1996; **110**: A1006.
7. Gore RM, Cohen MI, Vogelzang RL *et al.* Value of computed tomography in the detection of complications of Crohn's disease. *Dig Dis Sci* 1985; **30**: 701–709.
8. Tio TL, Mulder CJJ, Wijers OB *et al.* Endosonography of peri-anal and pericolorectal fistula and/or abscess in Crohn's disease: a study of 36 patients. *Gastrointest Endosc* 1990; **36**: 331–336.
9. Bluth EI, Ferrari BT, Sullivan MA. Abscess drainage with the aid of pelvic real-time ultrasonography. *Dis Colon Rectum* 1985; **28**: 262–263.
10. Millward SF, Ramesewak W, Fitzsimons P *et al.* Percutaneous drainage of iliopsoas abscess in Crohn's disease. *Gastrointest Radiol* 1986; **11**: 289–290.
11. Doemeny JM, Burke DR, Meranze SG. Percutaneous drainage of abscesses in patients with Crohn's disease. *Gastrointest Radiol* 1988; **13**: 237–241.
12. Felder JB, Adler DJ, Korelitz BI. The safety of corticosteroid therapy in Crohn's disease with an abdominal mass. *Am J Gastroenterol* 1991; **86**: 1450–1455.
13. Lévy E, Frileux P, Cugnenc PH *et al.* High output external fistulae of the small bowel: management with continuous enteral nutrition. *Br J Surg* 1989; **76**: 676–679.
14. Rinsema W, Gouma DJ, Von Meyenfeldt MF *et al.* Primary conservative management of external small-bowel fistulas. *Acta Chir Scand* 1990; **156**: 457–462.
15. Kelly JK, Preshaw RM. Origin of fistulas in Crohn's disease. *J Clin Gastroenterol* 1989; **11**: 193–196.
16. Driscoll RH Jr, Rosenberg IH. Total parenteral nutrition in inflammatory bowel disease. *Med Clin N Am* 1978; **62**: 185–201.
17. Von Meyenfeldt MF, Meijerink WJHJ, Rouflart MMJ *et al.* Perioperative nutritional support: a randomised clinical trial. *Clin Nutr* 1992; **11**: 180–186.

18. Korelitz BI, Present DH. Favorable effect of 6-mercaptopurine on fistulae of Crohn's disease. *Dig Dis Sci* 1985; **30**: 58–64.
19. Present DH, Lichtiger S. Efficacy of cyclosporine in treatment of fistula of Crohn's disease. *Dig Dis Sci* 1994; **39**: 374–380.
20. Nubiola P, Sancho J, Seguira M *et al.* Blind evaluation of the effect of octreotide, a somatostatin analogue, on small bowel fistula output. *Lancet* 1987; **ii**: 672–674.
21. Scott NA, Finnegan S, Irving MH. Octreotide and gastrointestinal fistulae. *Digestion* 1990; **45**: 66–71.
22. Rinsema W, Gouma DJ, Von Meyenfeldt MF. Reinfusion of secretions from high-output proximal stomas or fistulas. *Surg Gynecol Obstet* 1988; **167**: 372–376.
23. McIntyre P, Ritchie J, Hawley P *et al.* Management of enterocutaneous fistulas: a review of 132 cases. *Br J Surg* 1984; **71**: 293–296.
24. Gouttebel MC, Saint Aubert B, Colette C *et al.* Intestinal adaptation in patients with short bowel syndrome. *Dig Dis Sci* 1989; **34**: 709–715.
25. Nightingale JMD, Lennard-Jones JE, Walker ER, Farthing MJG. Jejunal efflux in short bowel syndrome. *Lancet* 1990; **336**: 765–768.
26. Nightingale JMD, Lennard-Jones JE, Gertner DJ *et al.* Colonic preservation reduces need for parental therapy, increases incidence of renal stones, but does not change prevalence of gall stones in patients with a short bowel. *Gut* 1992; **33**: 1493–1497.
27. Royall D, Thomas MS, Wolever BM, Jeejeebhoy KN. Evidence for colonic conservation of malabsorbed carbohydrate in short bowel syndrome. *Am J Gastroenterol* 1992; **87**: 751–756.
28. Nordgaard I, Hansen BS, Mortensen NPB. Colon as a digestive organ in patients with short bowel. *Lancet* 1994; **343**: 373–376.
29. Woolf GM, Miller C, Kurian R, Jeejeebhoy KN. Nutritional absorption in short bowel syndrome. *Dig Dis Sci* 1987; **32**: 8–15.
30. Woolf BM, Miller C, Kurian R, Jeejeebhoy KN. Diet for patients with a short bowel: high fat or high carbohydrate? *Gastroenterology* 1983: **84**: 823–828.
31. McIntyre PB, Fitchew M, Lennard-Jones JE. Patients with a high jejunostomy do not need a special diet. *Gastroenterology* 1986; **91**: 25–33.
32. Lennard-Jones JE, Wood S. Coping with the short bowel. *Hosp Update* 1991; **17**: 797–807.
33. Matuchansky C, Messing B, Jeejeebhoy KN *et al.* Cyclical parenteral nutrition. *Lancet* 1992; **340**: 588–592.
34. Griffin GE, Fagan EF, Hodgson HJ, Chadwick VS. Enteral therapy in the management of massive gut resection complicated by chronic fluid and electrolyte depletion. *Dig Dis Sci* 1982; **27**: 902–908.

35. Newton CR, McIntyre PB, Lennard-Jones JE *et al.* Effect of different drinks on fluid and electrolyte losses from a jejunostomy. *Proc Roy Soc Med* 1985; **78**: 27–29.

36. Nightingale JMD, Kamm MA, Van Der Sijp JRM *et al.* Disturbed gastric emptying in the short bowel syndrome. Evidence for a 'colonic brake'. *Gut* 1993; **34**: 1171–1176.

37. Newton CR. Effect of codeine phosphate, Lomotil and Isogel on ileostomy function. *Gut* 1978; **19**: 377–383.

38. Tytgat GN, Huibregtse K, Dagevos J, Van Den Ende A. Effect of loperamide on fecal output and composition in well-established ileostomy and ileorectal anastomosis. *Am J Dig Dis* 1977; **22**: 669–675.

39. McIntyre PB. The short bowel. *Br J Surg* 1985; **72**: S92–S93.

40. Pelemans W, Vantrappen G. A double blind crossover comparison of loperamide with diphenoxylate in the symptomatic treatment of chronic diarrhea. *Gastroenterology* 1976; **70**: 1030–1034.

41. Cortot J, Fleming CR, Malagelada JR. Improved nutrient absorption after cimetidine in short-bowel syndrome with gastric hypersecretion. *Med Intell* 1979; **300**: 79–81.

42. O'Keefe SJD, Peterson ME, Fleming CR. Octreotide as an adjunct to home parenteral nutrition in the management of permanent end-jejunostomy syndrome. *J Parent Ent Nutr* 1994; **18**: 26–36.

43. Cooper JC, Williams NS, King RFGJ, Barker MCJ. Effects of a long-acting somatostatin analogue in patients with severe ileostomy diarrhoea. *Br J Surg* 1986; **73**: 128–131.

44. O'Keefe SJD, Haymond MW, Bennet WM *et al.* Long-acting somatostatin analogue therapy and protein metabolism in patients with jejunostomies. *Gastroenterology* 1994; **107**: 379–388.

45. Gasche C, Reinisch W, Lochs H *et al.* Anemia in Crohn's disease. Importance of inadequate erythropoietin production and iron deficiency. *Dig Dis Sci* 1994; **39**: 1930–1934.

46. Schreiber S, Howaldt S, Schnoor M *et al.* Recombinant erythropoietin for the treatment of anemia in inflammatory bowel disease. *N Engl J Med* 1996; **334**: 619–623.

47. Dohil R, Hassall E, Wadsworth LD, Israel DM. Recombinant human erythropoietin for anemia of chronic disease in children with Crohn's disease. *Gastroenterology* 1996; **110**: A897.

48. Webberley MJ, Hart MT, Melikian V. Thromboembolism in inflammatory bowel disease: role of platelets. *Gut* 1993; **34**: 247–251.

49. Chamouard P, Grunebaum L, Duclos B *et al.* Biological manifestations of a prethrombotic state in developmental Crohn's disease. *Gastroenterol Clin Biol* 1990; **14**: 203–208.

50. Knot EA, Ten Cate JW, Bruin T *et al.* Antithrombin III metabolism in two colitis patients with acquired antithrombin III deficiency. *Gastroenterology* 1985; **89**: 421–425.

51. Bohe M, Genell S, Ohlsson K. Protease inhibitors in plasma and faecal extracts from patients with active inflammatory bowel disease. *Scand J Gastroenterol* 1986; **21**: 598–604.
52. Verspaget HW, Sier CFM, Ganesh S *et al*. Urokinase receptor and plasminogen activator inhibitors in tissue of patients with inflammatory bowel disease. *Gastroenterology* 1996; **110**: A1039.
53. Hudson M, Chitolie A, Hutton RA *et al*. Thrombotic vascular risk factors in inflammatory bowel disease. *Gut* 1996; **38**: 733–737.
54. Perri F, Villani MR, Annese V *et al*. Anticardiolipin antibodies in inflammatory bowel diseases. *Gastroenterology* 1996; **110**: A989.
55. Turpie AGG. Hirudin and thrombosis prophylaxis. *Lancet* 1996; **347**: 632–633.

8

Malignancy complicating inflammatory bowel disease

COLORECTAL CANCER IN ULCERATIVE COLITIS

There is general agreement that colorectal carcinoma is more common in those with long-standing extensive ulcerative colitis. Historically, risks of 5–10% at 20 years rising to 12–30% at 30 years, and with an approximately 20-fold increased lifetime risk, have been suggested. It might be pointed out that the latter figure is discordant with the two former, and is not entirely internally consistent as this would lead to nearly two-thirds of all patients with unresected extensive colitis going on to develop malignancy. It has not been clear whether young age at onset is an additional risk factor, nor if colonic tumours arising in the context of ulcerative colitis have a worse prognosis than sporadic cancers. More recent data collected to try to answer these (and other) questions paint a somewhat less gloomy picture. Although accounting for 50% of all the deaths in one referral centre that could be attributed directly to ulcerative colitis (B.I. Korelitz, personal communication), the death rate in a Swedish population study was only three (not 20) times background [1], and in Denmark there is no longer an increased rate of colorectal carcinoma at 25 years of extensive colitis (probably at least in part because of an aggressive surgical policy) [2]. The more recent studies confirm the absence of increased risk if the disease remains confined to the rectum and sigmoid, and continue to place the patient with left-sided disease at intermediate risk [3]. A note of caution is required here given the possibility of proximal extension of colitis (Chapter 2).

When colorectal carcinoma complicates ulcerative colitis, it shares many features with its sporadic counterpart, but the St Mark's study of 157 tumours in 120 patients [4] illustrates some of the differences. The distribution of tumours was predominantly left-sided (56% recto-sigmoid, 12% descending/splenic flexure), but the 32% of lesions which were proximal is a higher figure than for most sporadic series; 67.5% of all patients had a recto-sigmoid tumour. The overall 5-year survival in the St Mark's patients of 59.4% is consistent with UK survival data for colorectal carcinoma in general. For each Dukes' stage too, results seemed comparable (Table 8.1).

COLORECTAL CARCINOMA IN CROHN'S DISEASE

In Crohn's disease one population study has shown an increased risk of colorectal cancer [5], while four population-based studies indicate no overall increase [6–9]. From the total of 373 individuals subsequently considered by the Copenhagen group [10], the relative risk for all colorectal carcinomas was a non-significant 1.1, and only slightly higher for colonic cancer at 1.7 (not significant). However, referral centre studies show more obvious increased frequencies of colorectal carcinoma, with relative risks varying between 3.0 and 20 [11–17]. Only two units report an absence of increased risk [18, 19]. Both Gillen [16] and Cohen [17] find – as in ulcerative colitis – an increase in patients with extensive colitis of long duration.

There is obvious uncertainty about the veracity of a major increased risk given the apparent conflict between population and referral centre data, but patients with Crohn's disease are certainly not protected from colorectal carcinoma (except those who have had proctocolectomy) and, when it occurs, a clinical course a little different from that seen in the general population seems to be followed. The median age at diagnosis of colorectal carcinoma in Crohn's disease is around 50 years, and approximately 40% of patients have right-sided lesions. Most patients have had their Crohn's for a prolonged period prior to the diagnosis of malignancy (median duration 15 years), but nearly a third have had Crohn's for less than 10 years. Presumably because early symptoms are attributed to exacerbations of Crohn's disease (and perhaps because of the excess of right-sided lesion), diagnosis tends to be late, and is often only made at surgery even now. The overall prognosis is poorer than for colorectal carcinoma unassociated with inflammatory bowel disease, with typical 5-year survivals in the region of 20%, and it is probable that Crohn's patients with colorectal carcinoma have a worse prognosis than

Table 8.1 Five-year survival data for patients with colorectal carcinoma complicating ulcerative colitis

Overall	59.4%
Dukes' A	90.6%
Dukes' B	87.8%
Dukes' C	28.3%
Disseminated	nil

n = 157 tumours in 120 patients [4].

patients with sporadic neoplasms matched for Dukes' stage [11, 13, 15, 18, 20].

Those with Crohn's predicted, by one or more studies, to be at substantially higher risk of colorectal carcinoma are those with prolonged disease, early disease onset (before 20 years or in childhood), those with extensive or stricturing disease, those with chronic fistulae and those with bypassed segments of intestine, although it is likely that the 30% risk attributed to the latter group reflects several of the other risk factors also [13, 15, 16].

PATHOGENESIS OF INCREASED COLORECTAL CARCINOMA IN INFLAMMATORY BOWEL DISEASE

Epidemiological considerations confirm that the increased rate of colorectal carcinoma in inflammatory bowel disease cannot be explained by simple coincidence of a relatively common cancer. An adequate understanding of the mechanisms that lead from chronic inflammation to neoplasia, which can account for the timing and distribution of tumours, does not yet exist. However, an interesting new link has been suggested [21] by study of the expression of the transforming growth factor regulatory peptides in inflammatory bowel disease. Transforming growth factor-α (TGF-α) is a member of the epidermal growth factor family and as such is probably of considerable significance in the response of the intestinal epithelium to injury, and perhaps also in the pathogenesis of neoplasia. Curiously, although TGF-α expression was indistinguishable from normal in Crohn's disease and in active ulcerative colitis, the levels were enhanced to up to three times control values in inactive ulcerative colitis. This phenomenon is not easily explained and requires confirmation by others, but if true may help us to understand the independence of cancer risk from the clinical severity of colitis, since chronic overexpression of TGF-α might be expected to provoke epithelial hyperproliferation and to be (partly) causative in the increased incidence of neoplasia. Some additional support for this view comes from the authors' observation that TGF-α expression was at its highest level in patients with the greatest duration of colitis (i.e. those at most risk of neoplasia).

CANCER SURVEILLANCE

Cancer surveillance in inflammatory bowel disease has become controversial in a way that simple follow-up has and would not. Although some managerial voices have been heard to question the need for hospital follow-up of inflammatory bowel disease patients, there can be little doubt that patients and their doctors see clear advantage in regular clinical assessment; this is a central plank of the recently devised guidelines on management from the British Society of Gastroenterology [22]. This routine, long-term management and supervision is of especial value when toxic or unfamiliar drugs are in use, and warrants a major proportion of patient care occurring in the hospital setting. Re-investigation of clinical changes is then straightforward and the 'obvious' benefits of such a strategy are probably sufficient to justify it. Cancer surveillance differs from this traditional follow-up model in several particulars and must be specifically considered.

Cancer surveillance must, in any context, satisfy a number of criteria if it is to be justifiable. It must be able to identify early cancers, or (better) high-risk lesions that will progress to tumours if left untreated. There must be curative therapy available for these early lesions when detected. The surveillance method must be safe and acceptable to the subjects to whom it is to be offered, who must in turn be available to the surveyors. To avoid the medical, emotional and financial problems that arise from false positive and false negative results, there should be perfect sensitivity and specificity, but as this will never be achieved the methodology should ensure that an appropriate balance is drawn, to ensure maximal benefit at minimal cost in terms of missed cancers, against prolonged and potentially hazardous further investigation in those not at risk. The ideal surveillance programme will not only lead to its subjects avoiding cancer, but will also save money for their health-care system. The operational criteria appropriate to a diagnostic test do not normally satisfy the more stringent requirements for a surveillance procedure. In inflammatory bowel disease we have an identifiable and medically accessible high-risk population for colorectal carcinoma, and in colonoscopy we certainly have a surveillance tool, but one that is only moderately satisfactory, being unpleasant, time-consuming, expensive and not without risk. The experienced colonoscopist will recognize almost all sporadic colorectal carcinomas and their premonitory polyps, but will miss a higher proportion of early lesions when they are present alongside the abnormal mucosa of inflammatory bowel disease. The colonoscopist is also most unlikely to recognize pre-malignant change from its macroscopic appearances. The surveillance tool to be considered then, is colonoscopy with histological examination of multiple colonic biopsies.

SURVEILLANCE IN ULCERATIVE COLITIS

Surveillance of patients with long-standing ulcerative colitis has been conducted over the past 20 years or so by many centres, on the *a priori* assumption that it would be obviously beneficial. However, the results have not been clear-cut, and the lack of controlled data from the time of its introduction is now greatly regretted. Axon's critical analysis from 1994 [23] attracted much attention and had a perhaps overly negative influence on surveillance strategy in many units. His key points deserve to be revisited. Twelve programmes including 1916 patients were included, from which 92 cancers were identified. Only 52 were 'successful' in the sense of being probably curable Dukes' A or B lesions. However, only 41 had a preoperative or ante-mortem diagnosis, and only 24 of these were truly asymptomatic with no 'incidental' positive tests (satisfying him that the colonoscopies were performed entirely for surveillance reasons). By excluding a further group of patients in whom tumours were found at the first 'screening' colonoscopy, Axon accepted only 13 individuals as truly within surveillance programmes (and discounted a further two because of colectomy for low-grade dysplasia – to which we will return). By his account 476 surveillance colonoscopies were therefore required for each useful result, consequently comparing poorly with the likely benefits from random surveillance of a middle-aged European population looking for adenomatous polyps and early cancers. He accordingly concluded that colonoscopic surveillance in ulcerative colitis was not justified. A number of important points arise from this analysis, to which can be added newer data unavailable at the time.

Axon plays down the value of a contribution from identification of dysplasia, recognizing that its detection is an imperfect science, with problems in its definition and with marked between-observer variation, the latter reaching to 66% in one series [24]. The newer, tighter, histological criteria for dysplasia reduce, but do not eliminate, these problems [25]. It will also be noted that some patients develop malignancy apparently without previous dysplasia. Despite double reporting by skilled gastrointestinal pathologists using standardized histological diagnostic criteria, in around 25% of colitis-related cancers, no dysplasia can be found at a site separate from the malignancy, even though the whole resected colon is available for examination [26, 27]. In Connell's study 18% had no evidence of dysplasia at the site of malignancy nor on any previous surveillance biopsy [26]. It is unclear whether prior dysplasia was truly absent at the tumour site or was simply missed in the pre-invasive phase of neoplasia, but in either case this is a practical failing of current surveillance protocols.

Many samples historically categorized as borderline and low-grade dysplasia are now down-graded. This has the effect of increasing the clinical significance of the smaller number that retain a diagnosis of low- or high-grade dysplasia. Although dysplasia is undoubtedly an informative marker for future malignancy [27], its predictive value even when high grade remains imperfect. Approximately half of those affected can be expected on statistical grounds to develop frank malignancy within 5 years if, for some reason, surgery is not performed [28]. The recognition, from several centres, that around a third of those with ulcerative colitis complicated by high-grade dysplasia are found to have otherwise unsuspected cancer in the resected colon is also of considerable importance.

Axon's dismissal of the significance of low-grade dysplasia is more jus-
tifiably questioned. Several centres have now reported on the frequency
at which low-grade dysplasia progresses to high-grade dysplasia or cancer [26–28]. In each case the risk has been substantial (>18%) and in one
case was over 50% at 5 years [26], so long as the newer histological criteria
for dysplasia are employed (see above). It is, accordingly, current practice
at St Mark's to advise colectomy for all patients with confirmed low-grade
dysplasia that has been identified on two occasions (or at two separate
sites on the same occasion).

The latest update on the St Mark's surveillance programme was published shortly after Axon's paper, reporting on 332 patients with macroscopically right-sided ulcerative colitis of more than 10 years' duration
[26]. All patients with radiological or macroscopic disease at endoscopy
extending to or above the hepatic flexure were invited to participate and
the 332 represent a substantial majority of those eligible. The programme
required full colonoscopy with multiple biopsies every 2 years, and a rigid
sigmoidoscopy and rectal biopsy in the intervening years. The overall colorectal carcinoma rate was 6.0% ($n = 20$), occurring at a median age of 51
in patients with colitis for a median of 21 years; 60% of the tumours were
in the recto-sigmoid. Only 11 of the tumours were detected by the surveillance programme (eight Dukes' A; one B; two C). Nine of these were
therefore 'useful' diagnoses, although the two Dukes' Cs were alive and
disease-free at 3 and 7 years. Surveillance missed six cancers, all of which
were advanced at the time of diagnosis (four Dukes' C; two disseminated),
with an interval of 10–23 months from the most recent colonoscopy. These
six patients were younger (median 38 years), but had the same median
duration of disease as the whole group of patients with tumours. Three
further cancers occurred in previously surveyed patients, after they had
left the programme for a variety of reasons.

Surveillance detected dysplasia in 21 patients, nine of whom had cancer; these cancers were found at the same colonoscopy in four, and only
after resection in five. Twelve patients with dysplasia had no cancer at
resection.

In summary, surveillance genuinely and usefully detected nine early
cancers, and a further 12 very high-risk patients. Benefit to these 21
patients required a total of 1316 colonoscopies, and as one diagnosis was
made by rigid sigmoidoscopy (in the alternate year between colonoscopies), 66 colonoscopies were required for each useful result, at a cost of
around £25 000 (>US$40 000) per case detected. There were no important
complications from colonoscopy in the series. As far as can be ascertained,
provision of surveillance colonoscopy (at St Mark's) is more beneficial
than harmful to the individuals included, but it cannot be considered
mandatory.

The latest data from Sweden, which approach surveillance from an epidemiological standpoint, await full publication but are supportive of the endeavour [29]. The study base comprised all patients with ulcerative colitis for the Stockholm and Uppsala areas (for 1955–84 and 1965–83, respectively), representing around 6000 prevalent cases in a population of 3 million. Cases of fatal colorectal carcinoma occurring after 1975 were identified from cancer registry data (almost 100% inclusive), and were included if ulcerative colitis had been present for 5 years or more prior to cancer death. Forty such patients were found, and 102 colitic controls matched for age, sex, disease duration and disease extent were selected. It was required that controls were still alive at the time of death of the matching case, and had not undergone pancolectomy in the 5 years prior to the case's cancer diagnosis. Cases were then compared with controls for the utilization of surveillance colonoscopy. Colonoscopies performed for diagnosis, index examinations and those for clinical indications were excluded. These assessments were made retrospectively from clinical notes and may not be entirely free from error and/or bias. Although just failing to reach statistical significance, the results are nevertheless impressive. Only 2 of the 40 cancer patients had ever received a surveillance colonoscopy (5%) compared to 18 of the 102 controls (17.6%) (odds ratio, 0.25; CI, 0.05–1.11). Furthermore, 12 controls, compared to only one case, had received more than one surveillance procedure (OR, 0.18; CI, 0.005–1.19), indicating a 'dose-response'.

How can surveillance be improved?

It is evident that colonoscopic surveillance is imperfect, and should not be considered mandatory for patients with long-standing extensive colitis, but it is unlikely that any major centre will now feel able to sanction its controlled trial against routine care. However, strategies intended to improve the performance of surveillance can, and should, be tested in controlled fashion. There is little potential for improved colonoscopy, although doubtless it will become easier and more comfortable with the continual improvements in endoscopic technology and training. A higher yield of tissue will help the pathologist, but it is currently impractical to consider more than 15–20 biopsies per examination. Performing colonoscopy at greater frequency might help to improve the positive pick-up rate, and switching to annual colonoscopy is a rational response to the failings of the St Mark's 1994 analysis. This would be unlikely to have identified all five of the tumours missed between 12 and 24 months and could not have influenced detection of that at 10 months. It also has very major implications in terms of numbers of procedures (and therefore the cost of the programme) (see below). Accordingly, we should be looking for alternative means to supplement the existing data, aiming to identify patients at an especially high risk who can be most aggressively targeted, and conversely to identify those at relatively low risk in whom efforts may legitimately be less (e.g. colonoscopy every 5 years).

Additional markers of malignancy and pre-malignancy

Potentially useful additional markers identified from their actual or putative value in sporadic colorectal carcinoma or other solid tumours, include the presence of aneuploidy, mutations of oncogenes (such as Ki-*ras* or c-*myc*), of tumour suppresser genes (such as *p53* or *apc*) or of mismatch repair genes (e.g. *mut-s*). There is reasonable evidence that aneuploidy is of predictive value in ulcerative colitis, but otherwise very little reliable information.

Aneuploidy (disturbance of the cell's normal diploid state) can be demonstrated in colonic biopsies from patients with dysplasia and/or malignancy. Most authors favour a progressive sequence: aneuploidy preceding dysplasia, itself in turn preceding carcinoma [30]. This is evidently a generalization, however, with some carcinomas apparently lacking either aneuploidy or dysplasia, and some patients moving from aneuploidy to carcinoma without ever exhibiting dysplasia [31]. Detection of aneuploidy could thus be comparably informative to low-grade dysplasia. There is usually a positive correlation with histological grading, and a high proportion of patients with aneuploidy and without dysplasia seem likely to progress relatively quickly (five of five within 2.5 years in Rubin's study [30]) but progression is not inevitable. It is possible that the apparent high degree of protection (good negative predictive value) for patients in whom there is no aneuploidy may be more valuable from a prognostic viewpoint. Controlled prospective assessment is required.

Inactivating mutations of the *p53* tumour suppressor gene are very frequent in most solid tumours. There has been debate as to the relative frequency of *p53* mutation in ulcerative colitis-related colorectal carcinoma, and whether changes at this locus occur sufficiently early in the neoplastic process to provide additional or earlier information than is possible from detection of dysplasia. A consensus appears to be emerging that *p53* mutations are strongly correlated with aneuploidy [32]. In a tightly matched study (11 cases and 11 controls with almost 1000 biopsies examined) Wang *et al.* [33] failed to find abnormal expression of *p53* in any of the control colitis samples, but 1.6% of the 503 biopsies from patients who went on to develop high-grade dysplasia or carcinoma previously overexpressed *p53* gene product. Although in most of these cases there was dysplasia in the same sample, *p53* mutation was the only abnormality found in two patients prior to demonstration of frank malignancy. Only a single patient in this series failed to exhibit either dysplasia or *p53* mutation. Similar data have been reported from other centres. Prospective assessment is needed to clarify whether a routine search for aberrant *p53* expression in surveillance biopsies is warranted.

Markers of proliferative activity in the colonic mucosa have also been examined. The Ki-67 antigen is a proliferation marker (expressed in all stages of the cell cycle except G_0) and is expressed most at times of maximal cell proliferation. Newer antibodies make its immunohistochemical evaluation in routine formalin/paraffin sections relatively straightforward. Nuclear antigens associated with cell proliferation have also been identified and can be demonstrated similarly, and in a single paper Kullmann *et al.* examine both Ki-67 and proliferating cell nuclear antigen (PCNA) in biopsies from patients with ulcerative colitis with and without dysplasia compared to normal controls [34]. Although there were strongly supportive trends and good statistical correlation, there was insufficient discrimination between the labelling indices for either marker used alone to be other than a further guide, these data favouring Ki-67 as the better option. There was more PCNA in high-grade than in low-grade dysplastic samples (PCNA index 81% v. 44%) and similarly for Ki-67 (55% v. 31%). However, although the authors defend their work on the basis of providing an aid to the pathologist when there is borderline low-grade dysplasia or borderline high-grade dysplasia, they diminish a potentially more important role. The study took dysplasia to be a gold standard, but this it is not. It will be instructive to examine proliferation markers as independent predictors of neoplasia, not least since there are possible routes to their therapeutic manipulation [35].

The mucin-associated carbohydrate antigen, sialosyl-Tn, which has been linked with sporadic colorectal carcinoma, was expressed more often in patients with carcinoma complicating ulcerative colitis (44% of biopsies) than in controls without carcinoma or dysplasia (11%) [36]. The antigen appeared up to 7 years before neoplasia and its expression was not compromised by active inflammation. In a prospective study of five patients who underwent colonoscopy on at least six occasions, and who at some time developed aneuploidy, a prevalence of sialosyl-Tn positivity of 10% was found – roughly double that of aneuploidy, with only two biopsies from one patient showing dysplasia [37]. In all but one instance the sialosyl-Tn expression preceded aneuploidy. These data suggest a complementary role in identifying the patients at highest risk, but prospective analysis is required; alone it is clearly an inadequate alternative to established methods. Curiously, this antigen is often expressed in uncomplicated Crohn's disease and at too frequent a rate to be useful in predicting risk of neoplasia in this context [38].

To date none of the above options has been adequately tested in the context of its impact on a surveillance programme, and specific controlled data to judge whether a programme including such additional markers is more effective than one without are lacking. Hopefully, the lessons to be learnt from the uncontrolled initiation of surveillance will ensure that changes in clinical and pathological practice follow such data collection.

Better targeting of colonoscopy in ulcerative colitis

Better targeting of colonoscopy – or at least the frequency at which it is performed – is desirable to maximize the cost-effectiveness of surveillance. The importance of long duration and the extent of colitis are built into all existing surveillance strategies, coupled now with evidence that confirmed dysplasia is a sufficiently valid measure of cancer risk to warrant surgical intervention. In sporadic colorectal carcinoma there are very clear links with the prior presence of adenomas and of a positive family history (at their most dramatic in the hereditary polyposis syndromes) [39]. Until very recently there have been scant data to indicate whether these factors apply equally in patients with ulcerative colitis, and they have not been included as separate risk factors in determining frequency or intensity of investigation in any of the surveillance programmes that have reported to date. The Mayo Clinic group has examined its own programme (which includes 203 patients with colorectal carcinoma complicating ulcerative colitis) in a case-control fashion which includes no population data, but controls for the high degree of selection in patients reaching this tertiary referral centre [40]. Recall bias was apparently slight as judged from their cross-checking search for familial stroke. A family history of colorectal carcinoma affecting a first-degree relative proved to be 2.4 times more common in colitis patients with neoplasia than in those without (CI, 1.1–5.8), a difference that was not explained by familial colitis. As they point out, this is the same order of proportional difference to that seen in the general population for those with colorectal carcinoma. It is therefore rational to include the family history in determining surveillance strategy, but the magnitude of the effect requires further analysis before changes are implemented.

It is probable that adenomas are associated with an increased risk of malignancy in colitis, but there are no reliable data. Sclerosing cholangitis (Chapter 6) appears to be a marker of increased risk in a majority of centres (see below), but to an extent that probably does not warrant changes in surveillance strategy.

Groups at lower risk have not been identified with any confidence, but anecdotal experience suggests that patients with inactive colitis and with virtually normal endoscopic appearances and persistently quiescent histology are under-represented amongst those with dysplasia and carcinomas. If this can be confirmed, it would permit a relaxing of the intensity of surveillance in this subgroup. In each case prospective, controlled data are needed.

Meta-analysis and modelling of surveillance strategy in ulcerative colitis

Provenzale *et al.* [41] have reviewed the existing literature and tried to determine the most cost-effective strategy based on current knowledge. A decision analytic model was employed and costings were based on those thought reasonable for a health maintenance organization. Prophylactic colectomy at 10 years' extensive colitis was compared to surveillance colonoscopy at 1- to 5-yearly intervals, with surgery subsequently performed for carcinoma or any grade of dysplasia, or only for carcinoma/high-grade dysplasia. Other than prophylactic colectomy, annual colonoscopy with colectomy for any dysplasia offered the most protection from malignancy, but this was also by far the most expensive option (US$247 200 per life year gained) and gained on average a mere four additional days of expected life compared to biennial colonoscopy (as practised at St Mark's), which was costed at US$159 500 per life year gained. Interestingly, 5-yearly colonoscopy with colectomy for any dysplasia had the potential to be highly effective and was also cheaper than prophylactic colectomy (US$40 700 v. US$60 400 per life year gained). The figure for 5-yearly surveillance is only a little higher than the costings for routine flexible sigmoidoscopy every 3–5 years currently advocated for the general middle-aged population in both North America and Germany.

CONCLUSIONS: ULCERATIVE COLITIS

The epidemiology of colorectal carcinoma surveillance in macroscopically extensive ulcerative colitis indicates a risk of carcinoma or of high-grade dysplasia in the region of 0.5% per year of follow-up after 10 years of disease. For every 100 patients in any given programme, one high-risk lesion or early cancer can be expected every 2 years (or approximately 1 per million population per year). A screening colonoscopy at 8–10 years is justified whether or not subsequent surveillance is intended, to check the extent of colitis (Chapter 2) and because an important proportion of high-risk lesions are found at this index examination in most surveillance series. High-grade dysplasia, DALMs and confirmed low-grade dysplasia warrant colectomy; the minimum response to a finding of low-grade dysplasia is 6-monthly colonoscopy for the patient who refuses colectomy. It is recognized that up to 25% of cancers will not be preceded (or detectable) by dysplasia, and that in this, and probably in other respects, tumours currently missed by surveillance are likely to be biologically different. Colonoscopic surveillance is expensive and of unproven value, indicating a need for better markers of high- and low-risk patients, but if it is to be done then it must be safe and proficiently performed to be well tolerated by patients. In the absence of controlled data or a clearly mandated decision based on clinical criteria, decisions are properly made on grounds of health economics. Colonoscopy every 2 years is thus a reasonable frequency for units planning to commence or continue surveillance outside a trial setting. It is less clear at what age surveillance should stop if commenced, and what, if anything, should be done for patients with less extensive disease; stopping at 75 years, and a rectal biopsy every 2 years from 10 years, respectively, are suggested.

CANCER SURVEILLANCE IN CROHN'S DISEASE

In extensive Crohn's colitis of more than 8 to 10 years' duration, regular clinical assessment, especially of the anorectum is warranted (see below), with a high index of suspicion and a low threshold for examination and biopsy under anaesthetic if strictures are present. Those in whom the disease began in childhood or adolescence, those with chronic fistulae and those with bypassed segments of intestine are probably those at greatest risk. There are as yet no data which firmly justify more than clinically prompted investigations.

Many of the problems associated with surveillance in ulcerative colitis apply equally to Crohn's disease. Dysplasia is probably a predictor of future malignancy, of similar robustness to dysplasia in ulcerative colitis, with a frequency of 80% or more in published series once malignancy has supervened [20]. However, the data are generally more sparse, and many fewer units have adopted a general policy of regular surveillance colonoscopy. A biennial colonoscopy surveillance programme commencing at 8 years in those with total or segmental Crohn's colitis began in New York in 1988, and provisional data have now been presented [42]. From the published abstract it appears probable that the index colonoscopy was included as well as the subsequent true surveillance examinations. Dysplasia or frank malignancy was found in 6% of cases; these patients were generally older, with disease for longer and more likely to have had previous partial colectomy. The colonoscopies were technically demanding and even with paediatric endoscopes were incomplete in 11%. The authors nevertheless advocate surveillance for those with long-standing total or segmental colitis. The arguments in favour of this approach must be considered even weaker than for extensive ulcerative colitis, especially since 35% of patients entered the programme because of new symptoms and accordingly represent a selected cohort, almost certainly at above-average risk of neoplasia. It is a great pity that the difficulties in interpreting ulcerative colitis surveillance programmes were not tackled in Crohn's disease by a more controlled comparison of surveillance with normal clinical practice.

NEOPLASIA IN PRIMARY SCLEROSING CHOLANGITIS

Colorectal carcinoma

The risk of colorectal carcinoma is of course increased in extensive long-standing ulcerative colitis (see above). Several centres have speculated on a possible influence of primary sclerosing cholangitis (PSC) on this risk, and detailed analyses are now available. However, the results are not concordant, and the earlier reports are perhaps best discounted on the grounds of inadequate numbers and selection bias. The association remains a relatively rare one, with still under 100 reported cases of PSC, ulcerative colitis and colorectal carcinoma in the same patient. The most recent publication of the Stockholm group [43] takes advantage of a series which is almost population-based and yet one in which neither clinically overt PSC nor inflammatory bowel disease was likely to have been missed. A careful retrospective analysis was performed from contemporaneous records. A relatively high proportion of the patients with PSC lacked inflammatory bowel disease (18 of 58), but in other respects the clinical features were typical of those in other centres. Eighty controls with colitis but without PSC were paired with the 40 with both diseases, matching for age and for the extent and duration of colitis. During follow-up, 16 patients with PSC developed colonic dysplasia or carcinoma (40%), compared to only 10 in the controls (12.5%; $p < 0.001$). The cumulative risk of colorectal neoplasia was 9% and 31%, at 10 and 20 years, respectively, compared to only 2% and 5% in the controls without PSC. Interestingly, both colorectal and biliary neoplasia coincided in seven cases. Brentnall *et al.* [44] have reported on a prospective series of 20 patients with extensive colitis and PSC, and saw nine patients with dysplasia (45%), compared to only 4 in 25 patients matched for their colitis but without PSC (16%). At the Mayo Clinic retrospective review of 178 patients with PSC led to almost opposite conclusions [45]. The relative risk for colorectal neoplasia (excluding dysplasia alone) was elevated to 10.3 times that of the general population of the USA, but this was not influenced by the presence or absence of PSC. However, the relative risk for colorectal neoplasia was numerically increased (though not significant) for patients with PSC without colitis, at 4.9 times, with confidence intervals between 0.1 and 27 times. Their subsequent analysis comparing cancer frequency in colitis patients with or without PSC also claims an absence of association, but there was a relative risk of 1.3 in those with PSC [46]. Reports in abstract form from other centres support an increased risk of colorectal carcinoma in patients with sclerosing cholangitis, but are subject to the same reservations as the published studies. Perhaps another important key to understanding these differences of opinion lies in the report from Johns Hopkins [47] in which dysplasia or carcinoma was found in 37% ($n = 35$), but in combination with a cumulative cancer incidence similar to historical controls. It is possible that PSC predisposes to dysplasia but not to invasive malignancy, and thus marks a group in whom dysplasia should be accorded lesser significance. However, biological support for this contention is entirely lacking, and we should continue to seek better data on which to base our clinical decisions. For the moment it seems reasonable to employ the same criteria for colonic surveillance in patients with extensive colitis, regardless of whether or not they have PSC, and to regard dysplasia with the same critical respect in whomsoever it is demonstrated.

Cholangiocarcinoma

To date it has not proved possible to predict a high-risk group for development of the cholangiocarcinomas, and clinicians must maintain a high index of suspicion if curative surgery is ever to be an option. This group of malignancies affects at least 5% of patients with PSC on a lifetime basis [43, 45], and a regrettably high proportion are still diagnosed at autopsy. Progression from PSC to carcinoma is almost always difficult to identify, as the symptoms, signs and investigation results are so similar, but may be suspected in the patient whose condition suddenly deteriorates or becomes progressive rather than episodic. Cholangiocarcinoma is usually seen in patients with colitis rather than in those with PSC without IBD [43, 48]. There are no reliable laboratory markers. Use even of serological tumour markers is greatly hampered by their frequent positivity in uncomplicated PSC. Positive cytological brushings or biliary biopsies obtained at endoscopic retrograde cholangiography (ERCP) are conclusive, but false negatives are frequent, in part because of the relatively fibrous nature of the tumours. Changes in the cholangiogram may sometimes help, especially when the axis of a strictured area of duct deviates from the general axis of the remainder of the duct; this strongly suggests neoplastic change. Conventional imaging with ultrasound and CT scanning has not proved sufficiently discriminatory, but endoscopic ultrasound (perhaps using intrabiliary probes) may make a increasingly useful contribution through its ability to demonstrate small mass lesions, themselves strongly indicative of malignant change. If surgery is contemplated, it needs to be radical if there is to be curative intent. Many transplant units have discontinued transplantation for preoperatively diagnosed cholangiocarcinoma because of the near 100% recurrence rate in the transplanted liver. However, this may reflect the influence of the biliary 'field defect' in such patients and could perhaps be avoided if a porto-enteric anastomosis were insisted upon rather than the usual distal biliary join between donor and recipient tissues.

OTHER NEOPLASTIC DISEASE IN PATIENTS WITH CROHN'S DISEASE

Small bowel cancer

Malignancy affecting the small bowel is almost certainly more common in Crohn's disease. A relative risk of 50 ($p = 0.001$) quoted for intestinal carcinoma in comparison to the general population must be somewhat tempered, however, by the recognition that these data reflect only two patients with both conditions [10], but a cumulative incidence of 0.6% is substantially higher than expected [18]. There were no cases identified in the St Mark's series of 2500 patients with Crohn's [19]. As with colorectal carcinoma, the small bowel cancers usually occur in those that have had Crohn's for 10 years or more, and again the diagnosis is often delayed and rarely made preoperatively. The prognosis is very poor, with a median survival as short as 6 months. Patients at most risk seem to be those with proximal and/or chronic unremitting disease; males are also over-represented [13, 18].

Anal carcinoma

Carcinoma of the anal canal and the transitional zone leading to the rectum is seen more often in Crohn's disease than in the general population with (for example) no fewer than five anal tumours in the St Mark's series of 2500 Crohn's patients compared to an expected frequency of less than one [19]. There were also seven tumours very low in the rectum, and in all 12 cases the patients had previously suffered from severe chronic anorectal disease. Although multimodality non-surgical therapy is now yielding good results for late-stage anal carcinoma, the awareness of this possible complication should lead to biopsy of any suspicious anorectal lesion that is not responding to medical therapy. This will usually require general anaesthetic to achieve adequate analgesia.

IATROGENIC MALIGNANCY IN INFLAMMATORY BOWEL DISEASE

Gastrointestinal malignancies are over-represented in patients with inflammatory bowel disease (see above), with most of this excess reasonably attributed to the disease process. There have also been concerns that diagnostic and therapeutic interventions may play a part, immunosuppressive drugs being particularly implicated, given their associations with malignancy when used for other indications. The best documented and most frequently observed examples occur with immunosuppression for the prevention of rejection of solid organ transplants, but concern in other contexts remains. No data exist for the agents newer to inflammatory bowel disease therapy, but some comments can be offered for the more established drugs.

Steroids

It is unlikely that exogenous corticosteroids influence the risk of neoplasia in inflammatory bowel disease, but it is difficult to distinguish any effect of treatment from that of the underlying disease. As steroid use is deliberately minimized in accordance with other well-rehearsed arguments, and steroids are generally used for relatively short periods in active inflammatory bowel disease, they need be considered no further.

Aminosalicylates

The aminosalicylate drugs probably have no important effects on systemic immune functioning, and no increased cancer risk has been attributed. On the contrary, a recent study strongly favours their use in ulcerative colitis with the aim, *inter alia*, of reducing cancer risk [49]. This case-control study in a defined population compared the pharmacological records of ulcerative colitis patients with complicating carcinoma to those of matched controls with no malignancy. There was a significant protective effect in those treated for at least 3 months with an aminosalicylate preparation, the relative risk for neoplasia being only 0.38 (confidence interval 0.20–0.69).

Azathioprine/mercaptopurine

Later neoplasia, especially non-Hodgkin's lymphoma, intestinal lymphoma, myeloma and skin cancers, prove over-represented in patients who have received immunosuppressants (mainly azathioprine and 6-mercaptopurine) for non-neoplastic disease [50, 51]. Few patients with inflammatory bowel disease were included in the earlier studies, but a multiplicity of published case reports, and a review of 26 Crohn's patients with colorectal carcinoma, two of whom had earlier had azathioprine [52], also suggested a greater than chance association. The much larger report of 723 inflammatory bowel disease patients treated with immunosuppressants, which demonstrated no excess risk, was therefore especially reassuring [53]. Azathioprine is, however, almost certainly genotoxic in man [54].

The influence of azathioprine on cancer risk in inflammatory bowel disease has been further explored at St Mark's in a series of 755 patients followed prospectively for a median of 9 years from the time of introduction of the drug [55]. A small overall increase in malignancies was detected, there being 31 malignancies compared to the 24.3 predicted by national mortality rates for the same age and sex distribution. However, this difference did not reach statistical significance ($p = 0.186$). There were no lymphomas, but a significant excess of colorectal and anal tumours was found. The only other tumours to appear more commonly than expected were cervical and gastric carcinoma. It was thought likely that the excess of colorectal and anal tumours (15 observed v. 2.27 expected: $p < 0.00001$) represented an effect of the underlying disease rather than a complication of treatment. An attempt to resolve this issue was made by comparing the azathioprine-treated patients with ulcerative colitis, to controls matched as nearly as possible for the nature of their disease but who had never received azathioprine. There were 86 azathioprine-treated patients with colitis of over 10 years' duration, for whom 180 colitis controls were identified. In the azathioprine group there were eight colorectal carcinomas (v. 0.26 expected) compared to 15 in the control group (v. 0.63 expected). The modest difference in relative risk (30.8 v. 23.8) was not significant (p = 0.54). It is thus probable that most of the increase in neoplasia in azathioprine-treated individuals is explained by those with more severe disease and a greater underlying risk of neoplasia being also those most likely to require immunosuppression.

Reassuring though the St Mark's data are, it must be recognized that although the period of follow-up was substantial (median 9.0 years), the period of azathioprine usage was not, with a median of only 12.5 months. We have since seen a patient with gynaecological malignancy (probable cervical primary) presenting after 11 years' azathioprine therapy for otherwise intractable Crohn's disease (treated elsewhere and therefore outside the St Mark's database). Clearly one should not be greatly influenced by an anecdote of this nature, but an increasing risk of neoplasia with greater durations of immunosuppression is not illogical; reassuring data from long-term follow-up of short-term treatment should not be extrapolated to complacency about the safety of longer-term treatment. The apparent loss of benefit after more than 4 years' therapy lends further support to planned drug withdrawal at this stage [56].

Cyclosporin

There is some concern that cyclosporin increases the incidence of lymphoproliferative disorders and skin cancers after transplantation [57, 58], but few data particular to inflammatory bowel disease exist. Continued monitoring is indicated, especially in patients treated for longer periods. It is disturbing [59] that colorectal carcinoma has occurred in no fewer than 3 of 27 patients with ulcerative colitis (and retained colons) within the first 14 months after liver transplantation for primary sclerosing cholangitis. These patients were immunosuppressed (conventionally) with prednisolone, azathioprine and cyclosporin, and clearly represent a highly selected group, not least since sclerosing cholangitis may be a risk factor for colonic neoplasia (see above). It seems wise to enter such patients into an accelerated colonoscopic screening programme, but whether the increased risk is primarily related to drug, transplant or disease remains unclear. Cyclosporin does appear to be exonerated from concerns of mutagenicity [54].

Methotrexate

The risk of malignancy complicating long-term methotrexate therapy is thought to be low or absent, because methotrexate neither reacts with, nor becomes incorporated into, nucleic acid [60]. To date, no carcinogenic effect of the relatively low doses of methotrexate typically used for non-malignant indications has been demonstrated, background neoplasia rates remaining unaltered [61, 62]. Again, data specific to inflammatory bowel disease are lacking.

Diagnostic imaging and risk of neoplasia

Many patients with inflammatory bowel disease have repeated radiological examinations over many years, raising the possibility that medical exposure to ionizing radiation might contribute to risk of neoplasia. Ultrasound and magnetic resonance imaging appear exonerated so far as can be told, and the exposure from scintigraphic imaging is reassuringly low (frequency and dosimetry), but conventional imaging (plain films, barium studies, fistulograms, etc.) and computed tomography deserve attention. The average total annual radiation exposure in the UK and other Western nations is about 2.5 mSv per person [63]. With approximately 500 radiological examinations for every 1000 individuals, around 12% of the total irradiation comes from medical sources (which in turn accounts for over 80% of all man-made radiation) [64]. Most of these examinations are of the chest or periphery, which expose the patient to a very low 'effective dose equivalent', when compared to a typical plain abdominal film at 1.14 mSv (10 mGy absorbed dose), a barium meal at 3.8 mSv and a barium enema at 7.7 mSv [65]. The much greater figure for barium enema is a combined result of longer screening times as the flow of barium around the colon is monitored, the greater need for full-sized abdominal films and, to some extent, the greater energy required for the image in the lateral view. Accordingly, although barium enemas account for only 0.9% of all radiological procedures, they contribute 14% of the medical radiation dose in the UK [63]. However, it should be noted that there is considerable variation in the radiographic technique and hence in the final absorbed radiation dose between different centres and between different radiologists.

Extrapolation from occupational exposure (as for example in uranium workers) predicts a roughly linear relationship between increasing radiation exposure and increasing risk of malignancy [66], with no minimum radiation dose below which there is freedom from this increased risk. These assumptions lead to between 100 and 250 fatal cancers being attributed to medical radiation each year in the UK (1.8 to 4.5 per million population). The approximate lifetime risk that a given procedure induces a fatal malignancy can be calculated to lie between 20 and 60 per million for abdominal radiography, 50–170 for barium meal and 100–350 for barium enema, with the rather higher figure for abdominal CT scanning of around 500 per million [63, 65]. There is a probable additional risk of gonadal damage promoting childhood malignancy in the children of both males and females exposed to medical radiation during the reproductive period. The radiation dose from most of the commonly utilized nuclear scans is much lower, and of proportionately lesser importance.

Could iatrogenic irradiation contribute to the increased risk of colorectal carcinoma in ulcerative colitis? A lifetime's investigation might perhaps encompass three barium enemas and up to 20 plain abdominal films (more will usually have led on to colectomy). Combining the additive risks of these procedures leads to an expected excess of roughly 1400 cancers per million patients ($3 \times 200 + 20 \times 40$). These radiation-induced cancers are unlikely to be colorectal, as occupational and atomic bomb data indicate that the gastrointestinal mucosa is a 'protected' site [65,66], but even if all excess cancers resulting from radiological investigation of colitis were in the large bowel, then radiation would account for only about 0.14% of colitis cancers – or around 1.5% of the excess relative to the general population.

The situation is less easily modelled in Crohn's disease given less certainty as to the excess cancer rate (see above), but a larger number of radiographic studies of the small bowel and CT scans are typical. The relatively extreme case of the patient in whom 20 small bowel series, two barium enemas and 10 CT scans had been performed, would be placed at an increased risk of fatal malignancy in the region of 7400 per million. This lifetime risk of nearly 1% should not be ignored when considering the need for radiological investigation, as Crohn's patients are usually young and likely to survive to be at risk, but can fairly readily be placed in perspective. Again these excess malignancies can be expected to be extra-intestinal.

The epidemiological data are concordant with these predictions. The US National Cancer Institute has examined pre-morbid radiographic history in over 1000 lymphoma, leukaemia and myeloma patients, in comparison with matched controls [67]. Only a small increase in the risk of myeloma (relative risk 1.14) could be clearly linked to prior radiation, and, encouragingly, myeloma is not over-represented in inflammatory bowel disease-related neoplasia [1, 67, 68] (and see Chapter 2). However, the small numbers of malignancies described from each centre should preclude complacency.

REFERENCES

1. Ekbom A, Helmick CG, Zack M *et al*. Survival and causes of death in patients with inflammatory bowel disease: a population-based study. *Gastroenterology* 1992; **103**: 954–960.

2. Langholz E, Munkholm P, Davidsen M, Binder V. Colorectal cancer risk and mortality in patients with ulcerative colitis. *Gastroenterology* 1992; **103**: 1444–1451.

3. Nugent FW, Haggitt RC, Gilpin PA. Cancer surveillance in ulcerative colitis. *Gastroenterology* 1991; **100**: 1241–1248.

4. Connell WR, Talbot IC, Harpaz N *et al*. Clinicopathological characterisitics of colorectal carcinoma complicating ulcerative colitis. *Gut* 1994; **35**: 1419–1423.

5. Ekbom A, Helmick C, Zack M, Adami HO. Increased risk of large bowel cancer in Crohn's disease with colonic involvement. *Lancet* 1990; **336**: 357–359.

6. Binder V, Hendriksen C, Kreiner S. Prognosis in Crohn's disease – based on results from a regional patient group from the county of Copenhagen. *Gut* 1985; **26**: 146–150.

7. Kvist N, Jacobsen O, Norgaard P *et al*. Malignancy in Crohn's disease. *Scand J Gastroenterol* 1986; **21**: 82–86.

8. Gollop JH, Phillips SF, Melton LJ, Zinsmeister AR. Epidemiological aspects of Crohn's disease: a population based study in Olmsted County, Minnesota, 1943–1982. *Gut* 1988; **29**: 49–56.

9. Fireman Z, Grossman A, Lilos P *et al*. Intestinal cancer in patients with Crohn's disease: a population study in central Israel. *Scand J Gastroenterol* 1989; **24**: 346–350.

10. Munkholm P, Langholz E, Davidsen M, Binder V. Intestinal cancer risk and mortality in patients with Crohn's disease. *Gastroenterology* 1993; **105**: 1716–1723.

11. Korelitz BI. Carcinoma of the intestiinal tract in Crohn's disease: results of a survey conducted by the National Foundation for Ileitis and Colitis. *Am J Gastroenterol* 1983; **78**: 44–46.

12. Weedon DD, Shorter RG, Ilstrup DM *et al*. Crohn's disease and cancer. *N Engl J Med* 1973; **289**: 1099–1103.

13. Greenstein AJ, Sachar DB, Smith H *et al*. A comparison of cancer risk in Crohn's disease and ulcerative colitis. *Cancer* 1981; **48**: 2742–2745.

14. Gyde SN, Prior P, Macartney JC *et al*. Malignancy in Crohn's disease. *Gut* 1980; **21**: 1024–1029.

15. Stahl TJ, Schoetz DJ, Roberts PL *et al*. Crohn's disease and carcinoma: increasing justification for surveillance? *Dis Colon Rectum* 1992; **35**: 850–856.

16. Gillen CD, Walmsley RS, Prior P *et al*. Ulcerative colitis and Crohn's disease: a comparison of the colorectal cancer risk in extensive colitis. *Gut* 1994; **35**: 1590–1592.

17. Cohen RD, Gordon DW, Argo CK, Hanauer SB. Risk factors for adenocarcinoma in ulcerative colitis and Crohn's disease: a retrospective, matched case-control study. *Gastroenterology* 1996; **110**: A505.

18. Michelassi F, Testa G, Pomidor WJ *et al*. Adenocarcinoma complicating Crohn's disease. *Dis Colon Rectum* 1993; **36**: 654–661.
19. Connell WR, Sheffield JP, Kamm MA *et al*. Lower gastrointestinal malignancy in Crohn's disease. *Gut* 1994; **35**: 347–352.
20. Richards ME, Rickert RR, Nance FC. Crohn's disease-associated carcinoma. *Ann Surg* 1989; **209**: 764–773.
21. Babyatsky MW, Rossiter G, Podolsky DK. Expression of transforming growth factors a and b in colonic mucosa in inflammatory bowel disease. *Gastroenterology* 1996; **110**: 975–984.
22. British Society of Gastroenterology. *Guidelines in Gastroenterology 4: Inflammatory bowel disease*. London: British Society of Gastroenterology, 1996.
23. Axon ATR. Cancer surveillance in ulcerative colitis – a time for reappraisal. *Gut* 1994; **35**: 587–589.
24. Dixon MF, Brown LJR, Gilmour HM *et al*. Observer variation in the assessment of dysplasia in ulcerative colitis. *Histopathology* 1988; **13**: 385–397.
25. Theodossi A, Spiegelhalter DJ, Jass J *et al*. Observer variation and discriminatory value of biopsy features in inflammatory bowel disease. *Gut* 1994; **35**: 961–968.
26. Connell WR, Lennard-Jones JE, Williams CB *et al*. Factors influencing the outcome of endoscopic surveillance for cancer in ulcerative colitis. *Gastroenterology* 1994; **107**: 934–944.
27. Woolrich AJ, DaSilva MD, Korelitz BI. Surveillance in the routine management of ulcerative colitis: the predictive value of low grade dysplasia. *Gastroenterology* 1992; **103**: 431–438.
28. Bernstein CN, Shanahan F. Are we telling patients the truth about surveillance colonoscopy in ulcerative colitis? *Lancet* 1994; **343**: 71–74.
29. Karlén P, Kornfeld D, Broström O *et al*. Colonoscopic surveillance reduces colorectal cancer in ulcerative colitis – a case control study. *Gastroenterology* 1996; **110**: A539.
30. Rubin CE, Haggitt RC, Burmer GC *et al*. DNA aneuploidy in colonic biopsies predicts future development of dysplasia in ulcerative colitis. *Gastroenterology* 1992; **103**: 1611–1620.
31. Befrits R, Hammarberg C, Rubio C *et al*. DNA aneuploidy and histologic dysplasia in long-standing ulcerative colitis. A 10-year follow-up study. *Dis Colon Rectum* 1994; **37**: 313–319.
32. Brentnall TA, Crispin DA, Rabinovitch PS *et al*. Mutations in the p53 gene: an early marker of neoplastic progression in ulcerative colitis. *Gastroenterology* 1994; **107**: 369–378.
33. Wang C, Cymes K, Young E *et al*. P53 overexpression in colonoscopic surveillance biopsies of patients with longstanding UC: a retrospective case-control study. *Gastroenterology* 1996; **110**: A611.

34. Kullmann F, Fadaie M, Gross V *et al*. Expression of proliferating cell nuclear antigen (PCNA) and Ki-67 in dysplasia in inflammatory bowel disease. *Eur J Gastroenterol Hepatol* 1996; **8**: 371–379.

35. Thomas MG, Nugent KP, Forbes A, Williamson RC. Calcipotriol inhibits rectal epithelial cell production in ulcerative proctocolitis. *Gut* 1994; **35**: 1718–1720.

36. Itzkowitz SH, Young E, Dubois D *et al*. Sialosyl-Tn antigen is prevalent and precedes dysplasia in ulcerative colitis: a retrospective case-control study. *Gastroenterology* 1996; **110**: 694–704.

37. Karlén P, Broström O, Löfberg R *et al*. Chronology of sialosyl-Tn (STn) antigen expression and aneuploidy in prospective colonoscopic biopsies from patients with long-standing ulcerative colitis. *Gastroenterology* 1996; **110**: A538.

38. Ta A, Harpaz N, Chen A *et al*. Expression of the tumor-associated sialosyl-Tn antigen in Crohn's colitis. *Gastroenterology* 1996; **110**: A599.

39. Rustgi AK. Hereditary gastrointestinal polyposis and nonpolyposis syndromes. *N Engl J Med* 1994; **331**: 1694–1702.

40. Nuako KW, Ahlquist DA, Schaid DJ *et al*. Familial predisposition as a risk factor for colorectal cancer in chronic ulcerative colitis: a case-control study. *Gastroenterology* 1996; **110**: A569.

41. Provenzale D, Onken JE, Wong JB. Prophylactic colectomy or surveillance for patients with ulcerative colitis – a cost-effectiveness analysis. *Gastroenterology* 1996; **110**: A34.

42. Rubin PH, Present DH, Chapman ML *et al*. Chronic Crohn's colitis: a 7 year experience with screening and surveillance colonoscopy in 113 patients. *Gastroenterology* 1996; **110**: A1005.

43. Broomé, U, Löfberg R, Veress B, Eriksson LS. Primary sclerosing cholangitis and ulcerative colitis: evidence for increased neoplastic potential. *Hepatology* 1995; **22**: 1404–1408.

44. Brentnall TA, Haggitt RC, Rabinovitch PS *et al*. Risk and natural history of colonic neoplasia in patients with primary sclerosing cholangitis and ulcerative colitis. *Gastroenterology* 1996; **110**: 331–338.

45. Loftus EV Jr, Sandborn WJ, Tremaine WJ *et al*. Risk of colorectal neoplasia in patients with primary sclerosing cholangitis. *Gastroenterology* 1996; **110**: 432–440.

46. Nuako KW, Ahlquist DA, Siems DM *et al*. Primary sclerosing cholangitis as a risk factor for colorectal carcinoma in ulcerative colitis: a case-control study. *Gastroenterology* 1996; **110**: A981.

47. Gurbuz AK, Giardiello FM, Bayless TM. Colorectal neoplasia in patients with ulcerative colitis and primary sclerosing cholangitis. *Dis Colon Rectum* 1995; **38**: 37–41.

48. Wiesner RH, Grambsch PM, Dickson ER *et al*. Primary sclerosing cholangitis: natural history, prognostic factors and survival analysis. *Hepatology* 1989; **10**: 430–436.

49. Pinczowski D, Ekbom A, Baron J *et al*. Risk factors for colorectal cancer in patients with ulcerative colitis: a case control study. *Gastroenterology* 1994; **107**: 117–120.

50. Kinlen LJ. Incidence of cancer in rheumatoid arthritis and other disorders after immunosuppressive treatment. *Am J Med* 1985; **78**(suppl): 44–49.

51. Matteson EL, Hickey AR, Maguire L *et al*. Occurrence of neoplasia in patients with rheumatoid arthritis enrolled in a DMARD registry. *J Rheumatol* 1991; **18**: 809–814.

52. Zelig MP, Choi PM. Azathioprine or 6-mercaptopurine therapy and colon carcinoma in Crohn's disease. *Gastroenterology* 1992; 102: 1448 (letter).

53. Present DH, Meltzer ST, Krumholz MP *et al*. 6-Mercaptopurine in the management of inflammatory bowel disease: short- and long-term toxicity. *Ann Int Med* 1989; **111**: 641–649.

54. Olshan AF, Mattison DR, Zwanenburg TS. Cyclosporine A: review of genotoxicity and potential for adverse human reproductive and developmental effects. *Mutation Res* 1994; **317**: 163–173.

55. Connell WR, Kamm MA, Dickson M *et al*. Long-term neoplasia risk after azathioprine treatment in inflammatory bowel disease. *Lancet* 1994; **343**: 1249–1252.

56. Bouhnik Y, Lémann M, Mary J-Y *et al*. Long-term follow-up of patients with Crohn's disease treated with azathioprine or 6-mercaptopurine. *Lancet* 1996; **347**: 215–219.

57. Von Graffenried B. Sandimmun (cyclosporin) in autoimmune disease: overview on early clinical experience. *Am J Nephrol* 1989; **9**: 51–56.

58. Kurki PT. Safety aspects of long-term cyclosporin A therapy. *Scand J Rheumatol* 1992; **95**: 35–38.

59. Bleday R, Lee E, Jessurun J *et al*. Increased risk of early colorectal neoplasms after hepatic transplant in patients with inflammatory bowel disease. *Dis Colon Rectum* 1993; **36**: 908–912.

60. Turnbull C, Roach M. Is methotrexate carcinogenic? *Br Med J* 1980; **281**: 808.

61. Tishler M, Caspi D, Yaron M. Long-term experience with low dose methotrexate in rheumatoid arthritis. *Rheumatol Int* 1993; **13**: 103–106.

62. Weinblatt ME. Methotrexate for chronic diseases in adults. *N Engl J Med* 1995; **332**: 330–331.

63. National Radiation Protection Board. *Patient dose reduction in diagnostic radiology*. Documents of the NRPB. London: HMSO, 1990.

64. Mettler FA, Davis M, Kelsey CA *et al*. Analytical modeling of worldwide medical radiation use. *Health Phys* 1987; **52**: 133–141.

65. National Radiation Protection Board. *A national survey of doses to patients undergoing a selection of routine X-ray examinations in English hospitals*. NRPB-R200. London: HMSO, 1986.

66. Sevc J, Kunz E, Tomasek L *et al.* Cancer in man after exposure to Rn daughters. *Health Phys* 1988; **54**: 27–46.

67. Boice JD Jr, Morin MM, Glas AG *et al.* Diagnostic X-ray procedures and risk of leukemia, lymphoma, and multiple myeloma. *J Am Med Assoc* 1991; **265**: 1290–1294.

68. Sachar DB. Cancer in Crohn's disease: dispelling the myths. *Gut* 1994; **35**: 1507–1508.

9

Afterword

FUTURE TRENDS

It is wisely said that prediction is very difficult, especially when it concerns the future, but it will be instructive and – with the benefit of hindsight – no doubt entertaining to speculate on the important developments to be anticipated in the field of inflammatory bowel disease over the next few years.

I doubt that unequivocal single causes of ulcerative colitis and Crohn's disease will emerge, and although chastened by the experience with *Helicobacter pylori* and duodenal ulceration, it seems much more probable that we will continue to regard the inflammatory bowel diseases as responses to combinations of genetic and environmental factors. Equally, the remarkable progress in the knowledge of the human genome of the past few years is already identifying specific sites of major interest. The absence of individuals with an identified chromosomal deletion linked to inflammatory bowel disease (analogous to the major chromosome 5 defect that led to identification of the *apc* site coding for familial polyposis) suggests that the genes involved are at sufficiently crucial points in the genome to render major losses incompatible with life. The gene knock-out animal models described in Chapter 1 support this general contention, as do the many links to the HLA loci, and those to sites (on chromosome 16) near the genes for cell adhesion molecules. However, none of the foci identified – which by now should be most of those with a critical role if acting in isolation from other factors – can alone explain inflammatory bowel disease. Mechanisms for variation of the clinical phenotype are relatively obvious when different mutations of the same gene can be identified, but variation when the genetic defect is identical is less easily explained. Comprehensive analysis of polygenic inheritance also has some way to go.

It seems probable that a portfolio of inflammatory bowel disease-related genes will be accumulated, each with its own attributable risk for certain aspects of disease. What these may be must be speculative, but it would be reasonable to suggest that, for example, the tendency for Crohn's disease to form fibrous strictures might be coded by a specific genetic moiety. This allele (or mutation) could well be harmless, irrelevant or more probably of some evolutionary advantage, in the individual without Crohn's disease. It is easy to imagine that such a gene could promote life-saving, rapid, effective wound repair after trauma. Genome-wide searching would probably fail to identify its locus if it is common in the normal population, and although comparative studies within the inflammatory bowel disease population exploring genetic associations with phenotype might well be more productive, their recognition will be constrained by the reduced statistical power of smaller numbers.

It is important that the nature of the association between measles and Crohn's disease is rapidly clarified, and especially the postulated link to vaccination. The balance of risks currently points clearly towards continued global vaccination of infants, but the timing of this may be crucial if later Crohn's disease is not to be provoked. Is it fanciful to consider that an amended vaccination strategy or a modified vaccine might have the desirable opposite effect of protecting against later Crohn's disease?

The link between the 'normal' luminal flora and the development of inflammatory bowel disease has already been discussed at some length, and almost certainly reflects an interaction with the genetic profile of the human host. The relationship of diet to this, and to the consequent behaviour of the bowel, is probably very important but difficult to study in a controlled fashion. It is embarrassing how little useful advice we are able to give our patients, despite their conviction that diet is important, and our own recognition of the value (albeit a limited one) of nutritional therapy in Crohn's disease. There are a number of potentially useful leads including the responses to antibiotics, the influence of luminal short-chain fatty acids and the fermentation/hydrogen sulphide hypotheses. It is unlikely that a simple 'diet sheet' for inflammatory bowel disease will emerge, but it should be possible for us to identify helpful and harmful dietary habits a little more coherently than at present. A potential role for probiotic therapy also exists if we can demonstrate the safety of oral or rectal administration of live agents.

The pathogenesis of inflammatory bowel disease probably shares much with other chronic inflammatory disorders, and it is good to see (for example) the upsurge of interest in the arthropathy of gastrointestinal disease. Hopefully this will result in a greater cross-fertilization of research endeavour. Whatever triggers the inflammatory cascade in these conditions, it is probable that for some time to come we shall have to treat patients in whom inflammation has become established. It is encouraging, if surprising, that therapeutic agents such as antibodies to TNF-α, ridogrel or IL-10, active at a few specific points in inflammation, can seem to have a generalized beneficial effect in disease, but better results would be anticipated if interruption were possible at an earlier stage in the process. A fascinating paper in *Nature Medicine* suggests that this may soon be achievable [1]. The NF-κB family consists of macrophage and lymphocyte transcription factors that play an important and early part in the inflammatory response. They appear to regulate many of the cytokines and adhesion molecules with which we are more familiar, and their loss, in mutant animals with genetic disruption of NF-κB, leads to immunosuppression. A predominance of the p65 subunit of NF-κB in gastrointestinal inflammation seems likely, and it is strongly activated in inflammatory bowel disease. Neurath *et al.* have gone on to examine an antisense nucleotide directed against the NF-κB p65 translation site, which hence prevents the normal effects of NF-κB p65 on the target cell nucleus [1]. The antisense nucleotide was therapeutically effective in two very distinct animal models of colitis. It was active both topically and systemically, and proved of similar efficacy to, but of much greater duration of action than, steroids. Identical results were obtained in *in vitro* studies of lamina propria cells from patients with Crohn's disease. Although there might reasonably be concern about systemic use of potentially such a potent and long-acting immunomodulator, its topical application could very soon initiate a new era in targeted therapy.

Continued exploration of the sequence of events in the postoperative colitic who does or does not go on to develop pouchitis has the potential to be informative. Together with other high-risk individuals, such as those with resected Crohn's disease or apparently healthy relatives of those with inflammatory bowel disease, pouch patients constitute a circumscribed group in whom prophylactic strategies may be tested. Manipulations of epithelial integrity, of the luminal flora, and of the immune response are possible, but, with the exception of modest successes with the 5-ASA drugs (and stopping smoking in Crohn's disease), secondary prophylaxis is yet to be exploited.

Intestinal neoplasia is an emotive subject in inflammatory bowel disease circles, and only the debate about putative infective causes has been able to match the passions for and against surveillance colonoscopy. With luck, data already being collected will be adequately informative to allow us to be more precise in targeting surveillance to those most likely to benefit, and withdrawing it from those in whom it is an expensive and ineffectual intrusion. Without that luck, and in the absence of controlled data, we can expect another decade of frustration before molecular markers of neoplastic risk and early change are both sufficiently reliable and available to permit the replacement of colonoscopy with a simple series of serological and/or stool tests which could be applied to all patients with inflammatory bowel disease (and perhaps the population as a whole).

We very much need new ways of dealing with the more serious complications of extensive Crohn's disease such as enterocutaneous fistula and short bowel syndrome. Intestinal transplantation shows some promise for the latter, but its high morbidity and substantial mortality serve mainly to substitute for only one aspect of the condition – namely the provision of nutrients – and does not make it likely that the Crohn's patient will escape future illness nor the need for a stoma. Until the 1-year mortality is substantially less than 31% and the graft survival better than 65% [2] this can be advised only for the rare patient with major complications (particularly hepatic failure) in whom mortality is otherwise a possibility and yet in whom abdominal sepsis is absent. Whether concomitant bone marrow transplantation performed as a 'biological adjuvant' will live up to its initial promise remains to be seen [3]. Enterocutaneous fistulation and uncontrolled sepsis are infrequent but devastating when they occur. Improved understanding of wound healing should lead to better therapeutic options, and although I am not yet optimistic that this will be as rapid an advance as might be wished, there are promising signs from cell culture work on the fibroblast growth factors [4] which appear reliably to enhance intestinal epithelial cell restitution. It may in time prove possible to amend the determinants of fibrosis and those of 'penetration', such that pathological imbalance is remedied. Simple, carefully chosen pharmacological means would then permit the active closure of fistulae in one group of patients and help to prevent fibrostenotic strictures in another!

REFERENCES

1. Neurath MF, Pettersson S, Meyer von Büschenfelde K-H, Strober W. Local administration of antisense phosphorothioate oligonucleotides to the p65 subunit of NF-κB abrogates established experimental colitis in mice. *Nature Med* 1996; **2**: 998–1004.
2. Thompson JS, Langnas AN, Pinch LW *et al.* Surgical approach to short bowel syndrome. Experience in a population of 160 patients. *Ann Surg* 1995; **222**: 600–605.
3. Todo S, Reyes J, Furukawa H *et al.* Outcome analysis of 71 clinical intestinal transplantations. *Ann Surg* 1995; **222**: 270–280.
4. Dignass AU, Tsunekawa S, Podolsky DK. Fibroblast growth factors modulate intestinal epithelial cell growth and migration. *Gastroenterology* 1994; **106**: 1254–1262.

Appendix A

Scoring systems in inflammatory bowel disease

CROHN'S DISEASE

Crohn's Disease Activity Index (CDAI)

The CDAI score is derived from summation of information culled from a diary card completed by the patient for the preceding 7 days, together with current clinical data, as follows.

Days 1 to 7	Sum	× factor	Score
Number of liquid/very soft stools	...	2	...
Abdominal pain rating 0 = none; 1 = mild; 2 = moderate; 3 = severe	...	5	...

General well-being
0 = generally well; 1 = slightly under
  par; 2 = poor; 3 = very poor;
  4 = terrible
	...	7	...

Number of six listed categories patient
  now has:
    arthritis/arthralgia
    iritis/uveitis
    erythema nodosum/pyoderma
      gangrenosum/aphthous stomatitis
    anal fissure, fistula or abscess
    other fistula
    fever of >37.0°C in past week
	...	20	...

x factor

Taking opioids for diarrhoea – No = 0; Yes = 30   ...

Abdominal mass

0 = none; 20 = questionable; 50 = definite   ...

Haematocrit (%)   males: 47 – 'crit | 6   ...
                         females: 42 – 'crit |

Body weight (kg)
    %age below standard weight for
      height
    add if below standard weight;
      subtract if overweight   ...

Total = CDAI   ...

A score of <150 is usually taken to indicate a patient in remission. It can be seen that it is easily possible for a score in excess of 150 to be derived from the patient's symptoms alone without any more 'objective' evidence of disease.

Best WR, Becktel JM, Singleton JW, Kern F Jr. Development of a Crohn's disease activity index. National Cooperative Crohn's Disease Study. *Gastroenterology* 1976; **70**: 439–444.

The Modified/Simplified CDAI

For day before visit:

X1   Number of soft or liquid stools
X2   Abdominal pain rating
        0 = none; 1 = mild; 2 = moderate; 3 = severe
X3   Well-being
        0 = well; 1 = slightly below par; 2 = poor; 3 = very poor;
        4 = terrible
X4   Number of extra-intestinal manifestations (as for full CDAI)
X5   Abdominal mass
        0 = none; 2 = questionable; 5 = present

Score = 20(X1 + 2(X2 + X3 + X4 + X5))

The simplified index has the advantage that it permits scoring on the basis of the previous day's account only, and therefore is more applicable to regular clinic use. A score of <150 is taken as remission; 150–250 as mild; 251–400 as moderate; and >400 as severe disease activity.

Best WR, Becktel JM. The Crohn's disease activity as a clinical instrument. In: Pena A, Weterman IT, Booth CC, Strober W, eds. *Recent Advances in Crohn's Disease*, The Hague: Martinus Nijhoff, 1981: 7–12.

Harvey–Bradshaw Index

A five point score based on:

A	General well-being	0 = very well; 1 = slightly below par; 2 = poor; 3 = very poor; 4 = terrible
B	Abdominal pain	0 = none; 1 = mild; 2 = moderate; 3 = severe
C	Number of liquid stools per day	
D	Abdominal mass	0 = none; 1 = dubious; 2 = definite; 3 = definite and tender
E	Complications	Score 1 for each of arthralgia, uveitis, erythema nodosum, pyoderma gangrenosum, aphthous ulcers, anal fissure, new fistula, abscess

Comparison with the CDAI is good ($r = 0.93$; $p < 0.001$)

A CDAI score of 100 approximates to a Harvey–Bradshaw score of 2

150	4–5
200	6
250	7–8
300	9

Harvey RF, Bradshaw JM. A simple index of Crohn's disease activity. *Lancet* 1980; i: 514

The Van Hees or Dutch Index of Crohn's disease activity

The score is derived from nine objective parameters each with its own multiplier, as follows:

Albumin (g/l)	×	−5.48
ESR (mm/h)	×	+0.29
Quettelet index (BMI × 10)	×	−0.22
Temperature (°C)	×	+16.4
Sex (1 for male; 2 for female)	×	−12.3
Previous resection (1 for no; 2 for yes)	×	−9.17
Extra-intestinal manifestations (1 for no; 2 for yes)	×	+10.7
Stool consistency (1 for normal; 2 for soft; 3 for watery)	×	+8.46
Abdominal mass (1 for no; 2 for possible; 3		

for diameter <6 cm; 4 for diameter 6–12 cm;
5 for diameter >12 cm   ×   +7.83
Sub-total   A
Subtract constant   209
Final score   B

BMI, body mass index; ESR, erythrocyte sedimentation rate.

A score of <100 is considered normal; 100–150 to represent mild activity; 150–210 moderate activity; and >210 to represent severe disease.

Van Hees PAM, Van Elteren PH, Van Lier HJJ, Van Tongeren JHM. An index of inflammatory activity in patients with Crohn's disease. *Gut* 1980; **21**: 279–286.

ULCERATIVE COLITIS

The Baron Score

A four-point scale based on the sigmoidoscopic appearance, which is also used in modified form in the St Mark's score (see below).

0 = normal
1 = non-haemorrhagic – no bleeding spontaneously or on light touch
2 = haemorrhagic – bleeding to light touch but no spontaneous bleeding
3 = haemorrhagic – spontaneous bleeding proximal to the depth of insertion of the instrument

Baron JH, Connell AM, Lennard-Jones JE. Variation between observers in describing mucosal appearances in proctocolitis. *Br Med J* 1964; **i**: 89–92.

The St Mark's Score

A four-item scale permitting a score between 0 and 9 for ulcerative colitis, which may also be extended to include the erythrocyte sedimentation rate (ESR) (or an alternative biochemical marker of inflammation), derived from study of 10 parameters of potential clinical significance, including well-being, abdominal pain, stool frequency, consistency, bleeding, anorexia, nausea and vomiting, abdominal tenderness, extra-intestinal manifestations and pyrexia.

A   Limitation of activities   0 = none; 1 = impaired but able
                                                      to continue activities;

		2 = activity reduced; 3 = unable to work
B	Bowel frequency	0 = <3 per day; 1 = 3–6 times; 2 = >6 per day
C	Stool consistency	0 = normal; 1 = semiformed; 2 = liquid
D	Baron Sigmoidoscopy Score	0 = normal or grade 1; 1 = grade 2; 2 = grade 3

Powell-Tuck J, Day DW, Buckell NA *et al.* Correlations between defined sigmoidoscopic appearances and other measures of disease activity in ulcerative colitis. *Dig Dis Sci* 1982; **27**: 533–537.

Schroeder or Mayo Clinic Score

Stool frequency
> 0 = normal number of stools for this patient
> 1 = 1–2 stools/day more than usual
> 2 = 3–4 stools/day more than usual
> 3 = 5 or more extra stools each day

Rectal bleeding
> 0 = none
> 1 = streaks of blood with less than half the stools
> 2 = obvious blood with most stools
> 3 = blood alone passed

(Flexible) proctosigmoidoscopy findings
> 0 = normal or inactive disease
> 1 = mild disease (erythema/decreased vascular pattern/mild friability)
> 2 = moderate disease (marked erythema/absent vascular pattern/friability/erosions)
> 3 = severe disease (spontaneous bleeding/ulceration)

Physician's global assessment
> 0= normal
> 1 = mild disease
> 2 = moderate disease
> 3 = severe disease

The suggested grouping then is into four groups – inactive disease, mild, moderate and severe disease, but taking a greater account of the physician's global assessment as follows.

	Inactive	Mild	Moderate	Severe
Symptoms	0–2	1–3	3–6	>/=1
Endoscopy	0	1	1–2	>/=2
Physician's score	0	1	2	3
Total	0–2	3–5	6–10	>/=6

It may be argued that there is little point in calculating the score since the physician's global assessment effectively determines the grouping.

Schroeder KW, Tremaine WJ, Ilstrup DM. Coated oral 5-aminosalicylic acid therapy for mildly to moderately active ulcerative colitis. A randomized study. *N Engl J Med* 1987; **317**: 1625–1629.

ENDOSCOPIC SCORING SYSTEM FOR CROHN'S DISEASE

CDEIS

Score for each segment of bowel involved as follows: rectum; sigmoid/left colon; transverse; right colon; ileum.

Deep ulceration
      score 12 at each site present and summate (max. = 60)   Total 1

Superficial ulceration
      score 6 at each site present and summate (max. = 30)   Total 2
      (can coexist with a 12 score)

Surface involved by disease in centimetres for each site
   present and summate   Total 3
      = linear measurement of diseased bowel
      but to a maximum of 10 (representing 100% of surface)
      (max. overall therefore is 50)

Ulcerated surface area   Total 4
      expressed in same way as surface involved (max. = 50)

Total A = Total 1 + 2 + 3 + 4

Number of segments fully examined (1 to 5) = n

Subtotal = (Total A)/n = Total B

Add 3 if ulcerated stenosis anywhere
Add 3 if non-ulcerated stenosis anywhere

Total = CDEIS

CDEIS scores typically lie between 0 and 30. Further details in respect of definition of the various parameters are given in the full paper, but informal testing of experienced endoscopists indicates that consistent results may be achieved from a given operator's subjective interpretation of the criteria without special training.

Mary JY, Modigliani R, for Groupe d'Etudes Thérapeutiques des Affections Inflammatoires du Tube Digestif (GETAID). Development and validation of an endoscopic index of the severity of Crohn's disease: a prospective multicentre study. *Gut* 1989; 30: 983–989.

The Rutgeerts Ileitis Score

A simpler endoscopic score – the Rutgeerts score – is also in use for patients in whom the colon has been resected:

0	No lesion seen
1	Fewer than 5 aphthous lesions
2	More than 5 aphthous lesions with normal mucosa between them, or skip areas of larger lesions or lesions confined to the ileo-colic anastomosis (i.e. <1 cm in length)
3	Diffuse aphthous ileitis with diffusely inflamed mucosa
4	Diffuse inflammation with larger ulcers, nodules, narrowing or both

Rutgeerts P, Geboes K, Vantrappen G *et al.* Predictability of the postoperative course of Crohn's disease. *Gastroenterology* 1990; **99**: 956–963.

More general questionnaire formats for assessment are also in use. Probably the most relevant to inflammatory bowel disease are the following (discussed in Chapter 2):

1. Irvine EJ, Feagon B, Rochon J *et al.* Quality of life: a valid and reliable measure of therapeutic efficacy in the treatment of inflammatory bowel disease. *Gastroenterology* 1994; **106**: 287–296.
2. Stewart AL, Hays RD, Ware JE Jr. The MOS short-form general health survey: reliability and validity in a patient population. *Med Care* 1988; **26**: 724–735.

Appendix B

Useful addresses

PROFESSIONAL GROUPS

American Gastroenterological Association
AGA National Office,
7910 Woodmont Avenue,
7th Floor,
Bethesda,
MD 20814,
USA

American Society for Gastrointestinal Endoscopy
13 Elm Street,
Manchester,
MA 09144,
USA

British Digestive Foundation
3 St Andrew's Place,
Regent's Park,
London,
NW1 4LB,
UK

British Society of Gastroenterology
3 St Andrew's Place,
Regent's Park,
London,
NW1 4LB,
UK

Crohn's and Colitis Foundation of America
386 Park Avenue South,
17th Floor,
New York,
NY 10016-8804,
USA

SELF-HELP GROUPS AND SOURCES OF INFORMATION FOR PATIENTS

Associacion de Enfermos de Crohn Y Colitis ulcerosa (ACCU)
Suriname 36,
El Atabal – Puerto de la Torre,
E-29190 Malaga,
Espana

Association Français Aupetit (AFA)
Hôpital Rothschild,
33 Boulevard de Picpus,
F-75571,
Paris – Cedex 12,
France

Associazone per le Malattie Infiammatorie Croniche dell'Intestino (AMICI)
Via Adolfo Wildt 19/4,
I-20138,
Milano,
Italia

Australian Crohn's and Colitis Association
PO Box 201,
Moorolbark,
VIC 31 38,
Australia

Canadian Foundation for Ileitis and Colitis
387 Bloor Street East,
Suite 402,
Toronto ON,
M4W 1H7,
Canada

Colitis-Crohn-Foreningen (CCF)
Lyngevej 116,
DK-3450,
Allerod,
Denmark

Crohn's and Colitis Foundation of America
386 Park Avenue South,
17th Floor,
New York,
NY 10016-8804,
USA

Deutsche Morbus Crohn/Colitis ulcerosa Vereingung (DCCV) eV
Paracelsusstrasse 15,
D-51375,
Leverkusen,
Deutschland

European Federation of Crohn's and Ulcerative Colitis Associations
(EFCCA)
Düstere-Eichen-Weg 24,
D-37073,
Göttingen,
Deutschland

Ileostomy Association (Ileostomy and internal pouch support group) (IA)
PO Box 23,
Mansfield,
Nottinghamshire,
NG18 4TT,
UK

Insurance Ombudsman Bureau
135 Park Street,
London,
SE1 1EA,
UK

Irish Society for Colitis and Crohn's disease (ISCCD)
58 Limekiln Green,
Dublin,
Eire

National Association for Colitis and Crohn's disease (NACC)
PO Box 25,
St Albans,
Hertfordshire,
AL1 1AB,
UK

National Digestive Diseases Information Clearinghouse
Box NDDIC,
9000 Rockville Pike,
Bethesda,
MD 20892,
USA

Organ før Riksføbundet før Mag- & Tarmsjuka (RMT)
Box 9514,
S-10274,
Stockholm,
Sweden

Red Lion Group (Ileo-anal pouch support group)
20 The Maltings,
Green Lane,
Ashwell,
Herts,
SG7 5LW,
UK

South African Crohn's Disease Association
PO Box 2638,
Cape Town,
8000,
South Africa

Index